Plain Language

Health Literacy Strategies and Communication Resources for Common Pediatric Topics

MW00846297

Mary Ann Abrams, MD, MPH, FAAP

Benard P. Dreyer, MD, FAAP

Editors

American Academy of Pediatrics

141 Northwest Point Blvd

Elk Grove Village, IL 60007-1098

The development of this publication was supported in part by McNeil Consumer Healthcare. The translation of the plain language patient education handouts into Spanish was supported by Reach Out and Read, a pediatric literacy program.

This publication has been developed by the American Academy of Pediatrics. The authors, editors, and contributors are expert authorities in the field of pediatrics, health literacy, or plain language. No commercial involvement of any kind has been solicited or accepted in the development of the content of this publication.

The recommendations in this publication do not indicate an exclusive course of treatment or serve as a standard of medical care. Variations, taking into account individual circumstances, may be appropriate.

Please note: Listing of resources does not imply an endorsement by the American Academy of Pediatrics (AAP). The AAP is not responsible for the content of the resources mentioned in this publication. Phone numbers and Web site addresses are as current as possible, but may change at any time.

Note: Brand names are for your information only. The American Academy of Pediatrics does not recommend any specific brand of drugs or products.

Permission to duplicate the patient education handouts from this publication (hard copy and PDF) for distribution to patients for educational, noncommercial purposes is granted.

Printed in the United States of America.

Library of Congress Control Number: 2008931202

ISBN – 978-1-58110-265-9
MA0400

Authors/Contributors

From AAP Health Literacy Project Advisory Committee

Mary Ann Abrams, MD, MPH, FAAP (Editor)
Iowa Health System
Des Moines, IA

Benard P. Dreyer, MD, FAAP (Editor)
New York University School of Medicine
New York, NY

Barbara Bayldon, MD, FAAP
Children's Memorial Hospital /
Northwestern University Medical School
Chicago, IL

Carmelita Britton, MD, FAAP
Guthrie Family Health Clinic
Fort Drum, NY

Ellen Buerk, MD, MEd, FAAP
Oxford Pediatrics & Adolescents, Inc.
Oxford, OH

Steven G. Federico, MD, FAAP
Denver Health Medical Center
University of Colorado School of Medicine
Denver, CO

Shalini Forbis, MD, MPH, FAAP
Wright State University
Dayton, OH

Mariana Glusman, MD, FAAP
Children's Memorial Hospital /
Northwestern University Medical School
Chicago, IL

Perri Klass, MD, FAAP
New York University School of Medicine
New York, NY

Lee M. Sanders, MD, MPH, FAAP
University of Miami
Miami, FL

Joanne G. Schwartzberg, MD (AMA Liaison)
American Medical Association
Chicago, IL

Michael E. Speer, MD, FAAP
Baylor College of Medicine
Houston, TX

Rachel Téllez, MD, MS, FAAP
Community Clinic, Inc.
Takoma Park, MD

Teri Turner, MD, MPH, MEd, FAAP (APA Liaison)
Baylor College of Medicine
Houston, TX

Modena Wilson, MD, MPH, FAAP (AMA Liaison)
American Medical Association
Chicago, IL

Additional Authors/Contributors

Suzanne Boulter, MD, FAAP
NH Dartmouth Family Practice Residency Program
Capital Region Family Health Center
Concord, NH

William L. Cull, PhD
American Academy of Pediatrics
Elk Grove Village, IL

Martha Ann Keels, DDS, PhD
Duke University Pediatric Dentistry
Durham, NC

Audrey Riffenburgh, MA
Plain Language Works
Albuquerque, NM

Roger F. Suchyta, MD, FAAP
American Academy of Pediatrics
Elk Grove Village, IL

Adult Literacy Advocates

Debra Pettit
New Reader of Iowa
Winterset, IA

Archie Willard
New Reader of Iowa
Eagle Grove, IA

Staff Editors: Diane Beausoleil, Regina Moi Martinez

Copyeditor: Kate Larson

Developmental Editor: Amy Turnbull Clymer, Captus Communications, LLC

Marketing Manager: Kathleen Juhl

Production Manager: Shannan Martin

Design: Symmetry, DESIGNWORLD

Illustrations: Anthony Alex LeTourneau

Plain Language Consultants:

Audrey Riffenburgh, MA

Maria Collis, MFA

Aracely Rosales

Translation: Rosales Communications

Table of Contents

Introduction

We as pediatricians face growing pressures every day. We must care for patients, deal with insurers, advise parents, coordinate treatment with specialists, keep up with ever-changing procedures and advances, and deal with office administration. It can be difficult to slow down and, in addition to providing care, make sure that our messages to our patients and their families are clear, and that children and their caregivers understand the diagnoses we have delivered and the treatments we have prescribed.

But couple a rushed pediatrician—who doesn't take the time to make sure the parent understands his or her directions—with a parent whose health literacy is limited, and the results can be disastrous for the child.

What Is Health Literacy?

The capacity to obtain, process, and understand basic health information and services needed to make appropriate health decisions.

Source: Ratzan SC, Parker RM. Introduction. National Library of Medicine current bibliographies in medicine: health literacy. In: Selden CR, Zorn M, Ratzan SC, Parker, RM, eds. *Institute of Medicine Health Literacy: A Prescription to End Confusion.* Bethesda, MD: National Institutes of Health, US Department of Health and Human Services; 2004:v–vii.

Now, as everything in medicine seems to be growing in complexity, depth, and scope, and we need patients to understand us more than ever, health literacy is being recognized as a growing problem for Americans. Studies show that at least 90 million adults in the United States have limited understanding of basic health information and services.[1] Startlingly, half of all parents have difficulty reading and comprehending pediatric pamphlets,[2–5] and many struggle with understanding and remembering medical advice about how to care for their child.

It is important to note that, under the right circumstances, anyone can experience low health literacy, despite their education, background, or intelligence. Consider what it's like for a parent who is sleep-deprived after staying up all night with a sick child, worried about their ill child, concerned about missing work, and possibly trying to find child care for the other children in the family—all on top of ordinary daily stresses. Now they are being asked to undertake a complex management regimen that may or may not keep their child from being hospitalized later in the day. How can they actively (and reliably) participate in complex medical care decisions and manage acute health care for their child?

Through effective communication, you can help your patients and their families understand what they are facing and make informed health decisions. *Plain Language Pediatrics: Health Literacy Strategies and Communication Resources for Common Pediatric Topics* has been developed to jumpstart this process and bridge the communication gap between pediatrician and patient or family. This publication seeks to

- Identify pediatric-specific health literacy issues.
- Tailor promising practices in general health literacy to the pediatric health environment.
- Provide pediatric health literacy tools and resources.
- Offer techniques that will improve both verbal and written communication with patients.
- Include a practical, user-friendly compilation of general and pediatric interventions.
- Model the acceptability and use of plain language.

We hope you come to see *Plain Language Pediatrics: Health Literacy Strategies and Communication Resources for Common Pediatric Topics* as an essential tool—a way to help your practice address health literacy and improve communication so that you can more effectively care for your patients and their families.

Organization

Plain Language Pediatrics: Health Literacy Strategies and Communication Resources for Common Pediatric Topics is divided into 2 parts. In Part I we explore limited health literacy, including the scope of the problem, how it affects children in particular, and how pediatricians can address and overcome health literacy issues with patients and their caregivers. We highlight specific ways you can make changes in your practice today and offer effective techniques you can use to improve communication with your patients and enhance their understanding of medical diagnoses and treatments. We also describe a new line of American Academy of Pediatrics (AAP) plain language handouts that were developed in English and Spanish for this book.

> Improving communication with patients has been shown to better their understanding of the medical situation at hand, give them a more favorable impression of the physician, and even reduce lawsuits.
>
> **Source:** Levinson W. Physician-patient communication. The relationship with malpractice claims among primary care physicians and surgeons. *JAMA.* 1997;277(7):553–559

In Part II we highlight 17 topics—common pediatric conditions that we see with our patients every day. Within each topic, we discuss likely areas for miscommunication and provide solutions that you can use to explain the condition and management in a way parents and patients can understand and appreciate. We chose topics that address common acute, chronic, and preventive issues in ambulatory pediatrics for a wide range of patient ages.

Each topic includes

- A pediatric-specific patient story demonstrating missed opportunities for communication
- At least one *Ask Me 3* scenario that highlights key points that parents or patients should understand before the end of the encounter
- Suggested plain language alternatives to medical terms and jargon
- Talking points to use in discussing potentially confusing terms and concepts
- Ideas for teach-back approaches
- Information about cultural beliefs that may affect management of certain conditions
- Suggestions for integrating health literacy into efforts to encourage health-promoting behavior change among patients and their families
- Suggestions for how to involve a child in his or her own health care
- Key messages for all medical staff, so that everyone is delivering the same information
- Additional resources, both off-line and online, that you can consult or recommend to your patients and their families for more information
- Plain language patient handouts in English and Spanish and other selected handouts you can use in your practice

How to Use This Guidebook

This resource will save you time and improve patient satisfaction if used correctly and with some practice. It may help reduce the number of phone calls and unnecessary follow-up appointments, and it will save valuable staff time in fielding repeated questions from caregivers who need clarification, or who have simply forgotten a particular aspect of your advice or diagnosis. When patients and their families understand your first explanation, everyone benefits.

Learn the Basics of Health Literacy

Read up on health literacy issues and learn how your patients are affected when their literacy and health literacy are limited. Review the 17 topics, and discover new terms and tactics to use as you talk with your patients and their families about these common pediatric conditions.

Share This Guidebook With Your Staff

Use the plain language handouts and key message lists that come with each of the health topics in Part II to educate your staff, so that everyone communicates the same information to patients and their caregivers. Draw on the patient stories to role-play different scenes, so staff members can practice explaining various situations to a parent, a child, and an adolescent using the *Ask Me 3* and teach-back methods. Give all employees the opportunity to learn new plain language communication skills that can ultimately lead to improved health outcomes for the children in your practice.

Make Changes

Consider specific ways you can make changes to improve communication in your practice. Try your new skills with the last patient of the day, and focus on only 1 or 2 topics or conditions at a time. The interventions contained herein can be adapted to your practice's individual stage of change.

Too often there is a notable chasm between what is said by the doctor and what is understood by the patient or parent. And the result is poorer health care for our children. This book will help you close that gap and benefit everyone—children, parents, and the health care team.

Now, let's get started!

References

1. Nielsen-Bohlman L, Panzer A, Kindig DA. *Health Literacy: A Prescription to End Confusion.* Washington, DC: National Academies Press; 2004

2. Arnold CL, Davis TC, Frempong JO, et al. Assessment of newborn screening parent education materials. *Pediatrics.* 2006;117(5 Pt 2):S320–S325

3. Davis TC, Crouch MA, Wills G, et al. The gap between patient reading comprehension and the readability of patient education materials. *J Fam Pract.* 1990;31:533–538

4. Davis TC, Mayeaux EJ, Fredrickson D, et al. Reading ability of parents compared with reading level of pediatric patient education materials. *Pediatrics.* 1994;93:460–468

5. Davis TC, Bocchini JA Jr, Fredrickson D, et al. Parent comprehension of polio vaccine information pamphlets. *Pediatrics.* 1996;97(6 Pt 1):804–810

Part I Overview

Challenge of Low Health Literacy

The Institute of Medicine (IOM) defines health literacy as "the capacity to obtain, process, and understand basic health information and services needed to make appropriate health decisions."[1] More than the reading and computational skills that comprise general literacy, health literacy also includes writing, listening, speaking, conceptual knowledge, decision-making, and acting on information.[1]

Today, more than ever before, it is vital for patients to be health literate. With health care growing in complexity, pediatric patients (and their parents) serve alongside doctors as partners in their own health care. They must be able to follow detailed instructions from their physicians and manage their treatment at home. But for many patients and their families, limited health literacy is a major barrier to understanding and adhering to their physicians' advice.

Who Has Limited Health Literacy?

About half of the general US population—including at least 90 million adults—have limited health literacy.[2–5]

Inadequate health literacy affects all segments of the population, but it is more commonly represented in certain populations, such as the elderly, the poor, minorities, and people who did not speak English during early childhood.[6]

These people face challenges every day in understanding their health care and taking steps to improve it.

Table 1.1 Risk Factors for Low Literacy

Factor	% of All NAAL Population	% Below-Basic Group
High school education	15	55
Unemployed	5	51
Non–English-speaking prior to school	13	44
Elderly (65+)	15	26
Minority		
Black	12	20
Hispanic	12	39
Asian/Pacific Islander	4	4
Caucasian	70	37

Abbreviation: NAAL, National Assessment of Adult Literacy.
Source: Kutner M, Greenberg E, Baer J. *A First Look at the Literacy of America's Adults in the 21st Century.* Washington, DC: National Center for Education Statistics, US Department of Education; 2005.

Health Literacy and General Literacy

Because health literacy is highly associated with general literacy, it is useful to review the literature on general literacy in this country. According to the *2003 National Assessment of Adult Literacy*, 14% of adults older than 16 years in the United States have below-basic reading skills, and 22% have below-basic math skills. While limited literacy affects all ages, races, ethnicities, and classes, research shows that certain characteristics increase risk (Table 1.1).

- Having less than a high school education
- Using English as a second language at home
- Being a member of a minority group
- Suffering from hearing, vision, and/or learning problems or developmental delays

- Having immigrated to the United States after age 12 years
- Having Medicaid as the insurance provider
- Being unemployed
- Belonging to a single-parent family
- Being elderly[7,8]

The Price of Health Literacy

Limited health literacy costs the United States an estimated $106 to $230 billion a year.*

In one small study, the average annual health care costs for all Medicaid enrollees in one state was $2,891 per enrollee, but the annual cost for enrollees with limited literacy skills averaged $10,688.†

Sources:
*Vernon JA, Trujillo A, Rosenbaum S, DeBuono B. *Low Health Literacy: Implications for National Health Policy*. 2007. http://www.npsf.org/askme3/pdfs/case_report_10_07.pdf Accessed June 24, 2008.
†Weiss BD, Palmer R. Relationship between health care costs and very low literacy skills in a medically needy and indigent Medicaid population. *J Am Board Fam Pract*. 2004;17:44–47.

Conversely, it is important to note that 37% of those with literacy problems *do* have a high school education, 52% speak English *only*, and 54% have *no* physical or mental disabilities.[8] In addition,

- Caucasian and Hispanic Americans each represent more than one-third of those with below-basic literacy.[8]
- Fourteen percent of high school graduates have below-basic literacy.
- Fewer than half of adults with below-basic literacy have a disability.

Most importantly, families with both high and low literacy levels have been shown to lack knowledge regarding their children's health.[9,10] In one study, almost half of the parents interviewed did not know when the next well-child evaluation was scheduled. And, although most (80%) understood the purpose of their child's medication, only 52% to 74% knew the name of the medication and instructions for taking it.[9]

Why Is Health Literacy Important?

General Ramifications

Today's society demands a high degree of literacy to negotiate everyday life. At every turn, people are expected to follow directions, heed warnings, make decisions, and take actions that will protect them, their families, and their communities, whether such information is presented verbally or visually, through pictures or in writing.

With each year, the complexity of medical care increases, widening the base of people who are not health literate; where, at one time, a person's level of health literacy may have been adequate, medical advances have left them behind. The impact of low health literacy grows as fewer and fewer laypeople are able to follow increasingly complex medical advice. The escalating prevalence of chronic illnesses and conditions, growing number of treatment options, need for lifestyle-related behavior change, and emphasis on shared decision-making also contribute to the problem.

Day-to-Day Impact

When people have difficulty understanding health-related issues, they experience a ripple effect daily at home, at work, in schools, and in communities. Examples of such decision points may include

- Reading nutrition labels at the supermarket
- Selecting and using over-the-counter medications safely
- Determining medication dosage based on weight

- Accurately measuring liquid medicine for young children
- Understanding whether medicine must accompany a child to school, what the school's policy is, and how to give correct instructions for the medicine to be administered at school
- Using medical devices (such as inhalers, apnea monitors, and nebulizers) appropriately and safely
- Deciding which medicines children should take to prevent problems and which should be used to treat problems (such as confusion about when to use inhaled steroids and inhaled bronchodilators for chronic asthma)
- Deciding whether a child can participate in school or community activities

Even those who are highly educated or who have no trouble dealing effectively with many aspects of their lives may have difficulty obtaining, understanding, and integrating health information, especially when the information is presented using complex terms, dense text, and medical jargon.

With the increasing emphasis on behavior change as a critical means for prevention and treatment of such conditions as obesity, attention-deficit/hyperactivity disorder, and asthma, a lower level of literacy interferes with many tasks critical to achieving healthy goals. Understanding the relationship between behavior and outcomes can be undermined by low health literacy because a patient whose literacy skills are limited is likely to have difficulty

- Appreciating which outcomes are optimal and which suggest the need for a different course of treatment
- Grasping the outcomes that are likely to result from current behavior patterns and understanding what they need to do to make healthy changes

- Accepting the advantages of proposed behavior changes

Further, the increasing importance placed on physicians' partnering with patients or families means the latter are increasingly expected to seek out and understand medical information, and tackle the often complex responsibilities that come with effective self-management and comanagement of diseases and conditions. This task, made more difficult by the complex language on documents (eg, medical release and informed consent forms, small-print inserts that accompany medications, or applications for children's health insurance), can be arduous or even impossible for those with limited health literacy.

Pediatric Health Literacy

In pediatric health care, health literacy is a family issue. The care of each pediatric patient is affected by the health literacy skills of many people: the patient (after a certain age), primary caregivers, siblings, grandparents and other family members, child care providers, babysitters, teachers and school personnel, coaches, and friends. As the child and his or her family grow and develop, so should the depth and breadth of the family's collective health literacy.

The skills that lead to strong health literacy begin to develop early in life (Table 1.2). Emergent literacy skills—such as letter recognition, phonologic awareness, and book-handling—take shape during an infant's first year. Children usually begin to talk with adults about their health by about the age of 4 years, and children with chronic illnesses begin to participate in the management of their own health care needs by age 7 years.[11–13] While comprehensive health literacy curricula that infuse reading, writing, and mathematics instruction with practical health-related information are available for elementary and secondary school grade levels, they are not universally used.

By the same token, barriers to health literacy also develop early in life. Reading aloud to young children—the most important contributor to emerging literacy—does not occur in 20% of households in the United States.[14] And, almost half of all first-graders read below grade level.[15]

Research presented at the *2006 Surgeon General's Workshop on Improving Health Literacy* suggests that at an early age, children have the ability to evaluate sources of information and grasp cause-effect explanations. If we give children cause-effect explanations (as opposed to lists of behavioral "dos and don'ts"), we increase their understanding and reasoning, and prepare them to make good judgments about risk in novel situations, underscoring that children can and do play an important role in maintaining their own health, one that can be enhanced through optimizing health literacy–related skills.[16]

Health Disparities

Race and ethnicity have been found to correlate with persistent, and often increasing, health disparities among populations in the United States.[17] One of the 2 overarching objectives for *Healthy People 2010* is to "eliminate health disparities among different segments of the population that occur by gender, race or ethnicity, education or income, disability, geographic location or sexual orientation."[18]

Consider the following facts reported by the IOM in *Unequal Treatment: What Healthcare Providers Need to Know about Racial and Ethnic Disparities in Healthcare*[19]:

- Racial and ethnic minorities experience a lower quality of health services and are less likely to have routine medical procedures.
- Minorities are less likely to be given cardiac medications, undergo bypass surgery, receive kidney dialysis, or receive transplants.
- Minorities are more likely to receive lower limb amputation for diabetes than other groups.

¿Cómo?

Spanish-speaking patients who reported being comfortable speaking English were still at greater risk of giving medications improperly.

Source: Leyva M, Sharif I, Ozuah PO. Health literacy among Spanish speaking Latino parents with limited English proficiency. *Ambul Pediatr.* 2005;5:56–59.

Statistics about children's health disparities are even more shocking.

- Infant mortality among African Americans in the United States occurs more than twice as frequently as it does among white babies.[20]
- African American children are 3 times as likely as non-Hispanic white children to be hospitalized for asthma.[21]
- Lower socioeconomic status is associated with significantly higher risks of child behavior problems and oral health problems, and lower overall health status.[22–24]

The IOM attributes these health disparities to a variety of factors, including differences among patients' help-seeking behavior and their attitudes regarding treatment; cultural and linguistic barriers; mistrust of the health care system; and discrimination on the part of health care providers, including biases, stereotyping, and hesitancy.[19]

Research specific to children's health disparities shows that additional factors are at work, further thwarting their optimal health care.

- Family issues, which can involve a lack of social support or limited English proficiency
- Community limitations, which can include poor access to care, often caused by geographic isolation or a certain population's overall lack of insurance

Table 1.2 Health Literacy Skills for Each Developmental Stage[16]

Stage	Skills
Toddlers and preschool age	• Know body parts. • Know healthy vs non-healthy foods. • Talk to the doctor.
School age	• Learn basic human biology. • Read and understand nutrition labels. • Measure medication doses with the supervision of parents. • Know proper use of 911. • Provide a history of present illness to the doctor. • Answer questions and be able to teach back some key self-management information. • Adopt and practice healthy lifestyle choices.
Adolescence	• Learn advanced human biology in school curriculum. • Understand and execute preventive physical, dental, and mental health care behaviors. • Take increased responsibility for managing self-care for acute and chronic conditions. • Establish self-efficacy in practicing healthy lifestyle choices and resisting peer pressure. • Read and understand sexual health information. • Understand the indications and use of over-the-counter medications. • Access health care resources at school and in the community. • Complete office medical forms. • Provide medical history and family medical history to the doctor. • Participate in well-adolescent visit without parent present. • Ask questions when prompted by health care provider. • Teach back key health information. • Develop capacity to assent to medical treatment.
Young adulthood	• Independently seek preventive, acute, and chronic health care. • Elicit teach-back from health care provider. • Read and complete health insurance forms. • Read and complete HIPAA documents. • Understand the patient's bill of rights. • Understand how to navigate the health system. • Develop the capacity to consent to medical treatment.
Parenthood	Same skills as those for "young adulthood" above, with the following additions: • Model good health communication skills. • Seek answers to *Ask Me 3* questions. • Navigate the health care system on behalf of their child. • "Stop the line" when communication is unclear. • Model and teach health-promoting behaviors to their child. • Promote emergent literacy through language and reading aloud to their child. • Read and understand parenting books from the American Academy of Pediatrics and other sources.

- An unhealthy physical environment, where housing density, soil contamination, air pollution, and other conditions can be detrimental to health

- An unhealthy social environment, where health care system inefficiencies, poor schools, income inequality, and racism can work against a child's receiving high-quality care[25-28]

Recall that the percentage of low literacy and low health literacy among certain minorities is higher than among those who are white. This, coupled with health disparities experienced by minority groups, supports the need to optimize health literacy and health communication as one component of helping to reduce health disparities.

Low Health Literacy and Its Association With Health Outcomes

As noted previously, low literacy and low health literacy adversely affect the quality of health care provided to patients and families. Compounding this troubling situation is that not only do patients not receive optimal care from providers, but their ability to self-manage is also impeded. Many of those who don't understand a diagnosis or the importance of necessary treatment, or who can't decipher instructions to administer medications properly at home, do not fare as well as patients with high health literacy. Clearly, there is an association between lower health literacy and poor health outcomes.[3-5]

- Those with inadequate literacy are 2 times more likely to report poorer health[29] and are more likely to be hospitalized.[30]

- People with lower health literacy use health services more frequently and have worse control of their chronic illnesses.[31-33]

- A parent's low literacy correlates with diminished understanding of how ill a child is,[9] which might result in his or her not seeking care.

- Among patients with diabetes, those with inadequate health literacy were less likely than those with adequate health literacy to achieve tight glycemic control and were more likely to report having retinopathy.[34]

- Pregnant women with higher reading levels are significantly more likely to know about—and be concerned about—the effects of smoking tobacco during pregnancy.[35]

- Parents with lower health literacy lack knowledge regarding weight-based dosing of medications for children and are more likely to measure liquid medications with non-standardized dosing instruments.[36]

- Children with asthma whose parents had low literacy had worse outcomes, including a greater incidence of emergency department visits, more hospital admissions, and more days missed from school.[37]

While low health literacy on its own has not been shown to be a direct cause of poorer health outcomes,[38] it is clear that there is a strong association. While we strive to help patients achieve optimal care, we should be mindful of each patient's and each family's health literacy. As physicians, we should take steps to help those with low or limited health literacy improve their skills and understanding, with the hope and expectation that this will ultimately improve their health.

References

1. Ratzan SC, Parker RM. Introduction. National Library of Medicine current bibliographies in medicine: health literacy. In: Selden CR, Zorn M, Ratzan SC, Parker, RM, eds. *Institute of Medicine Health Literacy: A Prescription to End Confusion.* Bethesda, MD: National Institutes of Health, US Department of Health and Human Services; 2004:v–vii

2. Nielsen-Bohlman L, Panzer A, Kindig DA. *Health Literacy: A Prescription to End Confusion.* Washington, DC: National Academies Press; 2004

3. Comings J, Reder S, Sum A. *Building a Level Playing Field: The Need to Expand and Improve the National and State Adult Education and Literacy Systems.* Cambridge, MA: National Center for the Study of Adult Learning and Literacy; 2001. http://www.ncsall.net/fileadmin/resources/research/op_comings2.pdf. Accessed June 5, 2008

4. American Medical Association. Health literacy: report of the Council on Scientific Affairs. Ad Hoc Committee on Health Literacy for the Council on Scientific Affairs, American Medical Association. *JAMA.* 1999;281:552–557

5. Williams MV, Davis T, Parker RM, Weiss BD. The role of health literacy in patient-physician communication. *Fam Med.* 2002; 34:383–389

6. Weiss BD. *Health Literacy and Patient Safety: Help Patients Understand. Manual for Physicians.* 2nd ed. Chicago, IL: AMA Foundation; 2007:36

7. Kirsch I, Jungblut A, Jenkins L, Kolstad A. *Adult Literacy in America: A First Look at the Results of the National Adult Literacy Survey.* Washington, DC: National Center for Education Statistics, US Department of Education; 1993

8. Kutner M, Greenberg E, Baer J. *A First Look at the Literacy of America's Adults in the 21st Century.* Washington, DC: National Center for Education Statistics, US Department of Education; 2005

9. Moon RY, Cheng TL, Patel KM, et al. Parental literacy and understanding medical information. *Pediatrics.* 1998;102:e25

10. Spandorfer JM, Karras DJ, Hugher LA, Caputo C. Comprehension of discharge instructions by patients in an urban emergency department. *Ann Emerg Med.* 1995;25:71–74

11. Alderson P, Sutcliffe K, Curtis K. Children as partners with adults in their medical care. *Arch Dis Child.* 2006;91(4):300–303

12. Butz A, Pham L, Lewis L, et al. Rural children with asthma: impact of a parent and child asthma education program. *J Asthma.* 2005;42:813–821

13. Homer SD. Effect of education on school-age children's and parents' asthma management. *J Spec Pediatr Nurs.* 2004;9:95–102

14. Kridal B, Livingston A, Wirt J, et al. *The Condition of Education 2003.* Washington, DC: US Department of Education, National Center for Education Statistics; 2003

15. Denton K, West J. *Children's Reading and Mathematics Achievement in Kindergarten and First Grade.* Washington, DC: US Department of Education, National Center for Education Statistics; 2002

16. Keil FC. Meeting the literacy needs of young children. In: Proceedings from the Surgeon General's Workshop on Improving Health Literacy; September 7, 2006; Bethesda, MD.

17. Centers for Disease Control and Prevention. About minority health. http://www.cdc.gov/omhd/AMH/AMH.htm. Accessed April 22, 2008

18. US Department of Health and Human Services. A systematic approach to health improvement. http://www.healthypeople.gov/Document/html/uih/uih_bw/uih_2.htm#goals. Accessed June 5, 2008

19. Institute of Medicine. *Unequal Treatment: Understanding Racial and Ethnic Disparities in Health Care.* Washington, DC: National Academies Press; 2002

20. Miniño AM, Arias E, Kochanek KD, Murphy SL, Smith BL. Deaths: final data for 2000. In: *National Center for Health Statistics. National Vital Statistics Report.* Vol. 50, No.15. Washington, DC: Department of Health and Human Services, Centers for Disease Control and Prevention; 2002:100

21. Agency for Healthcare Research and Quality (AHRQ). *Selected Findings on Child and Adolescent Health Care from the 2004 National Healthcare Quality/Disparities Reports* [fact sheet]. Rockville, MD: AHRQ; 2005

22. Kahn RS, Wilson K, Wise PH. Intergenerational health disparities: socioeconomic status, women's health conditions, and child behavior problems. *Public Health Rep.* 2005;120(4):399–408

23. Hughes DC, Duderstadt KG, Soobader M, Newacheck PW. Disparities in children's use of oral health services. *Pub Health Rep.* 2005;120(4):455–462

24. Malat J, Oh HJ, Hamilton MA. Poverty experience, race, and child health. *Public Health Rep.* 2005;120:442–447

25. Marmot MG. Understanding social-inequalities in health. *Perspect Biol Med.* 2003;46(3):S9–S23

26. Newacheck PW, Rising JP, Kim SE. Children at risk for special health care needs. *Pediatrics.* 2006;118(1):334–342

27. Flores G, Abreu M, Tomany-Korman SC. Limited English proficiency, primary language at home, and disparities in children's health care: how language barriers are measured matters. *Public Health Rep.* 2005;12(4):418–430

28. Wise PH. The transformation of child health in the United States. *Health Aff.* 2004;23(5):9–25

29. Baker DW, Parker RM, Williams MV, et al. The relationship of patient reading ability to self-reported health and use of health services. *Am J Public Health.* 1997;87:1027–1030

30. Baker DW, Parker RM, Williams MV, Clark WS. Health literacy and the risk of hospital admission. *J Gen Intern Med.* 1998;13:791–798

31. Williams MV, Parker RM, Baker DW, et al. Inadequate functional health literacy among patients at two hospitals. *JAMA.* 1995;274:1677–1682

32. Gazmararian JA, Baker DW, Williams MV, et al. Health literacy among Medicare enrollees in a managed care organization. *JAMA.* 1999;281:545–551

33. Williams MV, Baker DW, Parker RM, Nurss JR. Relationship of functional health literacy to patients' knowledge of their chronic disease. *Arch Intern Med.* 1998;158:166–172

34. Schillinger D, Grumbach K, Piette J, et al. Association of health literacy with diabetes outcomes. *JAMA.* 2002;288(4):475–482

35. Arnold CL, Davis TC, Berkel HJ, et al. Smoking status, reading level and knowledge of tobacco effects among low literacy women. *Prev Med.* 2001;32:313–320

36. Yin HS, Dreyer BP, Foltin G, van Schaick L, Mendelsohn AL. Association of low caregiver health literacy with reported use of nonstandardized dosing instruments and lack of knowledge of weight-based dosing. *Ambul Pediatr.* 2007;7:292–298

37. DeWalt DA, Dilling MH, Rosenthal MS, Pignone MP. Low parental literacy is associated with worse asthma care measures in children. *Ambul Pediatr.* 2007;7:25–31

38. Yin HS, Forbis SG, Dreyer BP. Health literacy and pediatric health. *Curr Probl Pediatr Adolesc Health Care.* 2007;37:258–286

Common Approaches to Health Literacy for All Physicians

Today when we see patients in our practices, we rely on them (or their parents) to be partners in care. We ask for their help in pinpointing specifics of their health concerns, and we expect their help in managing the treatment protocols we prescribe. When our patients or their parents have low health literacy, they are less likely to understand our explanations or instructions, and we—and their child—lose this trusted partner, along with the assumption that our treatment plans will be followed.

As health care providers, we are in the unique position to recognize and help people with health literacy limitations. When we understand that a literacy problem exists, we are able to modify our communication techniques to meet the needs of the patient, and we are able to refer patients for outside help. Acknowledging and addressing these factors in the context of health literacy should be an integral part of health care management.

This chapter looks at specific areas of concern for patients with low health literacy and discusses successful practices that today's health care professionals can employ to help alleviate problems caused by limited health literacy. Factors and promising practices relating specifically to pediatric medicine are included Chapters 3, 4, and 5.

Need for Health Literacy in the Doctor's Office

One study found that up to 80% of patients forget what their doctor tells them as soon as they leave the doctor's office, and nearly 50% of what they say they recall is incorrect.[1] These statistics are likely compounded for patients and families whose understanding of medical conditions and treatment plans is already limited.

In its report, *To Err Is Human: Building a Safer Health System*,[2] the Institute of Medicine (IOM) discusses 2 processes that are significantly compromised by literacy limitations: safe care and customization.

Safe Care

This IOM report emphasizes the importance of safety (defined by the IOM as "freedom from accidental injury") and looks at cases where patient safety in health care organizations and institutions has been affected. The report concludes that medication-related errors and adverse events attributable to health care providers are due most often to the convergence of multiple contributing factors, including the health literacy of caregivers. "The problem is not bad people; the problem is that the system needs to be made safer."[2]

Similarly, children who are cared for at home are dependent on caregivers to administer medications and operate medical devices. When the person overseeing home care—whether that person is a parent, relative, babysitter, teacher, school nurse, child care attendant, or the child himself—lacks the level of health literacy necessary to provide appropriate care, there is a significant risk to the patient.

It is therefore incumbent on the health care professional to meet the health literacy needs of the child's caregiver and to be mindful of the affect that the caregiver's health literacy can have on the child's health outcome. Just as in health care institutions, "bad people" are typically not to blame for errors in care at home; rather, it is the system that needs to be reformed so that care can be made safer.

Customization or Patient-Centered Care

Patient-centered care is the term most commonly used to explain customization, which the IOM defines as "permitting the greatest responsiveness to individual values and preferences."[2] While institutionalizing this principle through policy directives is difficult, patient-centered care is integral to the medical home, and can and should be incorporated into general practices.[3]

In its 2003 summit report, *Health Professions Education: A Bridge to Quality*, the IOM identifies patient-centered care as one of the core competencies that should be integrated into health professionals' education to enhance quality of care.[4] The report describes patient-centered care as the center of overlapping competencies, including employing evidence-based practices, applying quality improvements, and using informatics.

Practicing patient-centered care includes

- Identifying, respecting, and caring about patients' differences, values, preferences, and expressed needs
- Listening to, clearly informing, communicating with, and educating patients
- Sharing decision-making and care management responsibilities

Identifying and understanding patients' health literacy are critical to ensuring that these principles are effectively integrated into health care practices at all levels of patient communication and care management.

Red Flags

Because low literacy is accompanied by stigma and shame,[5] those who struggle with reading often develop successful coping strategies to hide their disability.[6] It can therefore be difficult to identify patients with literacy problems because "you can't tell by looking," but there are red flags that can alert you that a family may require extra attention, including

- Appointment time errors
- Missed appointments
- Incomplete or slowly completed forms
- Forms where all yes/no responses are checked "no"
- A disinterested or angry demeanor
- Clues in the social history, such as a low income or not having a high school education
- Quick agreement to a plan, failure to ask questions
- Giving a poor, incomplete, or uncertain family history
- Medication refill requests either too early or too late
- Incorrect preparation for tests or procedures
- Lack of adherence

Another clue to parental literacy may come from simply handing the parent a book for the child during the visit and observing. Consider the parent's reaction: Does the father look uncomfortable with the book? Does the mother take the book away from the child or not give it to the child at all? These may be signs that the parent isn't comfortable reading and doesn't read regularly with the child, both of which can be the result of literacy limitations. This could also mean the child is not being exposed to books and language—troubling signs that early literacy skills are not being fostered and the legacy of low literacy is continuing.

If you notice any of these red flags, it is important to gently probe further, bearing in mind that they may be reluctant to share their reading difficulties, even with a physician.

Screening for Low Literacy

Most physicians do not ask patients about their reading ability.[7] This may be due to fear of offending or embarrassing patients, lack of knowledge of how to ask, uncertainty about what to do when a patient is identified as having limited literacy, or not recognizing the importance of literacy to health. As is the case for other uncomfortable topics that physicians are trained to discuss (eg, drug use, sexuality, domestic violence, gun ownership, etc), questions about literacy become easier to ask as the doctor becomes convinced of their worth and develops comfort with broaching the topic over time.

However, because ensuring understanding is critical to quality health care, and literacy and health literacy are key to understanding, it may be useful to inquire about parental literacy in a non-threatening, non-stigmatizing manner. Literacy-related questions can fit in the context of the social history, especially after discussing employment, the child's school performance, bedtime routines, or favorite activities, or when handing out educational material. You may begin with 1 or 2 of the following questions, and continue based on the parent's response and comfort:

- How comfortable are you with your reading?
- Have you ever had difficulty reading?
- Has reading ever been a problem for you?
- Have doctors ever been unclear when they explain things to you?
- How often do you need to have someone help you when you read instructions, pamphlets, or other written material from your doctor or pharmacy?
- How confident are you filling out medical forms by yourself?
- Have you ever had difficulty reading the materials that your doctor gives you?
- If you had the time, would you be interested in a program to help you read better?

At this time, however, there is insufficient evidence to recommend clinical screening for health literacy. Whereas brief literacy screening tools exist that, with further evaluation, could potentially be used to detect limited literacy in clinical settings, no screening program for limited literacy has been shown to be effective. Yet there is a noted potential for harm in the form of shame and alienation, which might be induced through clinical screening. There is fair evidence to suggest that possible harm outweighs any current benefit.[8]

Health Literacy Assessment Tools

The most common tools to measure health-specific literacy are the Rapid Estimate of Adult Literacy in Medicine (REALM) and the Short Test of Functional Health Literacy in Adults (S-TOFHLA). These are used primarily in research settings and may be difficult to use in a practice because they may offend patients and take valuable time that could be better used in other ways. A third test, the Newest Vital Sign, is a quick, newer alternative assessment tool.

- In the REALM test, the subject is given a list of 66 medical terms and is asked to read aloud as many as he or she can in 2 minutes. The examiner gives 1 point for each word pronounced correctly (according to standard pronunciation guides), and that total score is used to determine the subject's health literacy. For example, a subject who correctly pronounced up to 18 words is determined to have health literacy at the third-grade level or less; a score between 45 and 60 indicates a seventh- to eighth-grade health literacy level, and scores between 61 and 66 indicate health literacy at the high school level and above.[9] *Sample questions can be viewed online at http://www.hsph.harvard.edu/healthliteracy/doakab.pdf.*[10]

- The TOFHLA and the shorter S-TOFHLA include sets of questions that assess functional health literacy.[11,12] In the shortened version, subjects have 12 minutes to answer a short series of questions that measure the subject's ability to read and understand numbers, and then a longer section where the subject must complete health documents (eg, medication instructions) with multiple-choice responses.

  Sample questions can be viewed online at http://www.peppercornbooks.com/catalog/pdf/tofhla_eng_12pt_websmpl.pdf.

- A newer test that has been validated against the TOFHLA is the Newest Vital Sign,[13] a 3-minute test in which the subject is given a nutrition label for a carton of ice cream. The subject is then asked 6 questions to probe his or her understanding of a nutrition label, such as, "If you ate the whole container, how many calories would you have eaten?" (The subject is allowed to keep the label to answer the questions.)

  Test materials are available online at http://www.clearhealthcommunication.org/physicians-providers/newest-vital-sign.html.[14]

Researchers continue to look for quick, non-threatening ways to assess parents' health literacy. A possible promising pediatric screen is asking how many children's books are in the home.[15] One study showed that having 10 or more books had a 91% positive predictive value of adequate parental literacy. (More information on this question is included in Chapter 4.) It is important that efforts to assess parental literacy do not impede taking a universal approach to health literacy, working to communicate clearly with and ensuring understanding for all patients and parents.

The DIRECT Approach

The DIRECT approach, developed by Drs Mariana Glusman and Barbara Bayldon, can be a useful way to approach parents about literacy in the outpatient setting (Table 2.1). While it includes screening questions, it also takes a broader approach to the patient by considering the patient's full environment and suggests questions to ask the patient and family.

Table 2.1. The DIRECT Approach to Talking About Literacy

D	Ask about **difficulty** reading. *"Have you ever had a problem with reading?"*
I	Ask if they have an interest in **improving** their reading skills. *"Would you be interested in a program to help you improve your reading?"*
R	Have **referral** information for adult and family literacy programs ready to give patients and their caregivers identified with reading difficulty.
E	Ask **everyone** about their literacy skills. *Let patients know that it is your policy to ask all patients and families about their literacy skills.*
C	Emphasize that low literacy is a **common** problem and that they are not alone. *"Half of Americans have some difficulty with reading!"*
T	**Take down barriers.** To joining literacy classes—For example, you or your staff could help with the initial phone call, have informational sessions at your office, and make follow-up contact with patients to see if they were able to find the right class. To providing effective care—This is the most important part of the DIRECT approach: Ensure that patients understand the treatment plan, provide them with appropriate handouts, do "medication reviews," etc.

With regards to the "E" in the DIRECT approach, although Drs Glusman and Bayldon recommend excluding people you know can read, such as those with graduate or professional degrees, education level isn't a perfect indicator of health literacy. Remember, even parents with very high literacy may have difficulty understanding medical jargon and complex medical explanations and instructions.

How do parents like the DIRECT approach?

Responses to the DIRECT approach have been very positive, according to creators Mariana Glusman and Barbara Bayldon; no one has been upset or offended.

Some of their patients' responses have been

"I can read to myself, but have difficulty reading aloud."

"I want to improve my reading so I can help my kids with their schoolwork."

"I have no problems with my reading, but it's great that you ask your patients."

Drs Glusman and Bayldon say that since they began using the DIRECT approach at their inner-city clinic, they have gone from about 4 referrals to adult education per year to 2 or 3 referrals per *week.*

Making Changes in Your Practice

We as physicians have the unique opportunity to affect the lives of our patients every day in very meaningful ways. By adopting a generational approach to literacy in our practice—health literacy, emergent literacy, family literacy—we are able to improve the health, not just of today's patients, but tomorrow's as well. Success in improving the literacy of our current pediatric patients can ripple through generations, a tremendous professional legacy.

Survey your practice. A first critical step in any improvement plan is to survey the landscape.

Imagine that you are a new patient coming to your practice for a visit. Use a checklist to determine whether your practice is patient-friendly and what areas could be improved.[16] If English weren't your first language, could you be a patient in this practice or would it be too difficult? Consider how patients and families are greeted: the signs and maps you use to direct patients to your practice, the readability of your brochures and forms, and the interpersonal communication skills that you and your staff use to ensure patients and their families understand.

Build health literacy into your quality improvement plan. Quality improvement is a continuous process and part of lifelong learning.

In a follow-up report to *To Err Is Human,* the IOM identified health literacy and self-management support as cross-cutting priorities to transform health care quality in the United States for all ages and settings and for preventive, acute, and chronic care.[17] Engage all staff members regularly to determine specific targets for health literacy improvement. Make sure all members of the health care team recognize their responsibility to help ensure parents and patients have the information they need to safely and effectively manage their care. For example, all staff members could be assigned to read this publication's section titled Involve All Staff (page 17). They could then be asked to identify areas for change and develop possible interventions that they could share at a lunchtime meeting and then put into practice. Each month could bring a new topic for the luncheon gatherings.

Collaborate and network. Share success stories and build on ideas.

Create opportunities to network and collaborate with other practices; local, state, and national medical societies; health plans; and hospitals. Invite a colleague unfamiliar with your setting to do a "health literacy walk-through" or a navigational interview[18] to help identify opportunities for improvement. Find out how other pediatricians have successfully adopted health communication techniques like teach-back into their practice. Share sources for reader-friendly print materials.

Make a commitment. Your commitment will encourage buy-in from others.

To effect lasting and meaningful changes, there must be buy-in from everyone involved. Resistance to change is often related to lack of knowledge that a problem exists and concern about time. For example, suddenly deciding to simplify your intake forms and registration processes is likely to be met with some resistance at first, particularly for those who have grown comfortable doing things a certain way. However, if prior to instituting changes you meet with staff and explain that there is an increasingly recognized problem in pediatrics that we all have to address together, you're more likely to have staff who will work together to provide suggestions and solutions.

Review the resources listed at the end of many of the health topic sections of this handbook to identify tools you can share with staff to help everyone understand the extent of the health literacy problem and their role in addressing it.

Provide incentives and rewards.

After achieving a commitment to change, develop an action plan to implement these changes. Structure the practice environment with reminders and cues that prompt staff members to put into action these new changes. Start small. Use small tests of change or Plan-Do-Study-Act (PDSA) cycles to work out the bugs and build experience, confidence, and buy-in.[19] Try one new skill at a time and build up to bigger things. It takes at least 3 weeks for a change to become a habit, provided it is routinely employed. Set weekly goals; provide incentives to participate and rewards for success.

Then be sure to embed the changes in standard operating procedures like policies, checklists, job descriptions, and performance evaluations.

People will be tempted many times to do things the old way and may rationalize by saying, "Just this one time won't matter." And every time a deviation occurs, it will take longer for the change to become a habit. Part-time applications of changes do not result in development of new habits. New habits occur only as a result of consistent and persistent practice. Rewards and incentives can encourage persistent practice that can then be "hardwired" into the operations of your office or clinic.

Engage nontraditional partners.

Community volunteers and liaisons, especially people who have or have had lower health literacy skills, are invaluable consultants who can assist you in making change. Invite them to speak to your staff as part of the introduction of your new health literacy efforts. Their personal stories and passion about improving health communication can motivate your staff toward change.

Include the voice of the patient and adult learners.

Parents and families are the experts in what they need to know and understand in order to take action. Invite their input to help identify opportunities for improvement. These can include suggestion boxes, focus groups, navigational interviews, satisfaction surveys, formal communication assessments,[20] or patient and family advisory councils. Invariably, the input of parents, patients, and families contributes to improved communication and care.

Getting feedback from patients doesn't always have to be a formal process. For example, if you develop new written materials for patients, ask a few patients for feedback before finalizing them.

Adult learners or other nonclinical volunteers can help too. They can review written materials to help simplify them, participate in navigation interviews to help improve way-finding, share their experiences to raise awareness among staff, and serve as sounding boards for new ideas and spokespersons for improving health literacy.[21]

Just do it.

Try a new skill with the last patient of the day. Set a weekly goal to incorporate one new technique in your practice. Engage a partner in your endeavors to monitor progress.

Other Promising Practices

Involve All Staff

In medical settings, members of the office staff are usually the first line of contact for families and patients, many of whom are more comfortable disclosing personal health information to staff than to physicians. As such, it is absolutely critical to involve all staff members in initiatives to improve health literacy practices.

First, increase the staff's awareness and knowledge about literacy and health literacy, and their impact on health. Provide all employees with information on the scope of the problem in the United States and in your area (search https://www.casas.org/lit/litcode/Search.cfm for local statistics). Many programs and tools are available to assist in providing data on why literacy is important for health and examples of the kinds of barriers that parents with low literacy encounter when accessing and providing care for their children, including videos developed by the American Medical Association.[16] A powerful next step is to ask staff to then share stories from their own perspective about difficulties that arose from communication problems in the health care setting. This personalizes the issue and helps raise awareness that low health literacy can be a problem that anyone may experience.

Once awareness is improved, the next step is to increase the staff's acceptance of changes. Consider developing a work group to identify barriers to effective doctor-patient and staff-patient communication in your practice, and ask staff members to develop methods of implementing change.

The goal is for all staff members to be able to recognize potential signs of low literacy and communicate this information to doctors and nurses quickly and sensitively. To ensure the timely delivery of such critical information, be sure the lines of communication within your office remain open.

Create a Shame-free Care Environment

While it is incumbent on us to improve the ways we address the special needs of families with limited health literacy, for all patients and their families we need to create an environment that does not magnify the feelings of shame that come with limited literacy[6] or not understanding. A shame-free care environment is one where parents and patients feel comfortable saying they don't understand, asking questions, and talking openly about their health and concerns.

System changes should be put into place to help patients with low literacy overcome barriers to accessing care, such as displaying materials on literacy programs; reviewing the forms families are asked to complete; and creating an environment that encourages questions, offers proactive assistance, and provides confidential help when needed.

Maps and Directions. Studies have demonstrated that finding the way to a care facility—or navigating the facility once inside—can be difficult for some people with literacy problems.[22] To remove this barrier for your patients, consider the following ideas:

- Display signs with simple words and pictographs to help families find various departments or offices (such as billing or x-ray).

- Put maps on the back of appointment slips or referral forms.

- When giving a patient a complicated map of a hospital or other complex facility, first orient them to directions and where they currently are, then use a colored marker to trace the route from the front door to the appropriate department.

- Train all staff (not just those working at the information desk) on the layout of the hospital, the locations of various sites (eg, radiology, laboratory, cafeteria, etc), and how to give clear directions.[18] Remember that people in nonclinical roles, like housekeeping and transportation, may appear more approachable and be asked more questions.

Forms. As health professionals, we use forms to collect demographic data, insurance information, and personal and family medical history. To help patients and families with low literacy, keep forms to a minimum for everyone, avoid asking for duplicate information, and use forms that are short and contain simple words and phrases.[16] Regardless of the perception of a patient's literacy level, have staff offer to assist every patient with filling out the forms so that no one is singled out or made to feel embarrassed. Keep appointment cards and reminders simple as well.

Literacy referrals. Be prepared with a reader-friendly list for local literacy referral information so there is no delay when a patient seeks help—or even just seems open to accepting help—for literacy problems. Consider keeping a stack of these materials in each examination room so patients can take them without having to ask, which may embarrass them. The Web sites www.literacydirectory.org and www.proliteracy.org are useful in locating adult literacy programs near you.

Encourage questions to empower patients and caregivers. Foster an environment that encourages and expects questions from patients and family members. A change as simple as "Do you have any questions for me?" to "What questions do you have for me today?" creates an expectation of questions and removes the patient's usual response, "no," from the equation. *Ask Me 3* can be very helpful by making it clear that questions are welcome and expected, especially when all staff convey to patients that they want to make sure they get their questions answered.

Create confidential assistance opportunities. If you notice a red flag, it is important to find a private place to discuss the issue. Parents are often ashamed to admit their reading difficulties in front of their children, so consider creating a private interaction—without children present—to discuss literacy. Send the child to be weighed and measured by another staff member, for example, or take the parent to your private office or other confidential area so you can talk alone. And always be sure to address literacy issues in a sensitive, understanding manner.

References

1. Kessels RP. Patients' memory for medical information. *J R Soc Med.* 2003;96:219–222

2. Kohn LT, Corrigan JM, Donaldson MS, eds. *To Err Is Human: Building a Safer Health System.* Washington, DC: National Academy Press; 2000

3. American Academy of Family Physicians (AAFP), American Academy of Pediatrics (AAP), American College of Physicians (ACP), American Osteopathic Association (AOA). Joint principles of the patient-centered medical home. http://www.medicalhomeinfo.org/Joint%20Statement.pdf. Accessed June 5, 2008

4. Institute of Medicine. *Health Professions Education: A Bridge to Quality.* Washington, DC: National Academic Press; 2003

5. Institute of Medicine. *Health Literacy: A Prescription to End Confusion.* Nielsen-Bohlman L, Panzer AM, Kindig DA, eds. Washington, DC: The National Academies Press; 2004

6. Parikh NS, Parker RM, Nurss JR, Baker DW, Williams MV. Shame and health literacy: the unspoken connection. *Patient Educ Couns.* 1996;27:33–39

7. Braddock CH, Fihn SD, Levinson W, Jonsen A, Pearlman RA. How doctors and patients discuss routine clinical decisions: informed decision making in the outpatient setting. *J Gen Intern Med.* 1997;12:339–345

8. Paasche-Orlow MK, Wolf MS. Evidence does not support clinical screening of literacy. *J Gen Intern Med.* 2008;23(1):100–102

9. Davis TC, Long SW, Jackson RH, Mayeaux EJ, et al. Rapid estimate of adult literacy in medicine: a shortened screening instrument. *Fam Med.* 1993;25(6):391–395

10. Doak CC, Doak LG, Root JH. *Teaching Patients With Low Literacy Skills.* Philadelphia, PA: Lippincott Williams & Wilkins; 1996. http://www.hsph.harvard.edu/healthliteracy/doak/html

11. Parker RM, Baker DW, Williams MV, Nurss JR. The test of functional health literacy in adults (TOFHLA): a new instrument for measuring patients literacy skills. *J Gen Intern Med.* 1995;10:537–545

12. Baker DW, Williams MV, Parker RM, Gazmararian JA, Nurss J. Development of a brief test to measure functional health literacy. *Patient Educ Couns.* 1999;38(1):33–42

13. Weiss BD, Mays MZ, Martz W, et al. Quick assessment of literacy in primary care: the newest vital sign. *Ann Fam Med.* 2005;3:514–522

14. Pfizer Clear Health Communication Initiative. The newest vital sign: a new health literacy assessment tool for health care providers. http://www.clearhealthcommunication.org/physicians-providers/newest-vital-sign.html. Accessed May 22, 2008

15. Sanders LM. Number of children's books in the home: an indication of parent health literacy. *Ambul Pediatr.* 2004;4(5):424–428

16. American Medical Association. *Health Literacy and Patient Safety: Help Patients Understand* [videotape]. Chicago, IL: American Medical Association; 2007

17. Institute of Medicine. *Priority Areas for National Action: Transforming Health Care Quality.* Washington, DC: The National Academy of Sciences; 2003

18. Rudd RE. Navigating hospitals. *Lit Harvest.* 2004;11(1):19–24

19. Institute for Healthcare Improvement. Testing changes. http://www.ihi.org/IHI/Topics/ChronicConditions/AllConditions/HowToImprove/ChronicTestingChanges.htm. Accessed June 7, 2007

20. Makoul G, Krupat E, Chang CH. Measuring patient views of physician communication skills: development and testing of the Communication Assessment Tool. *Patient Educ Couns.* 2007;67(3):333–342

21. Osborne H. Health and Literacy Working Together: A Health Literacy Conference for New Readers & Health Professionals. http://www.ihconline.org/toolkits/healthliteracy/OsborneNewReadersConference.pdf. Accessed June 24, 2008

22. Klingbeil C, Speece MW, Schubiner H. Readability of pediatric patient education materials. *Clin Pediatr.* 1995;34(20):96–102

CHAPTER Unique Aspects of Health Literacy for Pediatricians

In pediatrics we have 2 patients: the child and the parent. We depend on parents to model and encourage healthy behavior in their children; bring them for well-child checks and sick visits when appropriate; and follow our instructions for treatment, management, and prevention. Both parents and patients must be active participants in the child's health care. Clear communication about key elements of health conditions and preventive services and encouragement to ask questions and raise issues are believed to have a positive impact on the quality of care delivered to children. But when parents don't understand the information they are given, children can miss appointments, skip vaccinations, undergo wrong treatments, or adopt poor health behaviors. Some may never make it to the pediatrician's office at all.

Consider these facts.

- Roughly 1 in 4 parents has low health literacy.[1]

- One in 3 adults of child-bearing age (aged 16–39) in the United States has limited literacy skills.[1]

- About 1 in 10 adults (aged 16–39) has below-basic reading skills (meaning they are unable to read TV listings), and an additional 1 in 4 has basic reading skills (meaning they can read somewhat, but they are unable to consult a nutrition label to determine which foods contain a particular vitamin).[2]

This chapter discusses the impact that limited health literacy has on children. We look at how children are affected when there is limited literacy in the family, and interventions that we as pediatricians can use to help our patients and their families improve their understanding in the office and their literacy skills at home.

The importance of health literacy is growing as we address the major emerging threats to children's health today—the "new morbidities"[3]—such as obesity; injuries; and tobacco, alcohol, and other substance abuse, many of which are related to behavior. Altering the trajectory depends on parents and patients having the knowledge, tools, and skills to make prudent short- and long-term choices.

The epidemic of childhood obesity is a problem where parents and children need to be equipped to process and judge the validity of multiple sources of health information, read and interpret food nutrition labels, know how much and what kinds of physical activity are needed, understand how near-term choices impact long-term health, and have confidence in their ability to set and achieve small goals for behavior change.

Health literacy and consumers' ability to manage their health (patient activation) both contribute to health behaviors, health choices, and health outcomes. Health literacy allows more choices and more educated decisions, while activation contributes to improved health behavior. When it comes to being able to understand health information, several factors come into play: the complexity of the information and the way it is presented, and the skill and motivation of the user. Health information and messages should be tied to both health literacy and patient activation levels. Tailoring materials so that they support patients with lower literacy and include strategies to increase activation is believed to contribute to improved health outcomes.[4]

The importance of health literacy to patient safety cannot be emphasized enough. Patients are considered important partners in safety. They are told to ask questions; point out differences in medications; inform us about the use of all over-the-counter and complementary and alternative medications; be responsible for knowing medication names, strengths, and doses; ask questions about the purpose of each medication to be used; and ensure that patient identity has been checked before medications are administered in the hospital.[5] But to fulfill these roles, parents must know and understand the necessary information and feel comfortable enough and encouraged to participate in such an active way.

- Data demonstrate that adults misinterpret and fail to understand prescription drug labels.[6] Because they are primarily responsible for administering medication to their children, this has major implications for medication safety.

- Parents with low literacy describe instances where they made mistakes administering their children's medications—resulting in serious side effects—because they did not understand the doctor's directions over the telephone.

Another important trend is that the proportion of children with special health care needs is growing.

- Thirteen percent of children have special health care needs.[7]

- A significant portion of patients discharged from the hospital are technology-dependent.[8]

Children with special health care needs usually have medical specialists and ancillary services that can make care coordination and treatment plans challenging even to the most literate. A multitude of new, often complex, treatments further increases the level of sophistication required of families to benefit from our health care system. From the complex care of preterm infants and critically ill children, to health maintenance issues of safety, nutrition, and vaccination, the decision-making process relies on understanding a wide field of information that is usually unfamiliar to a parent or patient.

Certainly, the stakes could not be higher when we depend on the parents of these children with special needs to act as true partners with adequate health literacy. But it is equally vital to the safety and health of children in America that we help their parents and other caregivers act as our partners in care, regardless of their current literacy level.

As such, we must deal with parental and familial literacy to provide the best possible care to our primary patients: children.

Relationship Between Health Literacy and Pediatrics

Pediatricians are wise to be concerned about the impact that a family's low health literacy has on children. Children with low literacy and children whose parents have low health literacy are at increased risk of poor health outcomes—even after controlling for parents' education and income.

- Globally, maternal illiteracy is closely associated with infant mortality.[9]

- Children whose caregivers have low health literacy have diminished access to primary health care and greater unmet health care needs.[10–12]

- Parents with low literacy are no more likely to smoke than parents with adequate literacy, but they are less likely to know about the health effects of smoking.[13]

- Among children with asthma, those with low-literacy caregivers are more likely to use the emergency department and to be hospitalized.[14]

- Among children with diabetes, those with low-literacy caregivers have worse glycemic control.[15]

- Compared with children who read at or above grade level, children who read below grade level are at twice the risk for exposure to physical violence and handling dangerous weapons.[16]

When a parent suffers from limited literacy or limited health literacy—or both—the child's health will almost certainly suffer (Table 3.1).

At least half of all parents have difficulty reading and understanding pediatric pamphlets—80% of which are written above the eighth-grade level.

Source: Arnold CL, Davis TC, Frempong JO, et al. Assessment of newborn screening parent education materials. *Pediatrics.* 2006;117(5 Pt 2):S341–S354.

Assessing for Low Literacy in the Pediatric Setting

While health literacy has been an emerging topic in internal medicine for the past decade, in pediatrics the subject is just beginning to be recognized. It is clear that low health literacy affects the whole family, but screening for it requires that pediatricians shift their focus from child to parent.

While Chapter 3 discusses screening adults for literacy problems, this section looks at modified, less formal ways to assess the literacy of parents and other adult caregivers. These questions can easily be inserted into conversation during the course of a regular office visit.

As discussed previously, one way to screen for literacy without directly asking about reading is to ask about the number of children's books in the home. The presence of more than 10 children's books at home has been found to be independently associated with adequate parental literacy (as measured by the S-TOHFLA).[17] Other possible screening questions to assess the literacy of household members (including the parent/guardian, extended family members, adolescent, and child) include

- How happy are you with how well you read?

- How do you like to learn new information? (Do you learn best through books, videos, or on the computer, or when somebody shows you how to do something?)

- What are your favorite things to do with your child? (Is reading one of them?)

- What are your child's favorite things to do? (Is reading one of them?)

- [For the child] What are your favorite things to do? (Is reading one of them?)

Discussions about children's school performance can also naturally lead to questions about the parents' reading abilities.

- Are you able to help your child with homework?

- Did you ever have difficulty in school?

- What was the highest grade you completed? (This is a helpful question to give you an idea if the parents dropped out of school early. However, educational level is not a reliable indicator of literacy level. Many people read several grade levels below their highest level of education, and some read at higher levels.)

Because the focus remains the care of a child, when pediatricians discuss literacy with parents, the goal is to help the whole family. To prevent the notion that the pediatrician is overstepping his boundaries, and to curtail any embarrassment that the caregiver may feel, the pediatrician should clearly explain that his or her concern is in meeting the health needs of the child—needs that cannot be met well if the caregiver isn't able to read, follow instructions, or communicate well.

Bringing up parental literacy in this context can also motivate parents to seek help. At first it may not feel natural for pediatricians to refer a parent to adult literacy, but it is imperative because it is a program that may help the parent care for their child and eventually help the child do better in school.

Child Health Literacy Interventions

There are few evidence-based approaches to addressing low pediatric health literacy in the pediatric setting. This may be partly because intervention research in the field is difficult to define; it can include work in such diverse areas as patient safety, health behavior research, and health services research.

Still, we do know that some health literacy interventions used with adults are applicable in pediatric settings. Pediatricians can, for example,

- Use teach-back and other time-efficient communication techniques.

- Develop, use, and mark up patient education materials written in plain language (such as those accompanying the topic sections in Part II of this publication).

- Provide and refer to simple pictures, drawings, and videos in the health care setting.

- Refer families to local or online educational resources, such as ESOL (English for Speakers of Other Languages) or ESL (English as a Second Language) classes and adult literacy and GED (General Educational Development/General Equivalency Diploma) high school equivalency education programs.

Table 3.1. Possible Pathways Between Health Literacy and Child Health Outcomes

Preventive Care
Adult primary caregiver with low health literacy → decreased ability to negotiate health system → limited access to child health services *and* limited practice of "recommended preventive health behaviors" → delayed preventive services and unmet health needs → poor child health outcomes
Child/adolescent with low health literacy → school failure → increased referrals for special education → personal and family frustration/stress → increased rates of violence, tobacco and drug use, and early sexual activity, reduced rates of seat belt use, and other risky health behaviors → increased injury, dependency, and sexual and mental health problems

Acute Care
Adult primary caregiver with low health literacy → decreased ability to understand prescription and follow-up instructions → errors in medication administration or follow-up care → poor child health outcomes
Child/adolescent with low health literacy → decreased ability to understand instructions from doctors and from caregivers → errors in medication administration and follow-up care → poor child health outcomes

Chronic Illness Care
Adult primary caregiver with low health literacy → decreased ability to accomplish multiple medical tasks *and* decreased coordination of services → decreased adherence → delayed preventive services and unmet health needs/increased need for services → poor health outcomes
Child/adolescent with low health literacy → decreased ability to communicate with caregivers about health needs → poor health behaviors and practices → poor health outcomes

Different settings require different types of interventions. Pediatricians working in outpatient clinics may consider

- Making disease managers or health coaches available to help families with special health care needs, both at home and in health settings

- Using plain language materials to improve self-management of common illnesses (eg, asthma action plans, American Dietetic Association diets, and medication schedules)
- Using plain language materials to encourage specific health-promoting behaviors (eg, breastfeeding, smoking cessation)

Providers serving in hospitals and emergency departments might

- Make case managers or patient navigators available to arrange follow-up care and help families understand discharge instructions.
- Give families plain language materials that explain common emergency department instructions (eg, head trauma, febrile seizures).
- Use plain language materials for common hospital discharge instructions (eg, newborn screening, jaundice).

Physicians working in nonclinical community settings could consider

- Supporting universal postpartum home-visiting services
- Improving health literacy education and training for children, parents, and teachers in child care centers, schools, and adult learning centers
- Using plain language materials for public health education (eg, letters about exposure to meningitis or pertussis/whooping cough) for use by child care centers, schools, and the general public
- Supporting policies to ensure the use of plain language in written health-related materials and the inclusion of health literacy in quality initiatives

Another unique way that pediatricians can incorporate adult literacy into their practices is by promoting programs that encourage children's emergent literacy, such as Reach Out and Read. Reach Out and Read trains practitioners to provide anticipatory guidance about the importance of reading books with children and to distribute books to patients at every well-child visit from 6 months to 5 years.[18] Many studies have demonstrated that Reach Out and Read is an effective program in increasing the amount of time that parents read with their children, improving both parents' and children's attitudes about reading (and making them more likely to say that reading is one of their favorite activities, both shared and individually). It has also been shown to raise children's receptive and expressive language scores.[19–30]

Let Them Be Children

As children acquire increased language and communication skills, new ethical and social issues emerge in the examination room.

In families where parental literacy or limited English proficiency—both general and health-related—can be a problem, children are inappropriately pressed into service as interpreters of spoken information.

Physicians should be aware of this issue, and be diligent not to cast children into these adult roles to meet the needs of their parents.

Communication Tips

Communicating With Children

In pediatrics, part of our responsibility is to track and assess children's communication skills and their understanding of health and bodily function as they mature, and to help them transition to adulthood and become capable consumers of health care. This is especially important for children who are being asked to monitor symptoms or to request as-needed medication. Studies of children with chronic conditions have found that even preschool-aged children can gain understanding about their conditions. And their understanding can help them contribute to improved disease management and treatment adherence.[31]

- Children as young as 8 years can reliably assess their own health and use simple scales related to health and well-being.[32]
- School-aged children with chronic illnesses, such as asthma, diabetes, and cystic fibrosis, can participate actively in their own care (although their understanding of the diagnosis will necessarily evolve over time).[33,34]
- One study found that among children aged 4 to 14 years with insulin-dependent diabetes mellitus and cystic fibrosis, older children assumed increasing responsibilities for self-care, although parents remained heavily involved into early adolescence.[35]

As we note that children are increasingly involved in their own care, we should engage in a kind of "double teach-back," in which both the parent and child are asked to articulate, in a shame-free manner, an understanding of instructions and important medical information in their own words. Alternate questions, first addressing the mother. For example: "How much medicine will you tell your husband Julie needs?" Then ask the child: "What will make you tell your father you're feeling worse?" Then back to the mother: "I want to make sure I told you this clearly. Remind me what I said about when you should call 911 for Julie if she has an asthma attack."

No matter what kind of information you need the child to understand, or how intellectually advanced they are, consider using these effective techniques when you communicate with children.

Ask open-ended questions. Elicit the child's own language and vocabulary to describe the illness, and then incorporate that terminology into your explanations and instructions. Determine the names used by the child (and the parent) for body parts and bodily functions; symptoms, pains, or troubling sensations; and treatments or responses to symptoms.

Offer age-neutral educational materials. Materials must use plain language and pictures, but should not make assumptions about the age of the child using the materials. If simple language is paired with illustrations of young children and is presented in a childish font, the materials aren't likely to be effective with older children. Text that looks formal and dense—and isn't broken up into small, digestible parts—will discourage younger children from getting information they need. Consider your audience when developing and distributing materials.

Use lists. Lists can be an effective part of health education materials for children from preschool age through high school. To communicate the importance of food and nutrition, for example, a younger child might be offered a simple list of foods to eat and foods to avoid, while an older child may be shown how to read food labels to evaluate nutritional content or avoid potential allergens. Lists that include pictures are very useful, not only for younger children, but also for older children whose literacy is limited and those who do not speak especially well.

Lists can be especially effective when developed with acronyms or other mnemonics that the child can remember. Following is an example from the American Lung Association of Washington.[36]

Could You Have ASTHMA?

Do you have **A**llergies?

Are you **S**hort of breath?

Is there **T**ightness in your chest?

Is it **H**ard to breathe while exercising?

Have you **M**issed work or school?

Are you **A**lways coughing?

Disseminate multimedia materials. Videotapes, comic books, magazines, and interactive computer activities can engage children and educate them about their condition in a fun, kid-friendly way. This can be an especially effective way to reach the increasing number of children who love computers or videogames. A recent review found 11 media-based interventions that were as effective as psychological counseling in improving child behavioral outcomes, such as sleep problems and conduct disorders. (The literacy of the study subjects, however, was not measured.)[37]

Children with chronic conditions that require self-monitoring and treatment—such as asthma, diabetes, and cystic fibrosis—need systematic teaching to help them understand their medical issues and allow them to move toward a higher degree of self-care and independence. Obviously, the more critical the self-monitoring and treatment, the more essential clear communication and teach-back become.

Communicating With Adolescents

Adolescents pose a special challenge in the area of health literacy and communication. While their literacy and health literacy skills should be nearing an adult level, they generally lack the experience, exposure, and vocabulary that help more experienced adults navigate health information. In this way, it is possible their health literacy skills may diverge from their general literacy skills.

Consider the following issues in communicating with adolescents:

- Adolescents, who are often resistant to any adult advice or expertise, are just as often motivated by peer group considerations or self-consciousness around medical problems.[38] Therefore, written health information may need to be tailored to appeal to the special concerns of this group.

- Novel education and communication strategies may be especially useful with this group; education sessions for parents and their children together have been shown to reduce risky behaviors in adolescents.[39]

- Confidentiality issues complicate medical communication with adolescent patients. The 3-way conversation—involving provider, parent, and patient—may be very difficult when the teaching is around adolescent risk behaviors and prevention. Critical topics, including contraception and substance abuse, may need to be discussed and may be presented more openly when only the physician and patient are present. All adolescents should have the opportunity to meet with the doctor without the parent present. As with all topics, it is essential for the physician to be fully aware of the patient's vocabulary and level of understanding.

- The increasing use of the Internet and other electronic communication with peers has the potential to affect adolescents' acquisition and use of health-related information. Studies show that children are inclined to doubt the truth of a message if it coincides with the speaker's self-interest,[40] suggesting that providing them with information about the people making health-related claims will make them better able to evaluate those claims.

Communicating With Parents

Think for minute what it might be like to be the parent of a child in your practice. Whether the patient is a newborn or a 15-year-old, there are many unexpected issues and concerns that can arise during pediatric office visits.

Remember: A parent's attention is divided because they have multiple responsibilities in addition to being information receivers. Children do not stop acting like children when seeing a doctor, and thus parents must still be parents. For the child who is worried or crying, the parent will console and comfort. For the child who is uncooperative or just a little too curious, the parent cajoles, distracts, and soothes or disciplines. For the child with questions, the parent has answers, and for the child who is bored, the parent must entertain.

The more roles the parent is playing at any time, the more his or her attention is divided, and the more difficult it becomes for him or her to listen and understand the messages you convey. The end result, unfortunately, is often that some information is missed, misunderstood, or not retained.[41–44]

Any relief you can provide to parents will increase the likelihood that information will be understood. Here is a quick list of some things you can try in your practice to free up some mental resources for parents.

Just wait. Sometimes it is clear that a parent is temporarily overwhelmed. For example, if a child is crying hard, 30 seconds may be all the time needed for the parent to console the child and refocus on your conversation.

Help out. At other times, you may want to step in and help the parent with one of their roles. For example, providing an interesting diversion for the curious or fussy child might be very helpful.

Set the stage. After seeing patient after patient every day, you are very familiar with what to expect within a specific medical appointment. For the parent, however, there is likely to be uncertainty about what will transpire. Take some time at the start of the visit to put the parent and child at ease. Tell parents you are there to help and that you will allot time to answer their questions. With this framework, parents can stop wondering when they can work in their questions.

Simplify. Most parents do not have any prior medical knowledge related to the topic you are discussing. While you need to explain the topic or diagnosis, keep it simple and limit the number of key messages to fewer than 5. You can always tell them more if they ask questions, and you can send them home with fact sheets and other handouts, but for starters, just tell them what they really need to know to keep their child healthy. For complex or technical topics, alternate forms of media, such as diagrams, pictographs, or anatomical models, can be helpful in breaking the topic down for parents.

Repeat. Even if the information is jargon-free, remembering information is not an easy task, particularly when attention is focused elsewhere. You cannot assume that information said only one time to parents will be remembered. Anything you feel is important for parents to know needs to be repeated. Encourage parents to take notes, or write down key pieces of information legibly for them. And review and mark important information on reader-friendly handouts or other, more detailed materials they can read when they can better focus their attention (eg, after the child has gone to bed) and share with family members.

Use multiple formats. Each person has a preference for the way he or she takes in information. Some people prefer written material, others visual, and others prefer to hear all new information. The general rule is that the more senses involved in receiving information (sight, hearing, and touch), the higher the likelihood that the information will be remembered. The use of illustrations and pictographs has been shown to improve patient comprehension.[45,46]

Focus, summarize, and check for understanding. There is a natural tendency to try to squeeze in as much information as possible within office visits. As the number of messages increases, the likelihood of the parent remembering each one decreases.[47] It is better to pick out the key messages that you feel are most important for a particular child and focus on them. You can always answer their questions or send them home with more information, but at the visit, keep your messages simple and summarize them at the end of the visit. Using teach-back also provides a great opportunity to check understanding, make sure they heard and internalized the important parts, repeat and expand on your messages, and transition into summarizing the key messages.

Consider group visits. Group visits are becoming a more common approach among pediatricians.[48,49] Within a group visit, there may be greater time to present information in multiple ways. Further, group discussion will naturally lead to certain topics being examined in greater depth. Parents will also teach each other, which may have an even greater impact on families than when the information is provided solely by the primary care physician.[50] Additionally, parents will ask questions that others may forget to ask or that may not have occurred to them.

References

1. Kutner M, Greenberg E, Baer J. *A First Look at the Literacy of America's Adults in the 21st Century.* Washington, DC: National Center for Education Statistics; 2005

2. US Department of Education, National Center for Education Statistics. *The Condition of Education 2003.* Washington, DC: NCES; 2003

3. American Academy of Pediatrics Committee on Community Health Services. The pediatrician's role in community pediatrics. *Pediatrics.* 2005;115:1092–1194

4. Hibbard J. Both health literacy and patient activation contribute to consumers' ability to manage their health. In: Proceedings from the Surgeon General's Workshop on Improving Health Literacy; September 7, 2006; Bethesda, MD

5. American Academy of Pediatrics Committee on Drugs and Committee on Hospital Care. Prevention of medication errors in the pediatric inpatient setting. *Pediatrics.* 2003;112:431–436

6. Davis TC, Wolf MS, Bass PF, et al. Literacy and misunderstanding of prescription drug labels. *Ann Intern Med.* 2006;145(12):887–894

7. The National Center of Medical Home Initiatives for Children with Special Needs. What is a medical home? http://www.medicalhomeinfo.org. Accessed May 22, 2008

8. Haffner JC, Schurman SJ. The technology dependent child. *Pediatr Clin North Am.* 2001;48:751–764

9. Grosse RN, Auffrey C. Literacy and health status in developing countries. *Annu Rev Public Health.* 1989;10:281–297

10. Broder HL, Russell S, Catapano P, Reisine S. Perceived barriers and facilitators to dental treatment among female caregivers of children with and without HIV and their health care providers. *Pediatr Dent.* 2002;24(4):301–308

11. Sanders LM, Lewis J, Brosco JP. Low caregiver health literacy: risk factor for child access to a medical home. Presented at: Pediatric Academic Societies; May 2005; Washington, DC

12. Sanders LM, Thompson VT, Wilkinson JD. Caregiver health literacy and the use of child health services. Presented at: Pediatric Academic Societies; May 2005; Washington, DC

13. Arnold CL, Davis TC, Berkel HJ, Jackson RH, Nandy I, London S. Smoking status, reading level, and knowledge of tobacco effects among low-income pregnant women. *Prev Med.* 2001;32(4):313–320

14. DeWalt DA, Dilling MH, Rosenthal MJ, Pignone MP. Low parental literacy is associated with worse asthma care measures in children. *Ambul Pediatr.* 2007;7(1):25-31

15. Ross LA, Frier BM, Kelnar CJ, Deary IJ. Child and parental mental ability and glycaemic control in children with Type 1 diabetes. *Diabetes Med.* 2001;18:364–369

16. Davis TC, Byrd RS, Arnold CL, Auinger P, Bocchini JA Jr. Low literacy and violence among adolescents in a summer sports program. *J Adolesc Health.* 1999;24(6):403–411

17. Sanders LM. Number of children's books in the home: an indication of parent health literacy. *Ambul Pediatr.* 2004;4(5):424–428

18. Reach Out and Read National Center. Making books part of a healthy childhood. http://www.reachoutandread.org. Accessed June 2008

19. Needlman R, Fried L, Morely D, Taylor S, Zuckerman B. Clinic-based intervention to promote literacy. *Am J Dis Child.* 1991;145:881–884

20. High P, Hopman M, LaGasse L, Linn H. Evaluation of a clinic based program to promote book sharing and bedtime routines among low-income urban families with young children. *Arch Pediatr Adolesc Med.* 1998;152:459–465

21. Golova N, Alario A, Vivier P, et al. Literacy promotion for Hispanic families in a primary care setting: a randomized, controlled trial. *Pediatrics.* 1999;103:993–997

22. High PC, LaGasse L, Becker S, et al. Literacy promotion in primary care pediatrics: can we make a difference? *Pediatrics.* 2000;105:927–934

23. Sanders LM, Gershon TD, Huffman LC, Mendoza FS. Prescribing books for immigrant children. *Arch Pediatr Adolesc Med.* 2000;154:771–777

24. Mendelsohn A, Mogliner L, Dreyer B, et al. The impact of a clinic-based literacy intervention on language development in inner-city preschool children. *Pediatrics.* 2001;107:130–134

25. Sharif I, Reiber S, Ozuah PO. Exposure to Reach Out and Read and vocabulary outcomes in inner city preschoolers. *J Natl Med Assoc.* 2002;94:171–177

26. Silverstein M, Iverson L, Lozano P. An English-language clinic based literacy program is effective for a multilingual population. *Pediatrics.* 2002;109:e76

27. Theriot JA, Franco SM, Sisson BA, Metcalf SC, Kennedy MA, Bada HS. The impact of early literacy guidance on language skills of 3-year-olds. *Clin Pediatr (Phila).* 2003;42:165–172

28. Weitzman CC, Roy L, Walls T, Tomlin R. More evidence for Reach Out and Read: a home-based study. *Pediatrics.* 2004;113:1248–1253

29. Needlman R, Silverstein M. Pediatric interventions to support reading aloud: how good is the evidence? *J Dev Behav Pediatr.* 2004;25:352–363

30. Needleman R, Toker KH, Dreyer BP, Klass P, Mendelsohn AL. Effectiveness of a primary care intervention to support reading aloud: a multicenter evaluation. *Ambul Pediatr.* 2005;5(4);209–215

31. Holzheimer L, Mohay H, Masters IB. Educating young children about asthma: comparing the effectiveness of a developmentally appropriate asthma education video tape and picture book. *Child Care Health Dev.* 1998;24(1):85–99

32. Rebok G, Riley A, Forrest C, et al. Elementary school-aged children's reports of their health: a cognitive interviewing study. *Qual Life Res* 2001;10:59–70

33. McNabb WL, Quinn MT, Murphy DM, Thorp FK, Cook S. Increasing children's responsibility for diabetes self-care: the In Control study. *Diabetes Educ.* 1994;20:121–124

34. Downs JA, Roberts CM, Blackmore AM, Le Souef PN, Jenkins SC. Benefits of an education programme on the self-management of aerosol and airway clearance treatments for children with cystic fibrosis. *Chron Respir Dis.* 2006;3:19–27

35. Drotar D, Ievers C. Age differences in parent and child responsibilities for management of cystic fibrosis and insulin-dependent diabetes mellitus. *J Dev Behav Pediatr.* 1994;15:265–272

36. American Lung Association of Washington. Asthma acronym. http://www.alaw.org/asthma/asthma_acronym/. Accessed June 8, 2008

37. Montgomery P, Bjornstad G, Dennis J. Media-based behavioural treatments for behavioural problems in children. *Cochrane Database Syst Rev.* 2006;(1):CD002206

38. Buston KM, Wood SF. Non-compliance amongst adolescents with asthma: listening to what they tell us about self-management. *Fam Pract.* 2000;17:134–138

39. Spoth RL, Redmond C, Shin C. Reducing adolescents' aggressive and hostile behaviors: randomized trial effects of a brief family intervention 4 years past baseline. *Arch Pedtiatr Adolesc Med.* 2000;154:1248–1257

40. Mills C, Keil FC. Knowing the limits of one's understanding: the development of an awareness of an illusion of explanatory depth. *J Exp Child Psychol.* 2004;87:1–32

41. Grover G, Berkowitz CD, Lewis RJ. Parental recall after a visit to the emergency department. *Clin Pediatr.* 1994;33:194–201

42. Heffer RW, Worchel-Prevatt F, Rae WA, et al. The effects of oral versus written instructions on parents' recall and satisfaction after pediatric appointments. *J Dev Behav Pediatr.* 1997;18:377–382

43. Moon RY, Cheng TL, Patel KM, Baumhaft K, Scheidt PC. Parental literacy level and understanding of medical information. *Pediatrics.* 1998;102:e25

44. Waisman Y, Siegal N, Chemo M, et al. Do parents understand emergency department discharge instructions? A survey analysis. *Isr Med Assoc J.* 2003;838:567–570

45. Austin PE, Matlack R II, Dunn KA, Kesler C, Brown CK. Discharge instructions: do illustrations help our patients understand them? *Ann Emerg Med.* 1995;25(3):317–320

46. Dowse R, Ehlers M. Medicine labels incorporating pictograms: do they influence understanding and adherence? *Patient Educ Couns.* 2005;58(1):63–70

47. Barkin SL, Scheindlin B, Brown C, Ip E, Finch S, Wasserman RC. Anticipatory guidance topics: are more better? *Ambul Pediatr.* 2005;5:372–376

48. Osborn LM. Group well-child care. *Clin Perinatol.* 1985;12:355–365

49. Jaber R, Braksmajer A, Trilling JS. Group visits: a qualitative review of current research. *J Am Board Fam Med.* 2006;19:276–290

50. Anderson, JE. Rejuvenate your practice with group visits. *Contemp Pediatr.* 2006;23(5):80–94

Effective Communication Techniques

Whether written or verbal, communication is the cornerstone of partnering with parents and patients in pediatric care. A child who doesn't know how to ask for help after a certain age, or a parent who can't understand the medication label—contribute to prolonged or worsened symptoms, and both need our help to keep children healthy. This chapter focuses on strategies and techniques that you can implement in your practice or clinic to help make sure that your messages are heard, understood, and retained by the patient and/or family.

The most important idea to remember is to practice patient-centered care. Patient-centered (or family-centered) care includes using a style of communication that gives the patient or family a larger role in the patient-doctor interaction and in the decision-making process. This approach has been shown to improve not only communication and compliance, but also patient satisfaction.[1-4] To practice this kind of care fully, however, you have to make sure your patients and their families have every opportunity to learn what they need to know to make informed decisions, regardless of their literacy levels. (For more on patient-centered care, see Chapter 3.)

This chapter includes some tips to remember when you're communicating with patients and their families, whether in writing or in conversation, as well as special sections on developing written materials and addressing special populations, such as the hearing impaired and those for whom English is a second language.

Use everyday words, or "plain language."

The language of medicine is so ingrained in us—from first learning the language in medical school to understanding how to use it during residency, and now using it in daily practice—that it can be easy to forget that patients don't understand medical terms and jargon. Always remember that none of your patients (and few of their parents) went to medical school, so they don't understand medical jargon any more than you may understand the language of your mechanic or electrician.

Using plain language (sometimes called "living-room language") can help bridge that communication gap, both in writing and in conversation. Presenting information in a way that makes it as easy as possible for every reader to understand; explain things in the way you would when talking with your grandmother, or to your neighbor. Here's how plain language is described by the Plain Language Information and Action Network, a group of federal employees from many different agencies and specialties that advocates for clarity in government

Plain language (also called Plain English) is communication your audience can understand the first time they read or hear it. Language that is plain to one set of readers may not be plain to others…. No one technique defines plain language. Rather, plain language is defined by results—it is easy to read, understand, and use.[5]

Plain language, as defined by the National Institutes of Health (NIH) Plain Language Coordinating Committee, involves using clear verbiage that conveys exactly what the audience needs to know "without unnecessary words or expression," with key features that include use of "common, everyday words, except for necessary technical terms." The NIH recommends written material be geared toward a fourth- to eighth-grade reading level.

Often, the plainest way to explain a complex concept is to use analogies. Analogies may help patients understand what is, to them, an abstract condition. For instance, instead of saying the child with asthma suffers from bronchoconstriction, say, "When Mary has an asthma attack it's like she is breathing through a tiny straw. She has to work very hard to get the air in and out."[6] (See the health topics in Part II for sample analogies you can use for common health conditions.)

A Little More Conversation

When developing materials for your patients and their families, write as if you were talking to friend.

A conversational style has a more natural tone and is easier to read and understand. Read aloud what you've written to see how it sounds.

Use: If you go near this chemical, you could get sick.

Avoid: Exposure to this chemical could cause adverse health effects.

Source: US Centers for Disease Control and Prevention. *Scientific and Technical Information Simply Put.* 2nd ed. Atlanta, GA: CDC Office of Communication; 1999. http://www.cdc.gov /od/oc/simpput.pdf. Accessed June 7, 2008

Slow down and allow the patient to talk too.

Providers may feel that they need to rush to cover as much as possible within each visit, but make an effort to slow down. Primary care is a longitudinal process (everything can't be covered every time), and doctors must have faith in the idea that all of the relevant topics will be covered over time—not during one visit. In fact, few people can remember more than 3 or 4 concepts at a time, so covering everything doesn't actually convey more information and therefore is not a wise use of time.

Prioritizing topics for each visit based on the child's age and history can help free up time that can be spent for meaningful discussion with patients. To help with this, the American Academy of Pediatrics developed Bright Futures materials that identify which priority health topics should be addressed at which visit from the prenatal visit to the late adolescent appointment.

One study compared the attributes of primary care physicians who had legal claims made against them and those who had not. It found that, on average, those with no claims spent 3 minutes longer with patients than the other physicians; they were more likely to be facilitating (including checking patients' understanding); and they laugh more.[7]

In addition to slowing down when *you* talk, slow the whole visit down so the *patient and family* can talk. Because of real and perceived time constraints, providers have a tendency to dominate their conversations with patients. Studies have shown that providers interrupt patients 30 seconds after they start speaking; however, if not interrupted, patients will speak less than 2 minutes.[8–10] So sit down, elicit patient concerns, ask open-ended questions, and engage in active listening.[11]

Focus your messages. Keep information simple and relevant, and repeat it.

Limit the amount of information provided at each visit, and focus your communication on the few most significant things the parent and patient need to remember. This is especially important on the first visit for a condition. When you initially diagnose a child with asthma, for example, you only need tell the family the most basic information on the condition and how it can be managed. Don't overwhelm them by explaining the physiology of asthma—focus more on explaining how to care for the child, manage the condition, and react in an emergency.

This will allow some time for the diagnosis to sink in, while the patient and caregivers start learning how to administer inhalers and other treatments. On subsequent visits, you can introduce additional—and increasingly more detailed and complex—information about the condition. If you add only a few messages at a time, the family is more likely to remember all of them.

You can also help patients retain information by having various members of the health care team (physicians, nurses, clerks and, in some cases, trained volunteers) reinforce information in different ways.[12] Under the Key Message section of each health topic discussed in Part II of this publication, you'll find lists of messages that will enable you to incorporate this idea into your practice. The key messages provide information that the entire staff should deliver consistently, so that a patient walking through your office will not get 5 conflicting messages from the 5 staff members he passes, and a sixth one when he calls in later with a question.

One way to foster communication, while ensuring families and patients retain the basic information they need, is to use the *Ask Me 3* tool.

Ask Me 3

Ask Me 3 was developed by communication and health literacy experts through the Partnership for Clear Health Communication as a tool to improve communication between providers and patients. This technique—adapted here with permission for pediatric patients—consists of 3 questions that help focus patient-provider communication so that the essential information is conveyed and understood.

- What is my main problem? (Or, What is my child's main problem?)
- What do I need to do?
- Why is it important for me to do this?

Ask Me 3 encourages patients to ask these questions and trains providers to ensure that patients know the answers before concluding the health care encounter. It is a useful tool to guide providers in identifying key messages and using plain language, and for empowering patients to ask questions and know what questions to ask. The following is an example:

- *What is Patricia's main problem?*

  A: Patricia has a urine infection.
- *What do I need to do?*

  A: I need to give her 1 teaspoon of medicine in the morning and another teaspoon in the evening every day for 10 days; take her temperature and call the doctor if it gets over 102 degrees; and give her clear liquids, like the ones listed on the handout the doctor gave me.
- *Why is it important that I do this?*

  A: If I stop giving her the medicine before 10 days, Patricia could have kidney problems. The liquids will help her bladder and kidneys get healthy again. A fever may mean she has something else wrong.

To learn more about this tool, go to www. askme3.org.

Learn from patients and families.

Get to know your patients. Address their concerns before giving advice, so you can alleviate any anxiety that may block their receptiveness to information.[13] Ask about their perceptions of any illnesses, their causes, and their treatments that you discussed during the visit, but do so with sensitivity and respect. (See Be sensitive to culture below.)

This can be a good way to find out about any cultural ideas or practices that may affect how your recommendations are implemented. Also, by broadening your cultural knowledge base, you can better treat other patients who share the same condition, background, or even neighborhood.

Along these lines, try to incorporate the family's treatment beliefs (such as herbal medicines and teas for some Latino and Asian patients) into your treatment plan, as long as doing so won't cause harm to the child. You'll be demonstrating respect for the patient's culture, and you might even discover a useful remedy.

Parents and families are the experts in what they need to know and understand in order to take action. Invite their input to help identify opportunities for improvement. Getting feedback from patients doesn't always have to be a formal process. For example, if you develop new written materials for patients, ask a few patients for feedback before finalizing them. Adult learners or other nonclinical volunteers can help too. They can review written materials to help simplify them.[14]

Be sensitive to culture.

Your patients likely come from a wide variety of cultural backgrounds. There are many cultural issues that might not occur to you as you develop written materials for your patients and their families. The Centers for Disease Control and Prevention offers some tips and examples to consider to avoid unintentionally offending readers.

- Use terms that your audience is comfortable, or at least familiar, with.

  Example: If your patients are disadvantaged and usually go to the health department for treatment, use "clinic" in your pamphlet about getting regular checkups, not "doctor's office."

- If you need to identify a group of people by race or ethnicity, use a term preferred by that group. Preferred terms may vary even within an ethnic or racial group, or they may vary by region.

  Example: One group may want to be identified as "African American." Another group may prefer to be identified as "black."

- Tailor messages to each cultural or ethnic group or subgroup. Groups may have different needs, values, and beliefs that will affect how they interpret your message. And minority groups often have subgroups that differ greatly from one another. What is effective for one minority group or subgroup may not work at all for another.

It would be impossible to know and understand all cultures in the world and tailor your materials to each of them, so focus on being sensitive and respectful of beliefs and practices that may influence the care of the child. Use staff members and even patients to help you. Talk to them before designing materials and let them review your drafts and provide feedback.[14]

Check your work.

As you figure out how your patients' families learn best and start to implement those methods, check to make sure patients and families have understood your important messages. You can be more confident that your message has been adequately conveyed and received only if you check. One effective method for this is the teach-back method.

Teach-back

In this method, the doctor, nurse, or other member of the health care team delivers a key message, then asks the patient (or caregiver) a question that causes the patient to respond by putting the message in his or her own words. The patient teaches back to the doctor what the doctor just taught the patient.

With this technique, the doctor is able to verify that the patient or parent understands the key points that the doctor intended to convey. It also allows the doctor to know which messages aren't resonating with the patient and therefore may need to be explained, repeated, or delivered in a new way.

The tricky part of teach-back is its delivery. It is crucial to introduce this concept in a respectful, nonconfrontational manner. You want to avoid the perception that you are quizzing the patient or that you think they aren't able or aren't smart enough to understand what you have said. In teach-back, put the onus on yourself. For example, after examining the patient and prescribing a course of action, a doctor might say

- I want to make sure I explained everything correctly. What will you tell your husband if he needs to give Jack his medicine?

- Let me make sure I told you everything. If you start wheezing, what will you do?

- Let's make sure this plan works for you. When you get home, what foods will you feed Quinn? How much will you give at a time?

- We went through a lot of information pretty fast, so I want to make sure I didn't leave anything out. What signs would mean you should take Emily to the hospital right away?

Notice that in each of these examples, the doctor is assigning the reason for the question to himself or herself and not to the patient's presumed lack of understanding.

While some physicians may resist using teach-back out of fear that it takes too much time, studies show this is not the case—the method generally adds fewer than 2 minutes to the discussion[15]; it is really just a different way of structuring the interview, so that there will be fewer last-minute questions. In addition, once teach-back becomes part of the usual way you explain things to patients, it becomes second nature and you get better at explaining things clearly up front, using plain language and focusing on the most important information the parent needs to know.

Written Techniques to Improve Patient-Doctor Communication

When patients are expected to learn more than 2 or 3 ideas in a single office visit—as is often the case—written reinforcement is necessary.[16] Written tools have been shown both to augment oral communication and improve the efficiency of information delivery.[17]

Problems arise, however, when written materials are not easy for patients and families to read and understand. Common pitfalls that make written materials less comprehensible—or even appealing—to patients include

- Using unfamiliar medical terms and jargon that can lead to misunderstanding

- Writing materials at a level of reading comprehension than is higher than the patient's

- Providing too much information

- Presenting text in a dense format that is not easy to digest

- Failing to take into account that the reader's attention is likely limited and his mental state is affected by dealing with an ill child; or he is likely to be worried, busy, sleep-deprived, or may be ill himself

Good written materials, on the other hand, allow readers to

- Find what they need.

- Understand what they find.

- Use what they find to meet their needs.[5]

The Plain Language Information and Action Network offers the following techniques that can help achieve these goals in written materials. Write materials using

- Logical organization with the reader in mind
- "You" and other pronouns
- Active voice
- Short sentences
- Common, everyday words
- Easy-to-read design features

Even good readers appreciate materials that are easy to read quickly.[18] For patients who have health literacy problems, and even for those who don't, handouts need to be simplified[19] (Table 4.1).

Addressing Special Populations

It is essential to identify special patient populations within your practice who may require additional assistance for doctor-patient communication to be successful. For these populations, encounters will require additional time, personnel, materials, and alternative methods of communication.

Table 4.1. Tips for Creating Easy-to-Read Handouts[a]

General Content
• Limit content to 2 or 3 key points that patients really need to know. Don't provide too much information or the patient will be overloaded.
• Use only words that are well-known to laypeople who don't have medical training. If you must use medical terms, explain them right away.
• Make sure content is age-appropriate and culturally appropriate to the target audience.
Text Construction
• Write at or below the 6th- or 7th-grade reading level.
• Use 1- and 2-syllable words, and keep paragraphs short.

• Write in active voice.
    Passive voice (wrong): One pill should be taken by the patient.
    Active voice (right): The patient should take one pill.

• Include only very simple tables and graphs and place clear explanations of them within the text, as well as in a legend adjacent to the table or graph.
Fonts and Typestyles
• Use large (but not too large) fonts. In blocks of text, the most comfortable font size to read is generally 11 or 12 points.
• Don't use more than 2 or 3 fonts on a page. Consistency in appearance is important.
• Use upper- and lower-case text: UPPER-CASE LETTERS CAN BE HARD TO READ.
• Avoid text colors that are too pale because they don't show up on black-and-white photocopies. And don't put text over red graphics because red comes out black in copies.
Layout
• Ensure a good amount of empty space on the page. Don't clutter the page with too much text or too many pictures. Too many elements distract from what's really important.
• Use headings and subheads to separate blocks of text.
• Bulleted lists are a good way to convey a lot of information without overwhelming the reader.
• Simple illustrations and pictograms are useful when they depict common, easy-to-recognize objects. Images should be age-appropriate and culturally appropriate to the target audience.

[a]**Source**: American Medical Association. Formatting checklist for easy-to-read written materials. In: Weiss BD, ed. *Health Literacy and Patient Safety: Help Patients Understand. Manual for Physicians.* 2nd ed. Chicago, IL: AMA Foundation; 2007:36.

Limited English Proficiency

For patients who do not speak or understand English well, health literacy is an especially difficult challenge. It's as if they must learn a third language based on their limited knowledge and understanding of English and health issues. Consider hiring bilingual staff and doctors, who can be particularly helpful for interpreting and translating complex information that cannot be explained in simple terms.

Bilingual staff members can help identify communications pitfalls and sort out misunderstandings that arise from differences between what is said and what is understood. But be sure nonclinical bilingual staff members are not used as interpreters for complex health information. Use only trained interpreters and do not use family members, especially children. Bilingual staff members can translate some fact sheets, instruction pages, and other patient handouts into other languages, but recognize that it is not easy to translate an English document with a high reading level into an easy-to-read version in another language. In addition, recognize that some people are not literate in their native language. Bilingual staff members can also alert you to cultural sensitivities and instill in patients a sense of trust in your practice.

Be sure that these and all staff members are aware of the risks of inadequate health literacy, and that they are trained on the teach-back method and *Ask Me 3*, because these can expose misunderstandings or misperceptions across language lines.

Hearing Impaired

It is especially important to explain information fully to a deaf patient. This is because many deaf people don't have the opportunity to gain incidental information that those with hearing have, and therefore may lack the common health knowledge that others have picked up along the way. In addition, deaf patients often don't receive adequate explanations about their illnesses or treatments because hospital staff members tend to talk to family members rather than to the deaf patient, even when the patient is an adult.[20]

When addressing patients who are deaf or hearing impaired, providers must first evaluate whether the preference is to use sign or spoken language. If sign language is the preferred choice of communication, seek out an interpreter and pay particular attention to the type of sign language used by the patient.

If the patient prefers spoken language, pay particular attention to the environment.

- Do not obscure your face with a mask, your hand, or anything else.
- Keep the room well lit and quiet.
- Don't stand in front of a bright window or light.
- Use appropriate plain language written information.
- Use teach-back, which may be of particular importance in this setting because a lot of medical terms look very much alike to a lip-reader.[21,22] Teach-back can help uncover such misinterpretations.

Other approaches for treating and advising patients with hearing impairment or other special communication needs include using pictographs, signs, videos with closed captioning, and phone reminders.

For more information on treating the deaf and hearing-impaired, visit the following Web sites:

- Association of Medical Professionals with Hearing Loss http://www.amphl.org
- Animated dictionary of the ASL (American Sign Language) http://where.com/scott.net/asl/abc.html
- Culture Clues and End-of-Life Care sheets http://depts.washington.edu/pfes/culture-clues.html

References

1. Svensson S, Kjellgren KI, Ahlner J, Saljo R. Reasons for adherence with antihypertensive medication. *Int J Cardiol.* 2000;76:157–163

2. Williams MV, Davis T, Parker RM, Weiss BD. The role of health literacy in patient-physician communication. *Fam Med.* 2002;34:383–389

3. Davis TC, Williams MV, Marin E, Parker RM, Glass J. Health literacy and cancer communication. *CA Cancer J Clin.* 2002;52:134–149

4. Winnick S, Lucas DO, Harman AL, Toll D. How do you improve compliance? *Pediatrics.* 2005;115(6):e718–e724

5. Plainlanguage.gov. What is Plain Language? http://www.plainlanguage.gov/whatisPL/index.cfm. Accessed June 7, 2008

6. American Medical Association. Health Literacy and Patient Safety: Help Patients Understand [videotape]. Chicago, IL: American Medical Association; 2007

7. Levinson W. Physician-patient communication. The relationship with malpractice claims among primary care physicians and surgeons. *JAMA.* 1997;277(7):553–559

8. Henbest RJ, Fehrsen GS. Patient-centeredness: is it applicable outside the West? Its measurement and effect on outcomes. *Fam Pract.* 1992;9:311–317

9. Marvel MK, Epstein RM, Flowers K, Beckman HB. Soliciting the patient's agenda: have we improved? *JAMA.* 1999;281:283–287

10. Langewitz W, Benz M, Keller A, Kiss A, Rüttimann S, Wössmer B. Spontaneous talking time at start of consultation in outpatient clinic: cohort study. *BMJ.* 2002;325:682–683

11. Lang F, Floyd MR, Beine KL. Clues to patients' explanations and concerns about their illness: a call for active listening. *Arch Fam Med.* 2000;9:222–227

12. Weiss BD, ed. *Health Literacy: A Manual for Clinicians.* Chicago, IL: AMA Foundation; 2003:3

13. Stewart M, Brown JB, Boon H, Galajda J, Meredith L, Sangster M. Evidence on patient-doctor communication. *Cancer Prev Control.* 1999;3:25–30

14. Osborne H. *Health and Literacy Working Together: A Health Literacy Conference for New Readers & Health Professionals.* http://wwwihconline.org/toolkits/healthliteracy/OsborneNewReadersConference.pdf. Accessed June 24, 2008

15. Schillinger D, Piette J, Grumbach K, et al. Closing the loop: physician communication with diabetic patients who have low health literacy. *Arch Intern Med.* 2003;163(1):83–90

16. Dewalt DA, Pignone MP. Role of literacy in health and health care. *Am Fam Physician.* 2005;72:387–388

17. Schmitte BD, Brayden RM, Kempe A. Parent handouts: cornerstone of a health education program. *Contemp Pediatr.* 1997;14(1):120–143

18. Weiss BD. *Health Literacy and Patient Safety: Help Patients Understand. Manual for Physicians.* 2nd ed. Chicago, IL: AMA Foundation; 2007:36

19. Centers for Disease Control and Prevention. *Scientific and Technical Information Simply Put.* 2nd ed. Atlanta, GA: CDC Office of Communication; 1999. http://www.cdc.gov/od/oc/simpput.pdf. Accessed June 7, 2008

20. University of Washington Medical Center. Communicating with your deaf patient. http://depts.washington.edu/pfes/pdf/DeafCultureClue4_07.pdf. Accessed May 22, 2008

21. Hudson R. Including deaf patients in the conversation. *Fam Pract Manag.* 2004;11(6):37–40

22. American Family Physician. Information from your family doctor. Deaf or hard-of-hearing: tips to share with your doctor. *Am Fam Physician.* 2004;69(5):1214

CHAPTER # New Line of AAP Plain Language Educational Handouts

Doctors, nurses, and other health care professionals often provide handouts or pamphlets to parents with the goal of informing them about actions they may need to take to promote their child's health.

While this seems simple, there are many barriers to making a successful transfer of knowledge from the written handout to the parent. For example, a parent may not be familiar with and therefore misunderstand key medical terms used in the handout. Another parent may not be a strong enough reader to understand text written at a high reading level. Still other parents may be strong readers, but may not choose to read the handout if there is too much information, or may not remember the most important points if they are buried within dense text.

The success of the educational effort also depends on the current frame of mind of the parent. A sleep-deprived parent, for example, may struggle to understand information that he or she might otherwise process easily. Similarly, one who is busy, worried, or distracted may miss important information.

There is growing recognition within the medical profession that it is challenging, yet vitally important, for patients to be informed, proactive, and empowered, and that the medical community must do a better job of communicating effectively. Within this book, we provide resources to pediatric health care professionals to help them communicate successfully. In Part II of the book, the resources are specifically targeted at various common pediatric topics.

The new line of 25 plain language handouts in English and Spanish is a cornerstone of this effort. These handouts are based on the content of existing American Academy of Pediatrics (AAP) patient education materials and cover acute, chronic, and preventive topics for a range of patient ages. The AAP is proud to make this new line of handouts available for your use.

Plain Language Background

As discussed in Chapter 4, the basic idea of plain language is to present information in a way that makes it as easy as possible for every reader to understand. The concept of plain language has been embraced as part of addressing health literacy within health care. The 2004 Institute of Medicine (IOM) report, *Health Literacy: A Prescription to End Confusion*,[1] found that there is a mismatch between the health information people receive and what they understand.

Several specific elements of plain language were focused on during development of this new line of handouts.

Reduced Medical Jargon

Whenever possible, we used everyday words instead of medical or scientific jargon. We made exceptions to this rule for medical words that we felt parents were likely to encounter outside the handouts, or from their child's doctor. These are listed in separate "Words to Know" sections, with simple definitions and pronunciation guides, when necessary.

Need-to-Know Information Up Front

It is common in the medical community to begin handouts with detailed explanations of medical topics that include complex biological information. Later, the reader is presented with the actions that he or she should take. To better focus parents on what they should do, the recommended actions are at the beginning of these handouts. This increases the chances that the need-to-know, rather than the nice-to-know, information will be remembered. It also makes it much easier for parents to return to the handout when needed and quickly locate the actions they should take.

Pronunciation Guide

Certain words are difficult to pronounce due to unconventional spelling. For words that may not be easily recognized, we inserted reader-friendly pronunciation guides.

Lower Reading Level

Reading level is primarily determined by the average length of the words and sentences. We aimed to limit the number of words with more than 2 syllables and keep sentences to 10 to 15 words. We also tried to keep paragraphs short. Medical information provided to patients often exceeds the 10th-grade level despite the fact that the average reading level of adults in the United States is below high school level. We strived for these handouts to be written below the 8th-grade level.

User-Friendly Layout

Within the handouts, we used headings, bullets, and larger fonts. We also highlighted information in sidebars, built in extra open—or white—space throughout, and kept all handouts to 2 pages. All of these design elements make information easier to access and comprehend. To further help make the handouts user-friendly, 2 individuals in adult literacy programs provided feedback concerning the general design and layout.

Simple, Purposeful Illustrations

Each handout is illustrated. We tried to make the illustrations simple and realistic. They depict a diverse population and reflect important content from the handouts. The illustrations either orient a reader to a topic area or make a point in support of the text, such as showing the correct way to perform an action. Detailed technical illustrations and nonrelevant illustrations were not included.

Measuring Reading Levels

The IOM health literacy report found that more than 300 studies demonstrate that health-related materials far exceed the average reading ability of US adults. It is generally accepted that health care materials should be written at the 8th-grade level or below, and this was our goal.

There are many different measures of readability, and the choice of measure can change the reading level by several grades. To be as transparent as possible, we computed 4 different measures of readability for each of the 25 handouts. They are presented in the table on page 41. In the first column is the Flesch-Kincaid, one of the most popular formulas because it is available in Microsoft Word. It tends to underestimate reading levels, but is included due to its popularity. The second measure is the Flesch Reading Ease. It scores text on a scale from 0 to 100, with 100 being easiest and 0 the most difficult. This is also in Microsoft Word and is more reliable than the Flesch-Kincaid. A third measure, the SMOG Grade Level, is also reliable and commonly used. Finally, as a fourth measure, an average reading level was computed based on the SMOG and 2 other reliable measures, the Fog Grade Level and the Fry. This combined measure is the most stable since it is based on 3 different measures and averages variations between measures that focus on slightly different aspects of the text.

Because readability formulas are designed only to be used on continuous, flowing text made up

Readability Scores on Plain Language Handouts				
Topic (title, if different from topic)	Flesch-Kincaid	Flesch Reading Ease (score converted to grade level)	SMOG	Average of Fog, SMOG, and Fry
ADHD (What Is ADHD?)	5	7	8	8
ADHD (What to Do for ADHD)	5	7	8	8
Asthma	4	6	8	8
Asthma (Asthma Triggers)	3	6	7	6
Bedwetting	3	6	7	5
Bronchiolitis (RSV, Bronchiolitis, and Your Baby)	5	6	7	7
Calcium	4	6	8	7
Constipation	5	6	7	7
Croup	3	6	6	7
Development (Start Reading to Your Child Early)	3	6	7	5
Development (What Is Your One-Year-Old Telling You?)	6	7	8	8
Fever	4	6	7	6
Fever (How to Take Your Child's Temperature)	4	6	8	9
Gastroenteritis (Diarrhea, Vomiting, and Water Loss)	5	6	5	7
Influenza (The Flu)	5	7	8	7
Medication (Prescription Medicines and Your Child)	5	7	9	8
Medication (Using Liquid Medicines)	4	6	8	7
Medication (Choosing Over-the-Counter Medicines for Your Child)	6	6	9	8
Medication (Using Over-the-Counter Medicines With Your Child)	6	7	9	8
Oral Health (Caring for Your Child's Teeth)	5	6	7	6
Otitis (Ear Infections)	4	6	8	6
Smoking (Secondhand Smoke)	5	7	8	7
Smoking (Teens and Tobacco)	5	7	8	9
Temper Tantrums	3	6	6	5
Upper Respiratory Infection (Colds)	5	7	7	8

Notes

- Text was "cleaned" before analysis so the samples contained only continuous, flowing text, which is considered best practice for reading level analysis.
- Scores were rounded to the nearest whole number since readability formulas are considered to be accurate only to + or − one grade level.
- SMOG scores are from the Web site of the formula's originator, Harry McLaughlin.
- SMOG, Fog, and Fry averages are derived using Readability Calculations software.
- Flesch-Kincaid and Flesch Reading Ease scores are from Microsoft Word.

of complete sentences, the text from the handouts was "cleaned" prior to testing for reading level. This included removing headings, sentence fragments, bulleted lists where the bulleted text was not a complete sentence, and extra periods that do not mark the end of a sentence (such as in "M.D." or "a.m."). This is a very important step for obtaining accurate reading levels.

The table above demonstrates the variability in reading grade level based on which readability measure is used. However, the new handouts meet our reading level target of 8th grade for nearly all topics and measures.

Plain Language Benefits All Patients

Up to 90 million adults in the United States have limited literacy skills. Providing plain language written materials to these individuals may be especially beneficial. It is a common misconception, however, that plain language materials only benefit individuals with limited literacy. It has been shown that for adults of all reading abilities, information written at the 6th- to 8th-grade level is most likely to convey the health message, and be remembered.

Furthermore, all people, even health care providers, in the context of worry, medication effects, unfamiliar settings, or preoccupation with other concerns, can experience difficulty in comprehension or memory. Making written information as accessible as possible benefits all users and is respectful to the reader.

Some fear that plain language handouts will oversimplify the material. We believe plain language focuses the reader on the important information and improves overall understanding. If you are not convinced, a simple solution may be to offer the choice of a plain language or a typical handout. You might be surprised how many people, of all educational backgrounds, will prefer plain language versions.

Using the Plain Language Handouts

We hope these handouts will help in your larger goal of communicating effectively with your patients. Here are some tips for working interactively with the handouts and getting the most out of these documents.

Highlight Key Points Using Distinctive Marks

One effective way to use the handouts to their best advantage is to explain a main idea to parents while pointing to that idea in the handout. Mark it with a distinctive marking while telling parents what you are doing. For example, "I'm putting a star by the things that would show an infection is starting." Then use a different mark while explaining the next point, "Here it tells you what kind of foods you can eat today and tomorrow. I'm circling this list."

This technique is very helpful for readers when they get home and need to find specific information quickly. They may remember what mark the doctor used for which information and be able to go directly to it. It makes it more likely that parents will use the print materials at home and builds in repetition for key messages, which is extremely important for understanding.

Write Notes in the Margins

In addition to making the information more inviting, having a lot of open space in the document allows room for you to jot down patient-specific notes for parents. When you do this, make sure you take the time to write clearly, or the notes will be of little use to parents.

Use Handouts as a Springboard for More Discussion

The handouts can provide a good way to open conversation with parents and make the visit more patient-centered. The handout may prompt the parent about concerns they want to discuss, and it will provide them with the opportunity to clarify exactly what they need to do after leaving.

Offer to Read Aloud

Parents with low literacy may be reluctant to take you up on this because of embarrassment. However, for the sake of their children's health, some parents who struggle with reading may appreciate the offer to read aloud.

Realize the Limitations of Handouts

No matter how well done any handout is, there will be some situations where the handouts cannot be expected to be effective. For example, if a gap in language and culture is too great, a handout will not be effective. In those situations, trained, professional interpretation is necessary, and other interventions and, perhaps, considerable time with the family may be needed.

In other situations, a parent may read at a very low reading level. Other approaches, such as use of video, pictographs, or even a simple diagram drawn on the examination table paper, may be more effective ways to support verbal communication.

Message to Parents

It is possible you are a parent who is reading this book. If so, we hope the information in the book and handouts is useful to you and helps you communicate more effectively with your child's doctor. We want you to feel comfortable asking questions and making sure you understand what you need to do for your child's health.

We also want you to know that the book and handouts should not take the place of talking with your child's doctor. Your child's doctor will tell you what's best for your child.

PDFs of Handouts

As you will see in Part II, photocopy-ready copies of all the English and Spanish handouts can be found within each of the topic-specific sections. If you prefer to use PDF files of the handouts for making copies of the handouts, please follow the following instructions:

1. Go to http://www.aap.org/pubserv /plainlanguage.
2. Enter the password easy123.
3. Click on the English or Spanish button next to the handout title to open the file.

Permission to duplicate the patient education handouts from this publication (hard copy and PDF) for distribution to patients for educational, noncommercial purposes is granted.

Reference

1. Institute of Medicine. *Health Literacy: A Prescription to End Confusion.* Nielsen-Bohlman L, Panzer AM, Kindig DA, eds. Washington, DC: The National Academies Press; 2004

Part II Common Pediatric Topics

Acute Otitis Media
Middle Ear Infection

Acute otitis media (AOM) is one of the most common reasons children are taken to the doctor's office. Three out of 4 children have had at least one ear infection by age 3. And almost half of those children will have 3 or more ear infections during their first 3 years.[1]

With otitis causing parents to seek medical attention on a frequent, often recurring basis, the information you and your staff give must be clear, concise, and consistent.

Issues that may complicate communication and effective treatment may include

- Belief that fever equals the need for antibiotics
- Lack of understanding the need to complete a course of antibiotics, if prescribed
- Unease with the concept of "watchful waiting"

Ask Me 3

During your patient encounter, you should communicate using plain language and health literacy principles, so that by the end of the visit, the parent or child will know the answers to the *Ask Me 3* questions.

A Patient Story. . .

Bryan is a 3-year-old whose mother has taken him to Dr Allen's office because he has a fever and has been tugging on his right ear. Examination showed acute otitis media.

His appetite is strong, he appears interested in his surroundings, and he smiles readily. Dr Allen tells Bryan's mother that he has a mild ear infection, but that it is probably due to a virus and that he will get better over several days.

Dr Allen then spends time talking about the pathophysiology of ear infections and gives Bryan's mother a handout on otitis media. Next, Dr Allen prescribes some eardrops for ear pain and tells the mother to give Bryan acetaminophen drops every 4 hours if his temperature increases to greater than 102°F. She also tells Bryan's mother to bring him back to the office for follow-up if he is lethargic or anorexic.

Also, Dr Allen counsels the mother to give copious fluids. Bryan's mother says she understands the instructions.

Four days later, Bryan is taken to the hospital's emergency department. He is dehydrated and his other symptoms are worse. His temperature is 103°F (39.4°C). His mother states he wanted to sleep "all the time."

- -

Providing more information than could be assimilated at one visit confused Bryan's mother. She had been putting the acetaminophen drops into the ear and did not know what "copious fluids" meant.

She also did not understand the terms "lethargy" or "anorexia." She didn't ask any questions, even though she didn't understand everything Dr Allen said.

Patient: Luke, 6-month-old boy with acute otitis media treated with antibiotics	
Ask Me 3 questions	**What the parent should understand at the end of the visit**
What is my child's main problem?	Luke has an ear infection. His fever will last at least 2 to 3 days, even though he is taking antibiotics.
What do I need to do?	• When I give the antibiotics to Luke, I need to make sure he swallows all of them. • I need to finish giving Luke all the doses of antibiotic the doctor told me to give him, even if he seems better after a few days. • I need to give him milk and other liquids as often as he will drink them, so he doesn't dry out. • If my baby gets worse or is not starting to feel better after 2 days, I need to call the doctor. • *If my baby doesn't wake up easily or starts vomiting, I need to have him seen by a doctor right away.*
Why is it important for me to do this?	• Finishing all of the antibiotics—not just stopping when Luke feels better—will make sure the infection is totally gone. • Giving him small amounts of liquid often will keep Luke's body from drying out.

Medical Terms and Plain Language Alternatives

Many of the medical terms we use every day don't mean much to many parents. Below is a list of medical terms that may be confusing or difficult to explain and suggestions for plain language alternatives.

Medical Terms	Plain Language Alternatives
Anorexia; loss of appetite	Not hungry; poor feeding; doesn't want to eat
Antibiotics	Medicine to get rid of the germs, called "bacteria," that cause infections. Antibiotics don't work against viruses.
Congestion	Stopped up or stuffy nose
Copious	Large amount; a lot
Dehydrated	Dry; dried out. The body needs water and other liquids to stay healthy; when it doesn't have enough, it dries out, or gets "dehydrated," which can be dangerous.
Hand hygiene	Keeping hands clean by washing them with soap and water
Insomnia	Trouble sleeping; can't sleep; wakes up a lot in the night
Lethargic	Tired, sleepy, weak
Mastoiditis	Infection in the bone behind the ear
Nasal congestion	Stuffy, runny nose
Otalgia	Ear pain or earache

Otitis media	Ear infection
Rhinorrhoea	Runny nose
Temperature; fever	The temperature is how warm or cold your body is. If the temperature is higher (hotter) than usual, you have a "fever."
Upper respiratory infection (URI)	Cold; the common sickness that gives you a cough, runny nose, and sometimes a fever or other symptoms.
Virus or bacteria	Germs that cause infections.

Confusing Terms and Concepts

With any condition, there are likely to be terms or concepts for which patients and families have a different understanding than a health care professional. These may include preventive strategies, complex disease processes, medication or treatment regimens, abstract laboratory results or measurements, technical terms, or words that have a different meaning in the health care arena than in everyday use. Cultural issues and misconceptions can also contribute to lack of understanding.

Consider the following when talking with parents about AOM:

Diagnosis

Some bouts of AOM are caused by viruses, but parents may not know what viruses are or that you do not treat a viral infection with antibiotics. In addition, even for bacterial causes, the American Academy of Pediatrics now recommends a "watch and wait" approach for children 2 years or older with mild disease.

- A virus is a germ that makes you sick and that antibiotics don't usually work for viruses.
- Even though the child may have been given an antibiotic for an earache previously, it may not be the right thing to do this time; watching and waiting is often all an earache needs to get better.

Remember, no one can understand more than 3 new concepts at any given time. Do not overburden parents with too much information.

Symptoms

Parents may not know the symptoms associated with AOM.

These are signs you can look for that the child may have an ear infection.

- She tugs at her ears.
- He cries more often than usual.
- Fluid is draining from an ear.
- She has trouble sleeping.

Management and Treatment

Make sure parents know how to give their child medication properly. Be very precise in your instructions. Consider adding details to your usual instructions, and demonstrate techniques when possible.

- To help his fever go down, give Ben the medicine [like this] and make sure he swallows all of it.
- The antibiotic must be swallowed in order for it to work.

Make sure the parent has a measured dosing instrument to give liquid medicines to the child and have parents demonstrate their understanding of measuring the correct dose. (See the "Medication and Dosing" topic on page 225 for more details on communicating about medication management.)

Stress the importance of completing a full course of antibiotics, because parents may not understand the concept of giving medicine to a child who feels fine.

- Ben must take all of the medicine [or take it for a certain number of doses or days] for the medicine to do its job and keep him healthy.
- Even though Lilly will start feeling better in 2 or 3 days, you must give her the medicine for 10 days straight (or 20 times) so we can make sure we kill all of the germs that made her sick.

Consider giving the parent a medication log to keep track of the course of medication. (See pages 237 and 238 for sample logs.)

Be clear in your instructions about dosage; telling parents to give a medicine 3 times a day is too vague. For medications that must be given multiple times in a day, work out a written schedule with the parents so the doses don't come too close together.

Avoid the more vague "breakfast, lunch, dinner, and bedtime" instructions because dinner and bedtime might be too close together, particularly for very young children. Instead, instruct them to give the medicine at 8:00 am, noon, 4:00 pm, and 8:00 pm.

To many, "day" refers to the time when it's light outside, so be sure to explain what you mean when you say "day"—24 hours or only during the part of the day before the child's bedtime.

Be sure to include instructions about pain management, and distinguish those instructions from medicine to treat the infection.

Especially with young children, parents may not be able to judge how much pain the child has. Make sure to be clear that the acetaminophen or ibuprofen is being given for fever and pain, and should be continued for at least 2 days.

If you are also giving anesthetic eardrops, make sure you explain that the eardrops are in addition to the oral pain medication and not a substitute for it.

Include instructions when to call or return for follow-up. Make a plan for the parent to contact you if the child's symptoms have not improved by then.

- The child's fever and ear pain should improve within 48 to 72 hours. Call me if she isn't feeling better.

While ear infections cannot be prevented altogether, there are things parents should know about what may increase or decrease a child's risk for ear infection.

Risk factors—The risk of acquiring otitis can be increased by child care attendance, allowing the child to bottle-feed while he is laying down or sleeping, letting the child use a pacifier, or exposing the child to tobacco smoke.

Risk reducers—Breastfeeding and immunization against pneumococcus and influenza can decrease the likelihood of an ear infection.

Cultural Beliefs

Families from different cultures may have their own ideas of what causes the symptoms of an ear infection and how to treat it. (See Cultural Spotlight.) Their beliefs can result in confusion and lack of adherence to suggested management if they are not understood.

Ask parents what they think is causing the ear symptoms and what they think will make it better. This will increase your understanding of their culture while uncovering possible roadblocks or cultural issues with treatment before they arise. Usually the parents' or families' beliefs will pose no harm to the child, but some herbal remedies do contain toxic substances (eg, lead). Try to incorporate their beliefs into your treatment plan when they are not harmful.

Some cultures oppose giving medicine to a child who doesn't feel or seem sick, and others don't want their child to take medicines for what they think to be too long a period.

Allay parents' fears by explaining that the medicines you have prescribed aren't addictive and they won't make the child feel "high."

For treatments that last significantly longer than the symptoms (such as a 10-day antibiotic course for a 2-day spike in symptoms), explain that just because the symptoms have gone away doesn't mean the child is completely healed. The child must take the recommended number of doses of medicine to make sure all of the germs that made her sick have been killed.

Worsening Condition

Using very clear terms, explain the signs that the child is getting worse and needs more or immediate medical attention. Be clear and tell them when and what triggers should cause a call to you.

- Call me immediately if Joy starts sleeping more than she usually does, or if she acts sleepy when she is awake, if she stops eating or eats less than usual, or if she throws up. Any of these signs could mean she has an infection all through her body, not just in her ear.

Similarly, explain the symptoms that should prompt a call to 911 or a visit to the emergency department. Tell them what to look for as signs of a more severe problem, such as meningitis. Give them a brochure to take home, if appropriate, and mark the important parts.

Parents may think that because they saw the doctor earlier in the day or yesterday, there is no need to check in again, even if the child seems worse. Make sure parents understand that if the child has any signs of worsening condition, they should call you (or 911), regardless of when you last saw the child.

Explain to parents that it doesn't take long for a serious problem to arise, so they should get help if they are worried about their child's condition.

Behavior Change

Behavior change is a key element in preventing and managing many pediatric conditions. Shifting from paternalistic advice that is either too vague or too complicated to a patient- or family-centered approach that incorporates elements of motivational interviewing and goal-setting, and that makes use of plain language, can be an effective way to empower patients and families to make changes and improve their health.

There are things family members can do at home to lessen the risk of a child acquiring otitis.

- Don't allow the child to drink from a bottle when she is sleeping or laying down.
- Breastfeed.

- Do not smoke in the home or car, or allow others to do so, even when the child isn't there.
- Keep the child's immunizations up to date, and get him a flu shot.
- Make sure everyone in the family keeps their hands clean, especially before and after diaper changing or going to the bathroom, and before preparing food or eating. Stress the importance of hand-washing in terms of making sure the rest of the family doesn't get sick too—not just with AOM, but with many common and potentially serious illnesses.

Ask the parents motivational interview questions to get the ball rolling toward positive behavior change.

- How convinced are you that you can get your mother to stop smoking in your house when she's watching Anna? What do you think might help her do that?
- What are you going to do when you see LaShay lay down with her bottle?
- How are you going to wean Bryce from his pacifier?

Child Involvement

Including the child, to the extent possible, is respectful and patient-centered and can contribute to developing health literacy skills as the child moves toward managing his or her own health as an adolescent and an adult. It can include direct, age-appropriate statements to the child, and also ways for the child to be involved in his or her health.

For example, beginning at preschool age, children with an ear infection can be told they need to take the medicine (eg, antibiotics) to get better and how to communicate their symptoms to you. And, even children younger than 2 years can be taught to cover their mouths with their sleeve when they cough and practice other healthful habits, such as washing their hands regularly so that they don't pick up the germs that cause colds and earaches. They can learn to wash their hands with soap and water using a simple familiar tune ("Happy Birthday" or "Twinkle, Twinkle Little Star," for example) to ensure they wash long enough.

Teach-back

The concept of teaching back entails asking parents or patients to demonstrate understanding *using their own words*, not simply asking whether they have questions or whether they understand, because that may not elicit lack of understanding. Having patients explain in their own words not only assesses their understanding, but it reinforces the information by repeating it and internalizes it for the patient. When there is a lot of information, go over each concept and elicit a teach-back before moving to the next idea.

When using teach-back, it's important to keep the burden on yourself. Avoid the perception that you are quizzing the parent or patient—emphasize that you want to be sure you've explained things clearly.

The practice of using teach-back can be especially important over the phone, because it may be the only way to gauge whether the parent or patient understands.

Here are some approaches to using teach-back when managing AOM.

- To make sure this plan works for you, when you get home, what medicines will you give Bethel, and how will you give them? How much will you give her at a time? And when?

- What will you tell your husband needs to be done to help Logan through this sickness?

- I want to make sure I was clear when I explained this to you. To check, can you tell me which symptoms of John's will make you call me back? What things might mean that he is getting worse?

- Some people may ask why Thomas isn't being treated with an antibiotic. How will you explain it to them?

Key Messages for Use by All Members of the Health Care Team

It is important to reinforce key messages for parents and children so they hear them more than once and recognize them as priorities in managing their health. In addition, families should not receive conflicting advice about their health and what to do.

Use the plain language handouts in this publication to educate your staff so that everyone communicates the same messages to patients. By delivering the same message, your staff can reemphasize the important core concepts. Review with staff the key concepts for AOM.

- Antibiotics are reserved for infants younger than 6 months and those with severe illness, defined as a temperature 39°C or higher and/or severe ear pain.

- Ear infections cause pain and giving medication for pain is very important, especially for the first 24 to 48 hours.

- At a well-baby visit, introduce and reinforce the ideas regarding risk reduction for AOM, particularly those involving hand-washing and avoidance of tobacco smoke.

For those who want to know more about their child's condition, in addition to explaining more information, here are 3 Web sites that present information on AOM at several different educational levels.

- National Institute on Deafness and Other Communication Disorders, National Institutes of Health: http://www.nidcd.nih.gov/health/hearing/otitismedia.asp

- Nemours Foundation: http://kidshealth.org/parent/infections/common/otitis_media.html

- New York State Department of Health: http://www.health.state.ny.us/nysdoh/antibiotic/tktintro.htm

Reference

1. National Institute on Deafness and Other Communication Disorders, National Institutes of Health. What is otitis media? http://www.nidcd.nih.gov/health/hearing/otitism.asp. Accessed April 9, 2008

Ear Infections

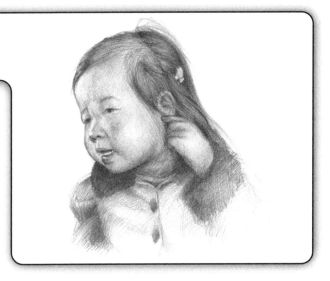

Ear infections (in-FEK-shuns) in children are common. Most kids get at least one ear infection by the time they are 3 years old. Most ear infections clear up without any lasting problems. Your child's doctor may also call an ear infection otitis (oh-TYE-tis) media.

Ear infections usually hurt. Older kids can tell you that their ears hurt. Little children may only cry and act fussy. You may notice this more when your child eats. That's because sucking and swallowing can make the pain worse. Children with an ear infection may not want to eat. They may have trouble sleeping. Ear infections also can cause fever.

What to Do for Ear Pain

Give your child **acetaminophen***or **ibuprofen*** for pain. They work well for pain with or without fever.

- Be sure to get your child the right kind for your child's age. Follow what the label says. Ask your child's doctor how much to give if your child is younger than 2 years.
- The pain may last up to 3 days. So it's fine to give medicine at the right dose during the day and at night for 3 days. Follow the label to see how often you can give it.
- There are also ear drops that can help with pain. Ask the doctor before you try them.

Call the Doctor If...

…your child has ear pain and any of these signs:

- Your child is younger than 2 years.
- Yellowish-white or bloody fluid is coming out of your child's ear.
- Your child is in a lot of pain.
- Your child is acting sick or can't sleep.
- Your child has trouble hearing. This could be from an ear infection. But it might be something else. It's important to get help if your child has a hearing problem.

- Your child has one ear infection after another for many months. It may be time to try a new treatment.

If your child is older than 2 years, you can wait 1 or 2 days to call the doctor if…

- Your child does *not* have a high fever (over 103°F or 39.4°C) AND
- Your child does not act sick.

What About Antibiotics?

The doctor may prescribe medicine for your child. This medicine will probably be an antibiotic (ant-uh-by-AH-tik). Antibiotics kill the germs that cause some infections.

Some ear infections will get better on their own. It's best for your child not to take an antibiotic unless it is needed. So the doctor may ask you to wait 1 or 2 days to see if your child gets better without medicine.

So when is an antibiotic needed? The doctor may prescribe an antibiotic if your child:

- Is very sick.
- Is younger than 2 years.
- Does not feel better 2 days after the ear pain began.

Make sure your child takes *all* the antibiotics. This may mean finishing the bottle. Or it may mean taking the medicine for a certain number

 Words to Know

acetaminophen (uh-set-tuh-MIN-uh-fin)—a medicine for pain and fever. Tylenol is one brand of acetaminophen.

ibuprofen (eye-byoo-PROH-fin)—a medicine for pain and fever. Advil and Motrin are brands of ibuprofen.

Continued on back

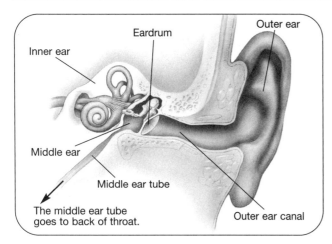

of days. Follow what the doctor says. If you stop the medicine too soon, some germs may still be left. That can make the infection start all over again.

If your child is taking antibiotics and isn't starting to get better after 2 days, call the doctor.

What *Not* to Do
- Don't give your child aspirin. It's dangerous for children younger than 18 years.
- Don't give your child over-the-counter cold medicines. They *don't* help clear up ear infections.
- Don't let your child swim or travel by plane right after an ear infection. Check with the doctor first.

What to Expect

With *any* ear infection:

- After 1 to 2 days, pain and fever should start getting better.
- After 3 days, pain and fever should go away.
- Call the doctor if your child doesn't start feeling better in 2 days.

Your child might feel a "popping" in the ears as the infection starts to clear up. This is a sign of healing.

Children with ear infections don't need to stay home if they feel OK. Just make sure your child keeps taking any medicine he or she needs.

How Your Child Can Get an Ear Infection

The ear has 3 parts—the outer ear, middle ear, and inner ear. A small tube, called the middle ear tube, connects the middle ear to the back of the throat. It's called the eustachian tube (yoo-STAY-shin toob). This tube can get blocked when a child is sick. Then fluid builds up in the middle ear. If germs get into the fluid, it can cause an infection. The inside of the ear may swell up and hurt.

How to Prevent Ear Infections

Here are some ways to lower your child's risk of an ear infection:

- Breastfeed instead of bottle-feed. Breastfeeding may help prevent colds and ear infections.
- If you bottle-feed, hold your child's head higher than the stomach during feedings. This helps keep the ear tubes from being blocked.
- Keep your child away from tobacco smoke, especially in your home and car.
- Some vaccines may help your child get fewer ear infections. These include vaccines to prevent flu and pneumonia (nuh-MOH-nyuh).

Other Causes of Ear Pain

Here are some other things that can make your child's ears hurt:

- An infection of the outer ear canal, often called "swimmer's ear" (Ask your child's doctor about home treatment for swimmer's ear.)
- Blocked or plugged middle ear tubes from colds or allergies
- A sore throat
- Teething or sore gums

To learn more, visit the American Academy of Pediatrics (AAP) Web site at www.aap.org.

Your child's doctor will tell you to do what's best for your child.
This information should not take the place of talking with your child's doctor.

Note: Brand names are for your information only. The AAP does not recommend any specific brand of drugs or products.

Adaptation of the AAP information in this handout into plain language was supported in part by McNeil Consumer Healthcare.

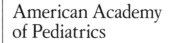

American Academy of Pediatrics

DEDICATED TO THE HEALTH OF ALL CHILDREN™

Infecciones de oído
(Ear Infections)

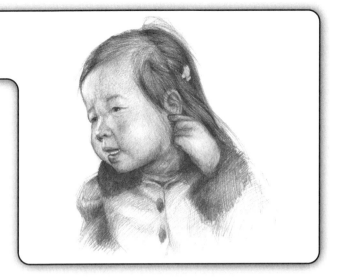

Las infecciones de oído en los niños son comunes. La mayoría de los niños sufren al menos una infección de oído antes de los tres años. Casi todas las infecciones de oído desaparecen sin ningún problema. El doctor de su niño también puede llamarle otitis media a la infección de oído.

Las infecciones de oído generalmente son dolorosas. Los niños mayores pueden decir que les duelen los oídos. Los bebés únicamente pueden llorar y ponerse inquietos. Puede ser que se note más el dolor cuando su niño come. Al succionar y tragar puede empeorar el dolor. Los niños con infección de oído tal vez no deseen comer y les puede costar dormir. Las infecciones de oído también pueden provocar fiebre.

Qué hacer con un dolor de oído

Cuando su niño sienta dolor déle **acetaminofén*** o **ibuproféno***. Ambos funcionan bien para dolores con o sin fiebre.

- Asegúrese de darle a su niño el tipo y la dosis correcta de medicina según su edad. Siga las direcciones de la etiqueta. Pregúntele al doctor de su niño la cantidad que debe darle si es menor de 2 años.
- El dolor puede durar hasta 3 días. Por lo tanto, está bien que le dé la dosis correcta de medicina durante el día y la noche por 3 días. Lea la etiqueta para saber con qué frecuencia se puede dar la medicina.
- También existen gotas para los oídos que pueden controlar el dolor. Pregúntele al doctor antes de usarlas.

Llame al doctor si…

…su niño tiene dolor de oído y alguno de estos signos:

- Es menor de 2 años.
- Le sale del oido un líquido con sangre o color blanco amarillento.
- Tiene mucho dolor.
- Luce enfermo o no puede dormir.
- Le cuesta oír. Podría ser a raíz de una infección de oído. Pero también podría ser algo más. Es importante que busque ayuda si su niño tiene un problema auditivo.

- Por muchos meses ha tenido una infección de oído tras otra. Tal vez es momento de probar un nuevo tratamiento.

Si su niño es mayor de 2 años, puede esperar 1 ó 2 días para llamar al doctor si…
- *No tiene* fiebre alta (más de 103° F ó 39.4° C)
- No sigue enfermo

¿Y los antibióticos?

El doctor puede recetarle medicina a su niño. Puede ser que esta medicina sea un antibiótico. Los antibióticos matan los gérmenes que causan algunas infecciones.

Algunas infecciones de oído mejorarán por sí solas. Es mejor que su niño no tome un antibiótico, a menos que sea necesario. Tal vez el doctor le pida que espere 1 ó 2 días para ver si su niño mejora sin tomar medicina.

¿Cuándo es necesario un antibiótico?
El doctor puede recetar un antibiótico si su niño:

- Está muy enfermo.
- Es menor de 2 años.
- No mejora 2 días después de que comenzó el dolor de oído.

Asegúrese de que su niño tome *todo* el antibiótico. Quiere decir que se debe terminar el antibiótico por completo. Hay que tomar la medicina durante cierta cantidad de días. Haga lo que el doctor le indique. Si el niño deja de tomar la medicina demasiado pronto, podrían quedar algunos gérmenes. Entonces podría volver a empezar la infección.

✳ *Palabras que debe conocer*

acetaminofén: Una medicina para el dolor y la fiebre. Tylenol es una marca de acetaminofén.

ibuprofeno: Una medicina para el dolor y la fiebre. Advil y Motrin son marcas de ibuprofeno.

Continúa atrás

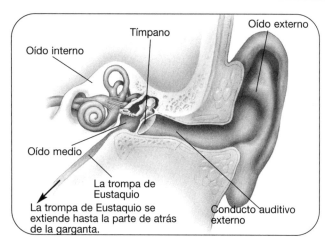

Labels in diagram: Oído interno, Tímpano, Oído externo, Oído medio, La trompa de Eustaquio, La trompa de Eustaquio se extiende hasta la parte de atrás de la garganta., Conducto auditivo externo

Si su niño está tomando antibióticos y no mejora después de 2 días, llame al doctor.

Qué no debe hacer

- No le dé aspirina a su niño. Es peligrosa para niños menores de 18 años.
- No le dé medicinas para la gripe de venta sin receta. Estas no combaten las infecciones de oído.
- No permita que su niño nade o viaje en avión justo después de tener una infección de oído. Consulte primero con el doctor.

Qué puede esperar

Con cualquier infección de oído:

- Después de 1 ó 2 días, el dolor y la fiebre deben empezar a mejorar.
- Después de 3 días, el dolor y la fiebre deben desaparecer.
- Consulte con el doctor si su niño no empieza a mejorar en 2 días.

Su niño puede sentir un "estallido" en los oídos, cuando la infección comience a desaparecer. Este es un signo de curación.

Los niños con infecciones de oído no necesitan quedarse en casa si se sienten bien. Sólo asegúrese de que su niño siga tomando la medicina que necesita.

Cómo es que su niño desarrolla una infección de oído

El oído tiene 3 partes: Oído externo, oído medio y oído interno. Un tubo pequeño, llamado tubo del oído medio, conecta el oído medio con la parte de atrás de la garganta. Se conoce como trompa de Eustaquio. Este tubo se puede tapar cuando el niño se enferma. El líquido se acumula en el oído medio. Si los microbios llegan al líquido, pueden provocar una infección. La parte interna del oído se hincha y duele.

Cómo prevenir infecciones de oído

Estas son algunas maneras de disminuir el riesgo de una infección de oído en su niño:

- Déle leche materna en lugar del biberón. De esta forma puede evitar resfriados y las infecciones de oído.
- Al darle el biberón, sostenga la cabeza de su niño más alto que su estómago. Así evitará que los tubos del oído se tapen.
- Aleje a su niño del humo del tabaco, especialmente en su casa y automóvil.
- Algunas vacunas podrían ayudar a que el niño tenga menos infecciones de oído. Estas incluyen las vacunas para prevenir la gripe y la neumonía.

Otras causas del dolor de oído

Estas son algunas otras cosas que pueden causar el dolor de oído en el niño:

- Una infección del conducto auditivo externo, también llamada "oído del nadador". (Pregúntele al doctor del niño sobre tratamientos en el hogar para este problema).
- Bloqueo o cierre de los tubos del oído medio provocado por gripes o alergias.
- Dolor de garganta.
- Dolor de encías o dientes.

Para aprender más, visite el sitio de la Academia Americana de Pediatría (AAP) en www.aap.org.
Su pediatra le dirá qué es lo mejor para la salud de su hijo.
Esta información no debe usarse en lugar de consultar con su doctor.
Nota: Los nombres de marca son para su información solamente. La AAP no recomienda ninguna marca o producto de medicina específicamente.
La adaptación de la información de este folleto de la AAP a lenguaje sencillo se hizo con el apoyo de McNeil Consumer Healthcare. La traducción al español fue patrocinada por Leyendo Juntos (Reach Out and Read), un programa pediátrico de alfabetización.

American Academy of Pediatrics
DEDICATED TO THE HEALTH OF ALL CHILDREN™

Asthma

This section focuses on asthma, which ranks among the most common chronic conditions in the United States, affecting an estimated 9 million children.[1] The burden of asthma has been increasing over the past 20 years, especially among children, according to the Centers for Disease Control and Prevention. The prevalence of asthma overall increased 75% from 1980 to 1994, and during the same period asthma rates among children younger than 5 years increased more than 160%.[2]

As the prevalence of asthma increases among children, so does the number of opportunities for misunderstanding the health care provider's directions for managing asthma, which can lead to prolonged or increasingly severe symptoms.

Common areas for miscommunication may include

- Diagnosis
- Recognition of symptoms
- Daily treatments
- Indicators that a child is getting worse and needs to step up management or see the doctor

Ask Me 3

During your patient encounter, you should communicate using plain language and health literacy principles so that by the end of the visit, the parent or child will know the answers to the *Ask Me 3* questions.

A Patient Story. . .

Li is a 5-year-old who coughs and has to stop every time he runs. He is brought in to see Dr Waylon because he now has a cold. He is breathing fast and cannot catch his breath. In the clinic, his doctor thinks he is wheezing and he is given albuterol with a spacer 3 times (repeated every 20 minutes) and he improves.

His father thinks he has used a medication like this before. Dr Waylon tells him to continue using the albuterol at home every 4 hours as needed, to take a steroid for 5 days, and then to come back and see her.

When Li returns 3 days later, Dr Waylon starts him on a daily medication to control the asthma and a rescue medication (albuterol) to be taken only when he has symptoms or before he exercises.

Three months later, Li comes back and he is no better. His father reports that he never filled the controller medication.

. . . .

Li's father did not understand that Li was supposed to use his asthma controller medication to prevent asthma attacks even when his symptoms got better.

It is possible that if Li had been using his controller medication correctly, he would not be sick today.

Health care professionals must help families understand the difference between medications that are used during an illness and medications that are used to avoid or prevent illness—and the importance of both.

Patient: Jonah, a 6-year-old with asthma (acute exacerbation)	
Ask Me 3 questions	**What the parent should understand at the end of the visit**
What is my child's main problem?	Jonah has swollen breathing tubes that are filling up with mucus, which makes it hard to breathe.
What do I need to do?	• I need to make sure Jonah uses his inhaler (puffer) every 4 hours. • I must give Jonah his other medicine (liquid/pills) once in the morning and once before bed. • I must call you or go to the emergency department if Jonah says his chest hurts, if he has trouble breathing, or if he is breathing fast.
Why is it important for me to do this?	If Jonah takes his medication, we can control his asthma and help him breathe normally. Without the medicine, he might have to go to the hospital, or he could even die.

Patient: Iris, a 12-year-old with asthma (chronic disease management)	
Ask Me 3 questions	**What the parent and/or patient should understand at the end of the visit**
What is my child's main problem?	The tubes that carry air to Iris' lungs get swollen and filled with mucus and make it hard for her to breathe.
What do I need to do?	Iris will get better if she uses the medicines. I need to make sure Iris and her other caregivers and teachers help her remember to do these things. • Iris needs to use her steroid inhaler (puffer) ____ times a day, even when she's not sick. • Iris needs her rescue medicine (albuterol) any time she has a cough or trouble breathing. It will help, but it only lasts for 4 hours. • We will follow the directions on the asthma action plan that we made with the doctor.
Why is it important for me to do this?	If she stops taking them, she will get sick again. By giving Iris the medicine to keep her breathing tubes clear she can go to school and play sports. If she doesn't use it, she might have to stay in the hospital.

Medical Terms and Plain Language Alternatives

Many of the medical terms we use every day don't mean much to many parents. Below is a list of medical terms that may be confusing or difficult to explain and suggestions for plain language alternatives.

Medical Terms	Plain Language Alternatives
Acute episode/asthma attack	When the child has severe difficulty breathing because the air tubes have become swollen
Asthma action plan	A plan you write with your child's doctor. It lists the medicines your child takes. It also tells what to do if your child has an asthma attack.
Beta-agonist	Rescue medication/quick-relief medicine
Bronchoconstriction	Breathing tubes getting tight/narrow
Controller	A medicine taken or used every day to keep the breathing tubes healthy and keep an asthma attack from happening
Metered-dose inhaler/inhaler	Puffer; a way to give medicine that gets it into the breathing tubes and lungs
Nebulizer	A machine that turns medicine or water into a mist that the child breathes in
Oral steroid	Pills that stop the breathing tubes from swelling during an asthma attack
Peak flow	Tool to measure breathing. It measures how easy it is for air to go in and out of the lungs.
Rescue medication	Medicine to help stop an asthma attack right away
Respiratory distress	Trouble breathing
Retractions	When the spaces between the ribs suck in from hard breathing
Spacer	Extra tube on the inhaler to help the medicine go in right
Steroid inhaler	A kind of medicine used every day through an inhaler to keep the breathing tubes healthy and keep an asthma attack from happening
Wheeze	A high-pitched whistling sound when breathing

Confusing Terms and Concepts

With any condition there are likely to be terms or concepts for which patients and families have a different understanding than a health care professional. These may include preventive strategies, complex disease processes, medication or treatment regimens, abstract laboratory results or measurements, technical terms, or words that have a different meaning in the health care arena than in everyday use. Cultural issues and misconceptions can also contribute to lack of understanding.

Consider the following when talking with parents about asthma:

Prevention and Health Promotion

Parents may not understand that there are many things that they can do to prevent some asthma attacks. Explain that while there is no cure for asthma, there are ways to prevent some asthma attacks. There are things called "triggers" that make the child's asthma worse. See the "Asthma Triggers" handout on page 75.

Triggers can include things the child is allergic to, like

- House dust mites, which are tiny bugs you can't see. They live in carpets, drapes or curtains, cloth furniture (like sofas), pillows, mattresses, and dust.
- Animal dander, which is made up of tiny flakes of skin from furry animals, including cats and dogs. You can't see animal dander.
- Cockroaches.
- Mold.
- Pollen, which is the dust from plants and flowers.

Triggers can also include things the child breathes in but might not be allergic to, like tobacco and other smoke, air pollution, cold or dry air, perfumes, chemicals, cleaning products, or fumes from gas or kerosene heaters and fireplaces.

Some people with asthma wheeze, cough, or get a tight feeling in their chest when they exercise. They can still be active, though—they just take certain medicines before they exercise.

While you can't keep a child away from all triggers, there is still a lot you can do.

- Don't smoke or let anyone else smoke around the child.
- Don't smoke or let anyone else smoke in the car or home, even when the child isn't there.
- Cover pillows and mattresses with allergy-proof covers.
- Wash the child's bedding and stuffed toys in hot water every week or two.
- Vacuum and dust often, and take any carpet out of the child's bedroom.
- Use a HEPA air filter in the child's bedroom to clean the air.
- If you have pets, and you can't part with them, keep them out of the child's room, and wash the animals often.
- Control cockroaches (without using bombs or bug sprays), and prevent mold from growing in the home by fixing leaks and cleaning the walls.
- Check the weather reports so you can keep the child away from pollen, and keep him inside when outdoor air quality is poor.
- Keep strong smells—like candles, mothballs, perfumes, and cleaning products—out of the house.

Diagnosis

Parents may not understand the diagnosis of asthma, so start with the basics.

- There is not a cure for asthma, but medicines can help children with asthma lead normal and healthy lives.
- Some children will have symptoms for only a short time, others for much longer.
- Nothing the parent or child did caused the disease, but you can help reduce the number and severity of asthma attacks.

Make sure families understand the potential severity of the disease and the importance of using the medicines correctly, as well as the need for an asthma action plan. (See below.)

Symptoms

Parents may have difficulty distinguishing which asthma symptoms are mild and which are severe.

Coughing is an important symptom, and families should keep track of frequency and severity of cough.

- Coughing at night is a sign that your child's asthma is not under control.
- Coughing with exercise may be a sign that your child needs more medication to control his or her asthma.

Families should be taught the signs of respiratory distress.

- If the child has to use his belly or shoulders to breathe, he should go to the doctor or hospital right away.

Management and Treatment

The most important messages you can deliver with regard to managing and treating asthma are the ideas of adhering to the medication regimen and knowing when and how to treat an acute episode (attack).

Adherence issues

It is imperative that parents and children understand the difference between rescue and controller medicines and the importance of each. If they don't understand that, they may not follow your treatment plan.

Adherence to the controller medications is about 50% in most studies. Issues include poor understanding of why the chronic medication is important, not filling or refilling prescriptions, insurance issues, transportation, and the medications' availability in pharmacies. (See Cultural Spotlight.)

Explain as simply and clearly as possible that the medicines must be taken all the time and according to your instructions—even when the child doesn't seem sick—so the child can continue breathing easily.

- Like a vitamin that you take even when you're well, these medicines will help the child stay healthy.
- The medicines are the reason the child is healthy now, but if the child stops taking them, he or she could get very sick, and possibly even die.

Work with the family to determine the best times of day to give the child the medicines, and write down a take-home schedule for them.

Some families may not be able to afford the medicines, so they don't fill the prescriptions you give them or they don't give the child enough medicine, hoping to stretch it out. Because they might not want to tell you that they can't afford the medicine, consider sending every patient home with a handout, which could include a message that tells them that if they can't afford their medicines, you and your staff will help them find free programs to help them get the medicines they need at reduced or no cost, and your office phone number and the name of your care coordinator or a local social worker.

Adherence to steroids is poor due to not filling the medication, general fear of giving the medicine, lack of understanding of steroids' effect and usage, and concerns about addiction or using medications when they are not needed. Explain that the kinds and amount of steroids you'll be giving the child are not the same as the steroids you hear about on the news.

- The child must have these medicines so he or she can breathe well and stay healthy.
- These steroids in this dosage are not harmful, and they do not make the child feel "high"—they open up the breathing tubes.

Safety issues

Make sure parents understand the condition and its seriousness, and the importance of treating it. If parents do not understand that asthma can be a serious disease with severe complications (including death), then they will not understand how important it is to treat an acute episode.

Also, if the parent doesn't understand the frequency and duration of medication usage, unintended side effects may occur, such as prolonged administration of steroids. And inappropriate usage, such as using an inhaled steroid rather than a beta-agonist as a rescue medication, results in ineffective treatment.

Cultural Beliefs

Families from different cultures may have their own ideas of what causes the symptoms of asthma. Extended family members may play an important role in decision-making and management, which can contribute to confusion or lack of adherence to suggested management.

Explore this by asking the parent what they think is causing the asthma and what they think will make it better. This will increase your understanding of their culture while uncovering possible roadblocks or cultural issues with treatment before they arise.

Usually the parents' or families' beliefs will pose no harm to the child. Try to incorporate their beliefs into your treatment plan, if possible.

Worsening Condition

Parents may not know what to look for when determining whether their child's condition is worsening; they may not know that breathing fast or shortness of breath or increased cough can indicate that a child is in distress.

Sometimes they may think that because they saw the doctor earlier in the day or yesterday there is no need to check in again, even if the child seems worse.

Be clear and tell them when and what symptoms should prompt a call to you. In particular, explain clearly what they should look for as signs of respiratory distress and give them a handout they can take home and mark the important parts.

Behavior Change

Behavior change is a key element in preventing and managing many pediatric conditions. Shifting from paternalistic advice that is either too vague or too complicated to a patient- or family-centered approach that incorporates elements of motivational interviewing and goal-setting, and that makes use of plain language, can be an effective

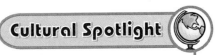

Cultural Spotlight

Issues for Asthmatics

It is important for the health care professional to be sensitive to cultural differences that come with the diagnosis of asthma.

"Asthma" is a scary word, and for many, giving their child medication for asthma means labeling the child with a disease that—prior to the development of inhaled steroids—was very limiting and potentially fatal. Beyond that, knowing what to take, what is safe, and when to take it can pose additional roadblocks to treating and managing the condition, and those roadblocks can be deeply rooted in cultural beliefs.

For example, while some cultures (Latino and Asian) are more likely to use alternative medicines, other culture groups (eg, African American) may not give their children medications if they think they are experimental or harmful.

Some cultures have no concept of chronic disease, and some are afraid of addiction to long-term medications or that the lungs will come to "need" the medication. For some families, taking a medication every day is an odd concept, especially when the child does not look sick.

At the time of diagnosis, the physician should assume that all parents will have concerns about the medications.

Most importantly, ask parents what they think is causing their child's asthma and what they have done to help it. This will start a conversation with the family about their health beliefs and complementary and alternative treatments they may be using. Try to incorporate their treatments into your treatment plan.

way to empower patients and families to make changes and improve their health.

Families with an asthmatic child should be aware of the triggers that cause the child to have an attack. While no one can get rid of all the triggers in the home, or protect their child from exposure at all times, there are things that can help.

- Don't smoke or let anyone else smoke in your home or car, regardless of whether the child is there at the time.
- Keep furry pets away from the child.
- Protect the child from dust and dust mites.
- Control cockroaches and mold.
- Keep the child away from heavy pollen and air pollution.
- Keep strong smells out of the house.

See the "Asthma Triggers" handout on page 75 and Prevention and Health Promotion on page 63.

Child Involvement

Including the child, to the extent possible, is respectful and patient-centered and can contribute to developing health literacy skills as the child moves toward managing his or her own health as an adolescent and an adult. It can include direct, age-appropriate statements to the child, and also ways for the child to be involved in his or her health.

School-aged children with asthma should know their medications and how to administer them, as well as be able to tell their parents, teachers, and coaches if they have symptoms or are having an attack. However, they should not be made totally responsible for their medications until high school or later.

Teach-back

The concept of teaching back entails asking parents or patients to demonstrate understanding *using their own words,* not simply asking whether they have questions or whether they understand, because that may not elicit lack of understanding. Having patients explain in their own words not only assesses their understanding, but it reinforces the information by repeating it and internalizes it for the patient. When there is a lot of information, go over each concept and elicit a teach-back before moving to the next idea.

When using teach-back, it's important to keep the burden on yourself. Avoid the perception that you are quizzing the parent or patient—emphasize that you want to be sure you've explained things clearly.

The practice of using teach-back can be especially important over the phone, because it may be the only way to gauge whether the parent or patient fully understands.

Here are some approaches to using teach-back with a child who has asthma.

In an acute scenario

- Now, can you tell me what you would do when you are having trouble breathing?
- I want to make sure I was clear when I explained this to you. Please show me how to use your inhaler.
- What would make you or your parents call me or 911?

Daily management of chronic symptoms scenario

- Can you please tell me when and how you will take each of these medications?
- Please show me how to use your inhaler.
- Can you tell me in your own words how often and when you need to use these inhalers?
- What will you tell your physical education teacher if you're going to be running outside during gym class?
- How will you help keep your room safe from things that can make your asthma worse?

Key Messages for Use by All Members of the Health Care Team

It is important to reinforce key messages for parents and children so they hear them more than once and recognize them as priorities in managing their health. In addition, families should not receive conflicting advice about their health and what to do.

Key concepts for asthma are

- Asthma cannot be cured, but its symptoms can be managed with medication and lifestyle/environmental changes.
- The child needs medicine every day, and without it could become very sick.
- If the child has an asthma attack and has to use his belly or shoulders to breathe, parents should take him to the emergency department right away.
- Keep the child away from smoke (from cigars, cigarettes, or any similar products), pet dander, dust, and other pollution in the home and car.

- If the child coughs a lot or during the night, or while exercising or playing, call the doctor.

Some health information is complicated but important. You can always explain more to parents if they are asking questions, or you can ask them if there are other questions that they have. But it is essential that all parents leave the office with the basic key concepts as noted above.

Miscellaneous

It is imperative that all patients with asthma (and/or their parents) leave your office with a *written* asthma action plan that should include the following:

Instructions on

- What to do when the child is having trouble breathing
- Whom to call when the child is having trouble breathing
- How to use an inhaler

Information about

- Avoidance of triggers and tobacco smoke
- The difference between a rescue medication and a controller (It is best to label them or talk about colors.)
- How often to refill the medications (inhaled corticosteroids are usually monthly)

A clear follow-up plan

- They should visit you at least every 3 months.
- Be sure to ask the family what they want to get out of the treatment, and write it on the plan too.

There are various asthma action plans available with varying formats and readability characteristics. It is important to develop the asthma action plan together with the parent or patient, to review it together and emphasize the most important information, and then to use teach-back to be sure they fully understand what they need to do.

References

1. Centers for Disease Control and Prevention. *Summary Health Statistics for US Children: National Health Interview Survey.* Series 10, No. 221. Atlanta, GA: Centers for Disease Control and Prevention; 2002:2004–1549

2. Mannino DM, Homa DM, Pertowski CA, et al. Surveillance for asthma—United States, 1960–1995. *MMWR CDC Surveill Summ.* 1998;47(1):1–27

Asthma

Asthma (AZZ-muh) is a disease of the breathing tubes that carry air to the lungs. The linings of the tubes swell, and they fill up with mucus (MYOO-kus). This is called inflammation (in-fluh-MAY-shun). It makes the tubes get narrow. This makes it hard to breathe.

Asthma can cause sickness, hospital stays, and even death. But children with asthma can live normal lives.

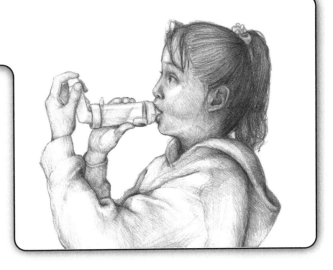

Signs of Asthma

Symptoms of asthma can be different for each person. They can come quickly or start slowly and they can change. Symptoms may include:

- Coughing.
- Trouble breathing.
- **Wheezing***.
- Shortness of breath.
- Tightness in the chest.
- Trouble exercising.

What to Do for Asthma

- There is no cure for asthma. But you can help control it. Your child will likely need one or more medicines. Using them right is **very** important.
- Make a plan for what to do for your child's asthma, wherever he or she is.
- Keep your child away from things that can make asthma worse (triggers).

Always Call the Doctor If...

- Your child has trouble breathing.
- Your child coughs, wheezes, or has a tight feeling in the chest more than once or twice a week.

Using Medicines

There are 2 kinds of asthma medicines:

- Quick-relief (rescue) medicines
- Controller medicines

Always use a spacer for medicines that are breathed in through the mouth. A spacer is a tube that you put between the medicine and the mouth. It helps get the medicine into the lungs (see picture above).

Quick-Relief Medicines

They work fast to open airways (the breathing tubes or bronchioles). They relieve tightness in the chest, wheezing, and feeling out of breath. They can also be used to prevent an asthma attack when exercising. They are called **bronchodilators***.

The most common quick-relief medicine is albuterol (al-BYOO-der-all). It comes in a form that can be breathed in.

If your child has a bad asthma attack, your child's doctor may also prescribe **steroids*** to be taken by mouth for 3 to 5 days.

✳ *Words to Know*

asthma action plan—a plan you write with your child's doctor. It lists the medicines your child takes. It also tells what to do if your child has an asthma attack.

bronchodilators (brahn-koh-DYE-lay-turz)—medicines that open up the breathing tubes in the lungs.

cromolyn (KROH-moh-lin)—an inhaled medicine that cuts down inflammation.

leukotriene receptor antagonists (loo-koh-TRY-een ree-SEP-tur an-TAG-uh-nists)— a kind of pill you take to prevent asthma symptoms.

steroids (STAIR-oydz)—a pill or liquid to take by mouth, or a spray you breathe in, to help prevent or get rid of asthma symptoms. It cuts down inflammation.

wheeze (weez) or **wheezing** (weez-ing)—high-pitched whistling sound when breathing.

Continued on back

Controller Medicines

Controller medicines are used every day. They don't take away symptoms. Instead, they keep them from happening. Some can be breathed in, and some can be swallowed.

Your child should take a controller medicine if he or she:

- Has asthma symptoms more than twice a week OR
- Wakes up with asthma symptoms more than twice a month.

There are several kinds of controller medicines:

- Steroids to breathe in
- Long-acting bronchodilators to breathe in
- *Both* steroids and bronchodilators in the same medicine to breathe in
- **Leukotriene receptor antagonists*** to take by mouth
- Other inhaled medicines like **cromolyn***

Make an Asthma Action Plan

Your child's doctor can help you write an **asthma action plan***. This lists:

- What medicines your child should take and how often.
- What to do if the symptoms get worse.
- When to get medical help right away.

You can check your action plan when you are not sure what to do for your child's symptoms.

Give a copy of the action plan to your child's school so they know what to do too.

What Are Asthma Triggers?

Things that cause asthma attacks or make asthma worse are called triggers. Common asthma triggers include:

- Tobacco and other smoke
- Dust and mold
- Cats and dogs
- Cockroaches
- Plant pollen (PAH-lin)
- Sinus (SYE-nis) and lung infections

Using a Peak Flow Meter

This is a tool that measures how fast a person can blow air out of the lungs. The peak flow meter has 3 zones—green, yellow, and red—like a traffic light. The different colors help show if your child's asthma is doing well or getting worse. Ask your child's doctor for help setting the green, yellow, and red zones for your child:

- Green—Asthma is under good control.
- Yellow—Your child may be having some asthma symptoms and may need to change medicines. Talk with the doctor and check your child's asthma action plan.
- Red—This is an emergency. Check your child's asthma action plan or call the doctor right away.

When to Use the Peak Flow Meter

- Each morning before taking any medicines.
- If symptoms get worse, or your child has an asthma attack. Check the peak flow before and after using medicines. This will help you see if the medicines are working.
- At other times if your child's doctor suggests.

Keep a record of your child's peak flow numbers each day. Bring this record with you when you visit your child's doctor.

When Your Child Is Away From Home

Children's asthma symptoms need to be controlled wherever they are.

Talk with teachers, the school nurse, office staff, and coaches. They need to know your child has asthma, what medicines your child takes, and what to do in an emergency. They need copies of your child's asthma action plan.

They also have forms for you to fill out and return:

- A medicine permission form from your child's doctor so your child can take medicines at school if needed
- A release form signed by a parent so the school nurse can talk with your child's doctor if needed

---

To learn more, visit the American Academy of Pediatrics (AAP) Web site at www.aap.org.

Your child's doctor will tell you to do what's best for your child. This information should not take the place of talking with your child's doctor.

Adaptation of the AAP information in this handout into plain language was supported in part by McNeil Consumer Healthcare.

American Academy of Pediatrics

DEDICATED TO THE HEALTH OF ALL CHILDREN™

Asma (Asthma)

El asma es una enfermedad de las vías respiratorias o los pequeños tubos que llevan el aire a los pulmones. Las paredes de estos tubos se hinchan y se llenan de moco. Esto se conoce como inflamación. El asma hace que estos tubos se vuelvan angostos. Esto dificulta la respiración en el niño.

El asma puede provocar malestar, hospitalización y hasta la muerte. Pero los niños con asma pueden llevar vidas normales.

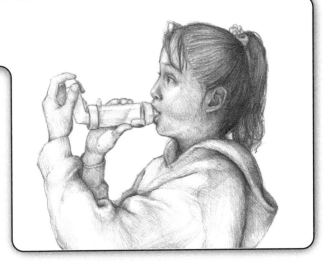

Las señales de asma

Los síntomas del asma pueden ser diferentes en cada persona. Pueden aparecer de repente o comenzar lentamente y pueden cambiar. Los síntomas del asma incluyen:

- Tos.
- Dificultad para respirar.
- **Silbido al respirar* (wheezing)** o ponerse ronco.
- Falta de aliento.
- Presión en el pecho.
- Dificultad al hacer ejercicio.

Cómo se trata el asma

- No hay cura para el asma. Pero se puede controlar. Es probable que su niño necesite una o más medicinas. Es **muy** importante que las use correctamente.
- Haga un plan sobre qué hacer por el asma de su niño en cualquier lugar donde se encuentre.
- Mantenga alejado a su niño de las cosas que le empeoran el asma.

Llame al doctor *siempre que...*

- su niño sienta dificultad al respirar.

- su niño tenga tos, silbido al respirar, o sienta presión en el pecho más de una o dos veces a la semana.

Medicinas que se usan para el Asma

Hay dos clases de medicinas para el asma:

- Medicina de alivio inmediato (rescate)
- Medicina de control

Siempre use un espaciador para las medicinas que se inhalan por la boca. Un espaciador es un tubo que se pone entre la medicina y la boca. Le ayuda a llevar la medicina a los pulmones. (Vea la ilustración de arriba).

Medicinas de alivio inmediato

Estas trabajan rápido para abrir las vías respiratorias (Los tubos respiratorios o bronquiolos). Estas alivian la presión en el pecho, el silbido al respirar y la falta de respiración. También se pueden usar para prevenir un ataque de asma cuando se hace ejercicio. Se les llama **broncodilatadoras***.

La medicina de alivio inmediato más común es el inhalador de albuterol. Si su niño tiene un ataque de asma fuerte, el doctor puede recetarle

---

✳ *Palabras que debe conocer*

plan de acción para el asma: Es un plan que usted y el doctor de su niño elaboran. En él se mencionan las medicinas que su niño debe tomar. También indica qué se debe hacer si su niño tiene un ataque de asma.

broncodilatadores: Son medicinas que abren los conductos respiratorios en los pulmones.

cromolyn: Un inhalador medicinal que reduce la inflamación.

antagonistas del receptor de leucotrienos: Una clase de pastillas que se toma para prevenir los síntomas del asma.

esteroides: Una pastilla o líquido que se toma, o que se inhala en forma de aerosol y es para prevenir o aliviar los síntomas. Reduce la inflamación.

silbido al respirar (sibilancias): Un sonido agudo en el pecho. En inglés se dice "wheezing".

Continúa atrás

esteroides* en pastillas o jarabe para tomar (por boca) de 3 a 5 días.

Medicinas de control

Las medicinas de control se usan todos los días. Estas no son para los ataques de asma y no quitan los síntomas. Algunas se pueden inhalar y otras se pueden tomar.

Su niño debe usar una medicina de control sí:

- Tiene síntomas de asma más de dos veces a la semana.
- Se despierta con síntomas de asma más de dos veces al mes.

Hay varias clases de medicinas de control:

- Los esteroides para inhalar.
- Los broncodilatadores inhalados de larga duración.
- La medicina combinada de los dos, esteroides y broncodilatadores, para inhalar.
- **Los antagonistas del receptor de leucotrienos*** que son para tomar por la boca.
- Otras medicinas para inhalar como el **cromolyn***.

Haga un plan de acción para el asma

El doctor de su niño puede ayudarle a escribir un **plan de acción para el asma**.

Este plan dice:

- Qué medicinas debe tomar su niño y cada cuanto tiempo.
- Qué hacer si los síntomas se empeoran.
- Cuándo pedir ayuda médica inmediata.

  Usted puede leer su plan de acción cuando no sabe que hacer con los síntomas de su niño.

¿Qué cosas empeoran el asma?

Estas son algunas cosas que causan ataques de asma o la ponen peor. Las más comunes incluyen:

- El tabaco y el humo
- El polen de las plantas
- Los gatos y perros
- Las cucarachas
- El polvo y el moho
- Las infecciones de los senos nasales (sinusitis) y de los pulmones

Dele una copia del plan de su niño al personal de la escuela para que sepan qué hacer.

Usar un flujómetro de pico
(peak flow meter)

Este es un aparato que mide qué tan rápido la persona puede soplar el aire de los pulmones. Tiene 3 zonas— verde, amarilla y roja—como un semáforo. Esto ayuda para ver si el asma de su niño está bajo control o no. Pídale al doctor de su niño que le ayude a definir la zona verde, amarilla y roja para su niño:

- Verde—El asma está bajo control.
- Amarilla—Su niño puede estar sufriendo síntomas de asma. Tal vez necesite cambiar la medicina. Consulte con el doctor de su niño y verifique el plan de acción de asma.
- Roja—Esta es una emergencia. Verifique el plan de acción de su niño o llame al doctor de inmediato.

Cuándo usar el flujómetro de pico

- Cada mañana antes de tomar cualquier medicina.
- Si los síntomas empeoran, o su niño tiene un ataque de asma. Use el medidor o flujómetro antes de usar sus medicinas. Esto le ayudará a saber si las medicinas están funcionando.
- Cuando el doctor de su niño lo sugiera.

Escriba todos los días el resultado de su medidor. Llévele este registro al doctor del niño en cada visita.

Consejos para cuando su niño no está en casa

Los síntomas de asma deben mantenerse bajo control en cualquier lugar donde esté el niño.

Hable con el entrenador de deporte, los maestros, la enfermera y el personal de la oficina de la escuela. Ellos tienen que saber que su niño tiene asma, que medicinas está tomando y qué hacer en caso de emergencia. Deles una copia del plan de acción para el asma de su niño.

También hay formularios que usted tiene que llenar:

- Un permiso del doctor de su niño para que pueda tomar medicinas en la escuela cuando lo necesite.
- Un permiso de los padres para que la enfermera de la escuela pueda llamar al doctor de su niño cuando se necesite.

Para aprender más, visite el sitio de la Academia Americana de Pediatría (AAP) en www.aap.org.
Su pediatra le dirá qué es lo mejor para la salud de su hijo.
Esta información no debe usarse en lugar de consultar con su doctor.
La adaptación de la información de este folleto de la AAP a lenguaje sencillo se hizo con el apoyo de McNeil Consumer Healthcare. La traducción al español fue patrocinada por Leyendo Juntos (Reach Out and Read), un programa pediátrico de alfabetización.

American Academy of Pediatrics

DEDICATED TO THE HEALTH OF ALL CHILDREN™

Asthma Triggers

Things that cause asthma (AZZ-muh) attacks or make asthma worse are called triggers. Asthma triggers can be found in your home, your child's school, child care, and other people's homes.

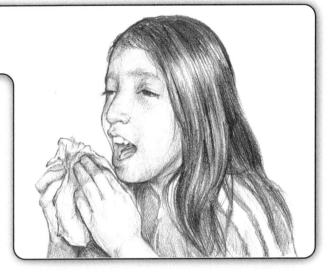

Common Asthma Triggers

Allergens (AL-er-jinz) are things your child may be allergic to.

- House dust mites—tiny bugs you can't see. They live in carpets, drapes, cloth furniture, pillows, mattresses, and dust.
- Animal dander—tiny flakes of skin from furry animals like cats and dogs. You can't see animal dander.
- Cockroaches
- Mold
- Pollen (PAH-lin)—the dust from plants.

Sinus (SYE-nis) **and lung infections.** The sinuses are spaces inside your head, behind your nose. They can get infected. Pneumonia (nuh-MOH-nyuh) is a kind of lung infection.

Things your child breathes in.

- Tobacco and other smoke
- Air pollution
- Cold or dry air
- Perfumes, chemicals, and cleaning products
- Fumes from gas or kerosene heaters and fireplaces

Exercise. Some people with asthma **wheeze***, cough, and get a tight feeling in the chest when they exercise. But they can still be active. There are medicines to use before exercise.

Avoiding Triggers

You *can't* get rid of *all* the asthma triggers in your home. But there's still a lot you *can* do. Here are some tips:

Don't smoke. And don't let anyone else smoke in your home or car.

Protect your child from dust and dust mites.

- Cover your child's mattress and pillows with allergy-proof covers.
- Wash your child's bedding in hot water every 1 to 2 weeks.
- Make sure your child's stuffed toys can be cleaned in a washing machine every 1 to 2 weeks. Check the label.
- Vacuum and dust often.
- Take carpet out of the bedroom.
- Use a HEPA air filter in the bedroom. This special kind of filter cleans the air. You can buy one at some drugstores.

Keep pets away.

- Try to find new homes for furry pets.
- Keep pets out of your child's bedroom.
- Wash pets often.

✳ Words to Know

asthma action plan—a plan you write with your child's doctor. It lists the medicines your child takes. It also tells what to do if your child has an asthma attack.

wheeze (weez) or **wheezing** (weez-ing)—high-pitched whistling sound when breathing.

Continued on back

Control cockroaches.

- Repair holes in walls, cupboards, and floors.
- Set roach traps.
- Don't leave out food, water, or trash.
- Don't use bug sprays or bombs.
- Call an exterminator (ex-TUR-muh-nay-tur).

Prevent mold. Floods, leaks, or dampness in the air can cause mold.

- Fix any leaks.
- Use exhaust fans in the bathrooms and kitchen.
- Use a dehumidifier (dee-hyoo-MID-uh-fye-ur) in damp parts of the house. A dehumidifier is a machine that takes dampness out of the air.
- Clean mold with water and detergent.
- Replace moldy wallboards.

Keep pollen away. If your child has hay fever:

- Find out when pollen is high in your area. Check with your child's doctor, your local newspaper, or the Internet.
- Put an air conditioner in your child's bedroom. Close the fresh air vent when pollen is high.
- Keep doors and windows closed.

Keep strong smells out of the house.

- Use unscented cleaning products.
- Avoid mothballs, air fresheners, perfumes, and scented candles.

Keep your child indoors when the air quality is very poor. Air quality is how clean or dirty the air is. It can change from day to day.

- Check weather reports or the Internet for air quality news.

What Is Asthma?

Asthma is a disease of the breathing tubes that carry air to the lungs. The linings of the tubes swell, and they fill up with mucus (MYOO-kus). This is called inflammation (in-fluh-MAY-shun). It makes the tubes get narrow. This makes it hard to breathe.

Asthma can cause sickness, hospital stays, and even death. But children with asthma can live normal lives.

Signs of Asthma

Symptoms of asthma can be different for each person. They can come quickly or start slowly and they can change. Symptoms may include:

- Coughing.
- Trouble breathing.
- **Wheezing***.
- Shortness of breath.
- Tightness in the chest.
- Trouble exercising.

What to Do for Asthma

- There is no cure for asthma. But you can help control it. Your child will likely need one or more medicines. Using them right is **very** important.
- Make a plan for what to do for your child's asthma, wherever he or she is.
- Talk with teachers, the school nurse, office staff, and coaches. They need to know your child has asthma, what medicines your child takes, and what to do in an emergency. They need copies of your child's **asthma action plan***.

To learn more, visit the American Academy of Pediatrics (AAP) Web site at www.aap.org.

Your child's doctor will tell you to do what's best for your child.
This information should not take the place of talking with your child's doctor.

Adaptation of the AAP information in this handout into plain language was supported in part by McNeil Consumer Healthcare.

American Academy of Pediatrics

DEDICATED TO THE HEALTH OF ALL CHILDREN™

Provocadores de asma
(Asthma Triggers)

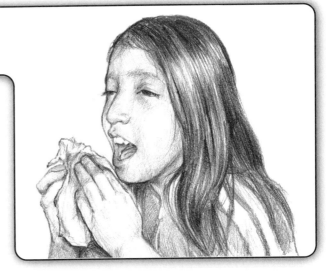

Los provocadores son cosas que causan los ataques de asma o la ponen peor. Estos se pueden encontrar en su casa, en la escuela, en el centro de cuidado del niño y en las casas de otras personas.

Provocadores comunes del asma

Los alérgenos son las cosas a las que su niño puede ser alérgico.

- Ácaros en el polvo de la casa—insectos pequeños que no se pueden ver. Viven en alfombras, cortinas, muebles de tela, almohadas, colchones y en el polvo.
- Caspa de animales—pequeñas escamas de piel de animales peludos como gatos y perros. La caspa de los animales no se puede ver.
- Cucarachas.
- Moho.
- Polen—el polvo de las plantas.

Sinusitis e infecciones en los pulmones.

Los senos nasales son espacios dentro de su cabeza, detrás de la nariz. Estos se pueden infectar. La neumonía es un tipo de infección de los pulmones.

Cosas que su niño inhala.

- Tabaco y otra clase de humo
- Aire contaminado
- Aire frío o seco
- Perfumes, químicos y productos de limpieza
- Humo de calentadores y chimeneas de gas o keroseno

El ejercicio. Algunas personas tosen, tienen **silbido al respirar*** (sibilancia), y sienten una sensación de opresión en el pecho cuando hacen ejercicio. Hay medicinas que se usan antes del ejercicio para evitar estos síntomas.

Cómo evitar los provocadores

Usted *no puede* librarse de *todos* los provocadores del asma en su casa. Pero hay muchas cosas que *puede* hacer. Aquí le damos algunos consejos:

No fume. Tampoco permita que nadie más fume en su casa o automóvil.

Proteja a su niño del polvo y de los ácaros del polvo.

- Cubra el colchón y los cojines (almohadas) de su niño con cobertores antialérgicos.
- Lave las sábanas de la cama de su niño en agua caliente cada 1 ó 2 semanas.
- Asegúrese de que los juguetes de tela de su niño se puedan poner en la lavadora cada 1 ó 2 semanas. Lea la etiqueta.
- Aspire y desempolve con frecuencia.
- Saque las alfombras del dormitorio.
- Use un filtro de aire tipo HEPA en el dormitorio. Este tipo especial de filtro limpia el aire. Puede comprarlo en algunas farmacias.

Aleje a las mascotas.

- Trate de encontrar nuevos hogares para las mascotas peludas.
- Mantenga alejadas a las mascotas del dormitorio de su niño.
- Bañe seguido a las mascotas.

✳ *Palabras que debe conocer*

plan de acción para el asma: Es un plan que usted y el doctor de su niño elaboran. En él se mencionan las medicinas que toma su niño. También indica qué se debe hacer si su niño tiene un ataque de asma.

silbido al respirar (sibilancia): Respiración **fuerte y ruidosa** o ponerse ronco. En inglés se la llama "wheezing".

Continúa atrás

Viene de la página anterior

Controle las cucarachas.

- Repare los hoyos en paredes, techos y pisos.
- Coloque trampas para cucarachas.
- No deje al descubierto la comida, el agua o la basura.
- No use aerosoles ni bombas para matar insectos.
- Llame a un exterminador.

Evite el moho. Las inundaciones, los escapes de agua o la humedad en el aire pueden causar moho.

- Repare cualquier escape de agua.
- Use ventiladores aspiradores en los baños y la cocina.
- Use un deshumidificador en las áreas húmedas de la casa. El deshumidificador es una máquina que quita la humedad del aire.
- Quite el moho con agua y detergente.
- Reemplace las paredes que tengan moho.

Manténgase alejado del polen.

- Averigüe cuando está alto el nivel del polen. Pregúntele al doctor, busque en el periódico de su área o en el Internet.
- Instale aire acondicionado en el cuarto de su niño. Cierre la rejilla del aire cuando el nivel de polen está alto.
- Mantenga las ventanas y puertas cerradas.

Evite los olores fuertes dentro de la casa.

- Use productos para limpiar sin olor.
- Evite las bolas de naftalina, los ambientadores del aire, perfumes y velas de olor.

Mantenga a su niño dentro de la casa cuando la calidad del aire sea mala.

Calidad del aire quiere decir qué tan limpio o contaminado está el aire del ambiente. La calidad del aire puede cambiar cada día.

- Averigüe cómo está la calidad del aire en el reporte del clima o las noticias en el Internet.

¿Qué es el asma?

El asma es una enfermedad de las vías respiratorias, que son pequeños tubos que llevan el aire a los pulmones. Las paredes que cubren estos tubos se hinchan y se llenan de moco. Esto se conoce como inflamación. El asma hace que estos tubos se vuelvan angostos. Esto dificulta la respiración.

El asma puede provocar malestar, hospitalización y hasta la muerte. Pero los niños con asma pueden llevar vidas normales.

Las señales de asma

Los síntomas del asma pueden ser diferentes en cada persona. Pueden aparecer de repente o comenzar lentamente y pueden cambiar. Los síntomas pueden ser:

- Tos.
- Dificultad para respirar.
- **Silbido al respirar* "wheezing"** o ponerse ronco.
- Falta de aliento.
- Opresión en el pecho.
- Dificultad al hacer ejercicio.

Cómo se trata el asma

- No hay cura para el asma. Pero usted puede ayudar a controlarla. Es probable que su niño necesite una o más medicinas. Es **muy** importante que las use correctamente.
- Mantenga alejado a su niño de las cosas que empeoran su asma (provocadores).
- Haga un plan de acción para saber qué hacer con el asma de su niño, en cualquier lugar donde el niño se encuentre.
- Hable con el entrenador de deporte, los maestros, la enfermera y el personal de la oficina de la escuela. Ellos tienen que saber que su niño tiene asma, las medicinas que está tomando y qué hacer en caso de emergencia. Deles una copia del **plan de acción para el asma*** de su niño.

Para aprender más, visite el sitio de la Academia Americana de Pediatría (AAP) en www.aap.org.
Su pediatra le dirá qué es lo mejor para la salud de su hijo.
Esta información no debe usarse en lugar de consultar con su doctor.
La adaptación de la información de este folleto de la AAP a lenguaje sencillo se hizo con el apoyo de McNeil Consumer Healthcare. La traducción al español fue patrocinada por Leyendo Juntos (Reach Out and Read), un programa pediátrico de alfabetización.

American Academy of Pediatrics

DEDICATED TO THE HEALTH OF ALL CHILDREN™

Attention-Deficit/ Hyperactivity Disorder *ADHD*

Age Group:	6 years and older
Preventive:	
Acute:	
Chronic:	✓

This section focuses on attention-deficit/hyperactivity disorder (ADHD), a chronic condition that makes it hard for children to pay attention and sit still.

One of the most common chronic conditions of childhood, ADHD is estimated to afflict between 3% and 5% of children—or about 2 million—in the United States. In other words, in a class of 25 to 30 children, it is likely that at least one will have ADHD, according to the National Institute of Mental Health.[1]

ADHD causes children to have chronic behavior problems that interfere with their ability to have good relationships with family and friends, and do well in school. But because all children have behavior problems at times, parents might not understand when intervention is needed, or they may mistake normal problem behavior for ADHD. Additionally, many parents are uncomfortable treating their children with the kind of medicines regularly used to help ADHD.

As such, there are many opportunities for miscommunication and misunderstanding, which can lead to delayed or inadequate diagnosis and treatment for the child, and frustration and anxiety for caregivers.

Common areas for miscommunication may include

- Diagnosis
- Frequency and severity of symptoms
- Management and treatment
- Cultural beliefs

A Patient Story. . .

Alex is a 6-year-old boy whose teacher reported as having frequent and severe temper tantrums, being unable to sit still, and not doing well in his schoolwork.

Alex's grandmother, who has custody of the child, said the school suspects Alex has ADHD, but she doesn't think there is anything wrong.

"That school just wants me to drug Alex so they won't have to work with him," she said, adding that she doesn't see anything in Alex but an active, energetic child. "Boys will be boys!"

After interviewing Alex and his grandmother, and giving Alex's grandmother and his teacher an ADHD scale to fill out, Dr Golden diagnoses the child with ADHD. He tells Alex's grandmother that the boy needs medication and behavior therapy. She refuses any treatment, saying that she is afraid the drugs are dangerous and may make Alex a "druggie."

A month later, she and Alex return: He has been held back a grade in school because of his inability to focus on his work.

. . . .

Alex's grandmother didn't understand the difference between normal high-energy behavior and inattentiveness and hyperactivity.

She wasn't clearly told that ADHD is a common condition, and that Alex could live a normal, productive life with it.

Further, she didn't know that the medications for ADHD are safe and very effective when coupled with behavior therapy. Dr Golden could have better explained what behavior therapy is so that Alex's grandmother wouldn't think the doctor was calling her grandson "crazy."

Finally, Dr Golden could have fully explained the relationship between Alex's ADHD symptoms and his school performance.

Ask Me 3

During your patient encounter, you should communicate using plain language and health literacy principles so that by the end of the visit, the parent or child will know the answers to the *Ask Me 3* questions.

Patient: Dana, a 10-year-old girl with ADHD	
Ask Me 3 questions	**What the parent and patient should understand at the end of the visit**
What is my child's main problem?	Dana has a condition that makes it hard for her to pay attention, sit still, take turns, and finish things.
What do I need to do?	• I will make a plan with Dana's doctor for helping Dana's ADHD, and I will make sure Dana's school is giving her all the extra help she needs. • The plan will probably include medicine to help Dana's brain work well, and behavior therapy that will show us and her teachers how to help Dana focus and behave better. • I will give (or Dana will take) her medicine the way the doctor told us, and tell the doctor how it's working and whether there are any side effects so the dose can be changed, if needed.
Why is it important for me to do this?	Dana needs treatment (medicine and behavior tips) to help focus her thinking, just like some people need glasses to help focus their eyes. This will help her do better in school and get along better with other children.

Medical Terms and Plain Language Alternatives

Many of the medical terms we use every day don't mean much to many parents. Below is a list of medical terms that may be confusing or difficult to explain and suggestions for plain language alternatives.

Medical Terms	Plain Language Alternatives
Behavior therapy	Tools to help the grown-ups around the child (like parents and teachers) relate to the child with ADHD. Behavior therapy teaches grown-ups how to set and keep rules that can help the child learn and act better.
Comorbid disorder	A problem that often occurs with ADHD, but is a separate problem and is not caused by ADHD or part of ADHD; examples are learning problems, anxiety, and depression.
Hyperactivity	Moves around a lot; trouble sitting still; squirms; talks too much
Impulsivity	Acts and talks without thinking; has trouble taking turns and interrupts a lot
Inattention	Can't pay attention; can't focus; daydreams; can't get organized and forgets things
Manage	Using medicines and behavior therapy or other ways to treat a health problem, or keep it under control, even if it can't be cured

Medication	Pills, drugs, medicine (Common brand names for ADHD medicines include Adderall, Concerta, Ritalin, and Strattera.) (See "stimulants" below, if appropriate.)
Side effects	Symptoms that come from taking a drug; they are not part of the treatment. For example, some medicines can make you feel sick to your stomach.
Stimulants	The safest, best types of medicines for most children with ADHD. They speed up the signals in the child's brain and help them focus. Examples include Adderall, Concerta, and Ritalin.

Confusing Terms and Concepts

With any condition, there are likely to be terms or concepts for which patients and families have a different understanding than a health care professional. These may include preventive strategies, complex disease processes, medication or treatment regimens, abstract laboratory results or measurements, technical terms, or words that have a different meaning in the health care arena than in everyday use. Cultural issues and misconceptions can also contribute to lack of understanding.

Consider the following when talking with parents about ADHD:

Diagnosis

Parents may be embarrassed or ashamed because they don't know how common ADHD is.

You may want to share statistics about the disorder. For example, in a class of 25 to 30 children, it is likely that at least one will have ADHD, according to the National Institute of Mental Health.[1] (Some estimate that the rate of children with ADHD is as high as 10%, meaning 3 children in a class of 30 will have the disorder.)

Some parents may blame themselves (or others) for the child's diagnosis.

- Parenting and discipline styles don't cause ADHD.
- ADHD does run in some families and not in others, but it also occurs in children whose family members don't have known ADHD.
- You didn't cause the ADHD, but you can help the child manage it by getting involved in the treatment, which means learning how to manage the child's behavior, making sure the child takes his or her medication as directed, and working with the school to help the child learn.

Take Another Look

Not all children with symptoms of ADHD turn out to have the disorder. Among possible causes of ADHD-like behavior are

- A sudden change in the child's life—the death of a grandparent; parents' divorce; a parent's job loss; a move to a new home
- Obstructive sleep apnea
- A middle ear infection that causes intermittent hearing problems
- Medical disorders that may affect brain functioning
- Underachievement caused by learning disability
- Anxiety or depression

Source: National Institute of Mental Health Web site. www.nimh.nih.gov/healthpublications/adhd/complete-publication.shtml. Accessed March 19, 2008.

It is imperative to explain that a diagnosis of ADHD doesn't mean the child is "crazy" or brain damaged. It's also important for parents to understand that ADHD isn't something the child can control by himself or herself. Getting these messages through will help with medication and treatment adherence, and shift potential blame away from the child. Removing the idea of mental illness at the outset may prevent possible stigmatizing and labeling of the child, which can hurt the child's self-esteem. Make sure to explain that ADHD is a chronic health condition, like asthma.

Explain that the child's brain just needs medicine to help it work properly. Consider explaining ADHD through similes and metaphors.

- Just like many people need glasses to focus their eyes, the child with ADHD needs medicine to focus his or her thoughts.
- Think of the child's brain as a car. On medication, the child is still driving, but the medicine will help the steering.
- Like a vitamin that you take every day to help the body stay healthy and work properly, medication for ADHD must be taken regularly, as directed, to help the child's brain stay healthy and work properly.

Symptoms

The key component of diagnosing ADHD is interviewing the child and parents or other caregivers about the child's symptoms. It is important to use ADHD scales given to parents and teachers to determine the types and severity of symptoms. ADHD scales use terms such as "sometimes," "often," and "very often." Parents and teachers may not understand these terms, or these words may have different meanings to parents and teachers than to doctors.

Ask parents or teachers what words like "sometimes" and "often" and "very often" mean to them. Consider defining the words for them after hearing their definition. For example, if a parent says that "sometimes" means several times a day, suggest that "sometimes" means several times a week and that "often" means several times a day.

Parents may not know what some of the words that describe behavior mean. For example, you may have to clarify what "focus" means. You may want to check with parents regarding their under-standing or say, "When we use the word 'focus,' we mean, 'Is the child able to give all his attention to his schoolwork without getting dis-tracted and to think only about the work he is doing?'"

Many cultures do not recognize the symptoms of ADHD as anything more than the child being active and energetic, or in the case of inattention, that the child just isn't good at schoolwork; they consider ADHD to be a myth. Ask what the parents believe is causing the

---

Did You Know...?

Distracted Driving

In their first 2 to 5 years of driving, teens with ADHD, especially when not on medication, have nearly 4 times as many automobile accidents, are more likely to cause bodily injury in accidents, and have 3 times as many citations for speeding as the young drivers without ADHD.

Source: Barkley RA. *Taking Charge of ADHD*. New York, NY: The Guilford Press, 2000:21.

---

problem and what they think is needed to make it better. This will help to inform you about what the parents' health beliefs are concerning ADHD.

Explain the condition to them in simple terms.

- ADHD is a very real condition that causes the child to be far more active and energetic than other children.
- The level of energy and activity that comes with ADHD is so high that it interferes with the child's activities, relationships, and schoolwork.
- The child could do much better in school if she could focus on her schoolwork and pay attention to what the teacher is saying.
- The child may get along better with friends, too, because treating the ADHD can help him be patient and take turns.

Management and Treatment

It is important for parents to know at the outset that most children with ADHD can succeed in regular classrooms with the help of parents and teachers who use certain techniques (such as positive reinforcement and instructional aids) and who teach organizational and study skills.

Explain to parents that while children with ADHD have difficulty paying attention to most tasks for extended periods, they can often concentrate on things that are interesting and stimulating to them.

Ask parents what activities the child is able to pay attention to and suggest a treatment plan around that activity. For example, for the video game or computer fan, educational computer games might hold the child's attention.

Or, you can suggest that parents use the child's interests as the theme for a reward chart. For example, if the child is interested in baseball, use a reward chart system with baseball-related stickers, or give the child tokens for good behavior that they can trade in for a new ball, or even game tickets.

Parents may resist the idea of putting their child on daily medication. Ask the parents what their concerns are about medication, and try to address these concerns very specifically.

Point out that we know more about the safety of stimulant medications than most other medications we give children. Medication can help improve the symptoms of ADHD in an estimated 70% to 90% of children with ADHD by helping them increase their focus and their ability to control their own behavior.

Another good thing about stimulants is that they work right away, on the first day they are taken by the child, and their effects are gone

Did You Know...?

Homework Hardship

For a child with ADHD, homework can pose a real struggle.

He or she will forget to write down assignments or leave them at school. They'll forget books or bring the wrong ones home. And once the homework is finished, it often has a lot of errors and corrections.

That's because deliberately focusing and paying conscious attention to organizing and completing a task or learning something new can be very difficult for a child with ADHD.

Parents and teachers can help the child by teaching him or her learning techniques and organizational skills and by tying lessons to activities that the child enjoys. Parents may need to take an active role in supervising their child's homework time.

Source: National Institute of Mental Health.

ADHD for Traditional Chinese

Families that believe in traditional Chinese medicine often believe in the yin-yang of disease. According to traditional Chinese health beliefs, diseases are caused by an imbalance of the yin (the passive, cold, and wet) and the yang (the hot, active, and dry). ADHD may be seen as an excess of yang.

Explaining how stimulants work to help ADHD, therefore, may be critical to acceptance of the medication by the family. Rather than say that the medication suppresses or controls the excess energy (decreases yang), it may be better to explain its actions as restoring the balance by increasing yin. Traditional Chinese medicine will generally use a cold or yin treatment to treat a disease caused by an imbalance of yang, and vice versa.

Traditional Chinese parents may also be concerned that Western medicines that suppress yang will cause damage to the brain because excess energy must be able to leave the body and not be kept in. In this case, you may want to explain that stimulants are allowing the excess energy to leave the body, not keeping it in.

Most importantly, start by asking the parents what they think is causing the problem, and try to elicit their beliefs concerning yin-yang before explaining how stimulants work to help ADHD. Ask what they have already done to treat the symptoms, and determine if they have used "cooling" remedies or "warming" remedies. This will help lead to a discussion of their health beliefs regarding ADHD.

If the parents want to use a "cooling" herbal tea as part of the treatment, be respectful and accepting of adding that to your treatment.

Finally, most traditional Chinese will want to stop a Western medicine, seen as potentially damaging, as soon as the symptoms seem better. You will need to explain that ADHD is a chronic disease that may need long-term treatment. Discuss their concerns about long-term medicines.

almost as soon as the child stops taking the medicine.

Explain the common side effects to parents, and answer questions about these side effects.

Make sure parents know that some side effects, such as headaches and stomachaches, are common but usually go away after several weeks. Explain that loss of appetite can be controlled by giving the medicine after breakfast and giving extra food at dinner, when the medicine has worn off.

Tell the parents that you will be working with them to help monitor and manage the side effects.

Parents may need help in understanding their child's right to special help in school. Make sure parents understand that federal laws say that public schools must pay for testing for a child with learning problems, use teaching methods that meet children's learning needs, and give extra help when needed. Parents also have a right to be involved with and approve any plan the school devises to help their child.

Cultural Beliefs

Families from different cultures may have their own ideas about how children should act and what—if anything—should be done about it. Explore this by asking the parent what they think is causing the condition and what they think will make it better. This will increase your understanding of their culture while uncovering possible roadblocks or cultural issues with treatment before they arise.

Studies have shown that Latina mothers are less likely to report their children's bad behavior, while African American mothers think their children are diagnosed (and misdiagnosed) with ADHD more often than white children. Explore these attitudes and concerns with parents.

Extended family members may play an important role in decision-making and management. This can result in confusion or lack of adherence to suggested management. Usually the parents' or families' beliefs or practices will cause no harm to the child, and may help. Try to incorporate their beliefs into your treatment plan.

Behavior Change

Behavior change is a key element in preventing and managing many pediatric conditions. Shifting from paternalistic advice that is either too vague or too complicated to a patient- or family-centered approach that incorporates elements of motivational interviewing and goal-setting, and that makes use of plain language, can be an effective way to empower patients and families to make changes and improve their health.

Parents have an important role in helping children with ADHD change their behavior. Discuss the following with parents:

- Setting goals for their child: For example, parents can set goals that relate to homework. Be clear and precise with parents. Make sure to communicate that goals should be small and specific, such as staying focused on homework for 15 minutes at a time.

- Praising their child for good behavior: Parents should try to find activities that their child does well so the child can experience success.

- Giving rewards and consequences: Help parents determine appropriate rewards (such as extra playtime or a special outing) for their child when he or she does the right thing, and consequences (such as losing privileges or not getting something he or she wants) for failing to meet agreed-on goals.

- Help parents learn how to organize their child through the use of charts and checklists.

Child Involvement

Including the child, to the extent possible, is respectful and patient-centered, and can contribute to developing health literacy skills as the child moves toward managing his or her own health as an adolescent and an adult. It can include direct, age-appropriate statements to the child, and also ways for the child to be involved in his or her health.

Most children with ADHD are school-aged or adolescents. They should be active participants in the plans to take medicines and behavior therapy. For example, when helping parents decide about rewards and consequences, involve the child or adolescent in the conversation and have them participate in picking appropriate rewards.

If the patient is an adolescent, speak directly with the patient, preferably with the parents not in the room, about their understanding of ADHD, how they are doing in school and with friends, their use of stimulant medication (including risk of abuse), and risky behaviors commonly seen in teenagers with ADHD.

Teach-back

The concept of teaching back entails asking parents or patients to demonstrate understanding *using their own words,* not simply asking whether they have questions or whether they understand, because that may not elicit lack of understanding. Having patients explain in their own words not only assesses their understanding, but it reinforces the information by repeating it and internalizes it for the patient. When there is a lot of information, go over each concept and elicit a teach-back before moving to the next idea.

When using teach-back, it's important to keep the burden on yourself. Avoid the perception that you are quizzing the parent or patient—emphasize that you want to be sure you've explained things clearly.

The practice of using teach-back can be especially important over the phone, because it may be the only way to gauge whether the parent or patient understands.

Here are some approaches to using teach-back when managing ADHD

- To make sure this works for Maggie, when you get home, what dose of medication will you give her, and when you will be giving it?

- What will you tell your husband needs to be done to help William do better in school?

- I want to make sure I was clear when I explained this to you. To check, can you tell me which side effects of the medication you will be looking for?

Key Messages for Use by All Members of the Health Care Team

It is important to reinforce key messages for parents and children so they hear them more than once and recognize them as priorities in managing their health. In addition, families should not receive conflicting advice about their health and what to do.

Key concepts for ADHD are

- ADHD, short for attention-deficit/hyperactivity disorder, makes it hard for children to sit still, pay attention, take turns, and finish things.

- The cause of ADHD is not clear. We know the brain works a little differently in a child with ADHD. We also know ADHD can run in families.

- While there is no cure, medication, behavior therapy, and working with the school will help most children lead normal and successful lives.

- Children have the right to free educational testing and special help from the school system. And parents have the right to be involved in any plans made by the school for their child.

- It is important for parents to learn how to help their children behave better and do homework by setting goals and using rewards and consequences to help children reach those goals.

Miscellaneous

Some health information is complicated but important. For example, some parents may think that special tests are needed to diagnose ADHD. You may want to explain to parents that there are no medical tests to diagnose ADHD. Blood tests, computer tests, x-rays, or brain-wave tests don't help. ADHD is diagnosed by doctors asking questions of parents and teachers, and having them fill out forms with questions about behavior.

You can always explain more to parents if they are asking questions or you can ask them if there are other questions that they have. But it is essential that all parents leave the office with some of the basic key concepts as noted above.

Reference

1. National Institute of Mental Health, National Institutes of Health. Attention deficit hyperactivity disorder. http://www.nimh.nih.gov/health/publications/adhd/complete-publication.shtml. Accessed March 19, 2008

What Is ADHD?

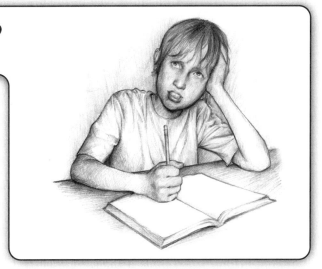

ADHD is short for **attention-deficit/hyperactivity disorder** (uh-TEN-shun DEF-uh-sit HYE-pur-ak-TIV-uh-tee dis-ORD-ur). ADHD makes it hard to sit still, pay attention, take turns, and finish things. It is one of the most common chronic (long-term) problems of childhood.

All children have problems behaving sometimes. Children with ADHD have a *very hard* time behaving a *lot* of the time. They usually have problems behaving in school and at home.

The cause of ADHD is not clear. We know the brain works a little differently in a child with ADHD. We also know it runs in families. There is no cure, but we are learning more every day. Children who get treatment can do very well.

Symptoms of ADHD

A child with ADHD may have one or more of these problems:

Inattention (IN-uh-TEN-shin)

- Has trouble paying attention
- Daydreams and is easily distracted
- Can't get organized and forgets things

Hyperactivity (HYE-pur-ak-TIV-uh-tee)

- Is moving almost all the time
- Has trouble sitting still, squirms, and talks too much

Impulsivity (IM-puhl-SIV-uh-tee)

- Acts and talks without thinking
- Has trouble taking turns and interrupts a lot

Hyperactivity and impulsivity go together. Or maybe the child just has trouble paying attention. Most children with ADHD have all the problems above.

Finding Out If Your Child Has ADHD

If your child has ADHD, the symptoms will:

- Happen in more than one place, like home, school, team sports, and camps.
- Be worse than in other children the same age.
- Start before your child is 7 years old.
- Last more than 6 months.
- Make it hard for your child to do well at school and in other group activities.

Call your child's doctor if you think your child may have ADHD. The doctor will talk with you both and check your child.

You should know:

- It is hard to diagnose ADHD in children younger than 6 years.
- The doctor will ask about how your child behaves at home, school, and other places. The doctor may have you or your child's teacher fill out a form to learn about your child's behavior.
- There are other problems that have the same symptoms as ADHD. And some children have ADHD with other behavior problems, like not obeying, anxiety, learning problems, or depression.

Are There Medical Tests for ADHD?

There is no proven medical test for ADHD at this time. Blood tests; computer tests; x-rays, like MRIs or CAT scans; or brain-wave tests don't help diagnose ADHD. Your child's doctor may have other reasons for ordering these tests. Ask the doctor if you have questions.

Continued on back

Continued from front

Treatment

There is no cure for ADHD. But there are many good treatments to help your child. As a parent, you are very important in the treatment process.

Your child's doctor will help you make a long-term plan for managing your child's ADHD. The plan will have:

- Goals (often called "target outcomes"). Example: better schoolwork
- Activities to help reach your child's goals. Examples: taking medicine, making changes at school and at home
- Ways to check your child's progress toward the goals.

Most ADHD plans include:

Medicine. For most children, drugs called stimulants (STIM-yuh-lints) are safe and work well. They speed up the signals in your child's brain. This helps your child focus and can help other symptoms too. There may be other medicines that the doctor suggests. The doctor may prescribe these *instead* of stimulants, or *together* with stimulants.

Behavior therapy. This helps parents, teachers, and other caregivers learn better ways to relate to the child with ADHD. You will learn how to set and enforce rules. And your child will learn better ways to control his or her behavior.

Working with the school. Treatment works best when everyone works as a team. The team should include doctors, parents, teachers, caregivers, and children themselves. Talk with the teacher or principal if you think your child needs more help.

By law, public schools must:

- Pay for testing for a child with learning problems.
- Use teaching methods that meet children's needs.
- Give extra help when needed.

It may take time to find the right treatment for your child. And treatment may not get rid of all the ADHD problems. But treatment with both medicine and behavior therapy helps most school-aged children with ADHD.

What Else Should Parents Know?

You are not alone. There are parent training and support groups for ADHD. These can be a great help. Being the parent of a child with ADHD can be hard. Seek counseling if you feel overwhelmed or hopeless. Ask your child's doctor where you can find this kind of help.

Answers to Common Questions

Will my child outgrow ADHD?
ADHD usually lasts into adulthood. People with ADHD can live good, productive lives. Having lots of energy can help in some careers.

Do children get "high" on stimulants?
Stimulants *don't* make children high. They don't make children sleepy or "dopey" either. But it's important for your child to get the right kind and amount of medicine for him or her. That's why regular doctor visits are important.

Do schools put children on ADHD medicines?
Sometimes teachers are the first to notice signs of ADHD. But only a doctor can say whether your child has ADHD and order medicine for it.

To learn more, visit the American Academy of Pediatrics (AAP) Web site at www.aap.org.

Your child's doctor will tell you to do what's best for your child.
This information should not take the place of talking with your child's doctor.

Adaptation of the AAP information in this handout into plain language was supported in part by McNeil Consumer Healthcare.

American Academy of Pediatrics

DEDICATED TO THE HEALTH OF ALL CHILDREN™

¿Qué es el déficit de atención con hiperactividad? (What Is ADHD?)

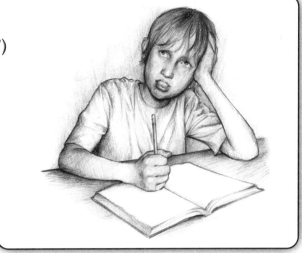

El déficit de atención con hiperactividad se conoce en inglés como ADHD. Las personas con ADHD tienen problemas manteniéndose sentados, prestando atención, esperando turno y completando actividades. Este es uno de los problemas crónicos (a largo plazo) más comunes de la niñez.

Todos los niños tienen problemas de comportamiento de vez en cuando. Los niños con déficit de atención con hiperactividad tienen *más problemas* de comportamiento la *mayor* parte del tiempo. Usualmente tienen estos problemas en la escuela y en la casa.

No se sabe bien cual es la causa del déficit de atención con hiperactividad. Sabemos que a todos los niños con esta condición, el cerebro les funciona de manera un poco diferente. También sabemos que se hereda de padres a hijos. No hay cura, pero todos los días aprendemos más. Los niños que reciben tratamiento responden muy bien.

Síntomas del déficit de atención con hiperactividad

Un niño con ADHD puede presentar uno o más de los siguientes problemas:

Distracción

- Le cuesta prestar atención
- Se distrae fácilmente y fantasea
- No puede organizarse y olvida las cosas

Hiperactividad

- Se mueve constantemente
- Le cuesta quedarse quieto, se retuerce y habla demasiado

Impulsividad

- Actúa y habla sin pensar
- Le cuesta esperar su turno e interrumpe con frecuencia

La hiperactividad y la impulsividad suceden juntas. Tal vez, al niño sólo le cueste poner atención. Pero la mayoría de los niños con ADHD tienen síntomas de distracción, hiperactividad e impulsivilidad.

Cómo saber si su niño tiene déficit de atención con hiperactividad

Los niños con ADHD:

- Son muy inquietos en varios lugares. Por ejemplo: en la casa, en la escuela y jugando deportes.
- Son más inquietos que otros niños de la misma edad.
- Empezarán antes de que el niño cumpla 7 años.
- Durarán más de 6 meses.
- Tienen dificultades en la escuela, con las tareas y con actividades en grupo.

Consulte al doctor si cree que su niño puede tener déficit de atención con hiperactividad. El doctor hablará con ustedes y evaluará a su niño.

Usted debe saber que:

- Es difícil diagnosticar la hiperactividad en niños menores de 6 años.
- El doctor preguntará sobre el comportamiento de su niño en la casa, la escuela y otros lugares. Es posible que le pidan al maestro y a usted que llenen un questionario para saber sobre la conducta del niño.
- Existen otros problemas que presentan los mismos síntomas que el ADHD. Algunos niños con este problema también pueden tener otros problemas de conducta. Por ejemplo: No obedecen o tienen ansiedad, depresión o problemas de aprendizaje.

¿Existen exámenes médicos para detectar la hiperactividad?

Por ahora no existen exámenes médicos eficaces para detectar este problema de salud. Las pruebas de sangre; las pruebas con computadoras; los rayos X, como el MRI o CAT Scan; o las pruebas de ondas cerebrales no ayudan a diagnosticar el ADHD. El doctor de su niño puede tener otras razones para ordenar estas pruebas. Si tiene dudas, pregúntele a su doctor.

Continúa atrás

El tratamiento

No hay cura para el déficit de atención con hiperactividad. Pero existen muchos tratamientos que son buenos para ayudar a su niño. Como padre, usted es muy importante en el proceso del tratamiento.

El doctor de su niño le ayudará a elaborar un plan a largo plazo para controlar el déficit de atención con hiperactividad de su niño. El plan de tratamiento tendrá:

- Metas (también conocidas como "objetivos a alcanzar"). Por ejemplo: mejores tareas escolares.
- Actividades para ayudar a alcanzar estas metas. Por ejemplo: tomar la medicina, hacer cambios en la escuela y la casa.
- Maneras de chequear el progreso de su niño hacia sus metas.

La mayoría de los planes para el déficit de atención con hiperactividad incluyen:

La medicina:
Para la mayoría de los niños, las medicinas que funcionan como estimulantes son seguras y efectivas. Estas aceleran las señales químicas en el cerebro de su niño. Además, le ayudan a concentrarse y a aliviar otros síntomas. Puede ser que el doctor le recomiende otras medicinas *en lugar* de los estimulantes, o *junto* con los estimulantes.

La terapia de conducta: Ayuda a que los padres, los maestros y otros cuidadores aprendan mejores formas de relacionarse con el niño con ADHD. Usted aprenderá cómo establecer las reglas y hacer que estas se cumplan. Su niño aprenderá mejores formas de controlar su conducta.

El trabajo en equipo con el personal de la escuela: El tratamiento funciona mejor cuando se trabaja en equipo. Este equipo debe incluir a los padres, los maestros, los cuidadores y al niño. Si usted cree que su niño necesita más ayuda, hable con su maestro o con el director de la escuela.

Por ley, las escuelas públicas deben:

- Pagar por las pruebas para evaluar los problemas de aprendizaje.
- Usar métodos de enseñanza que cumplan con las necesidades de los niños.
- Darle ayuda extra a los niños que la necesiten.

Puede que tome tiempo encontrar el tratamiento correcto para su niño. Es posible que este tratamiento no elimine todos los problemas del déficit de atención con hiperactividad. Pero la mayoría de niños de edad escolar con este problema se mejoran con la combinación de medicina y terapia de conducta.

¿Qué más deben saber los padres?

Ustedes no están solos. Existen cursos para padres y los grupos de apoyo. Ambos pueden ser de gran ayuda. Es difícil tener un niño con ADHD. Si se siente ansioso y desesperado, busque ayuda. Consulte con el doctor de su niño para encontrar este tipo de ayuda.

Respuestas a preguntas comunes

¿Superará mi niño el déficit de atención con hiperactividad?
Este problema generalmente se extiende hasta la edad adulta. Las personas con hiperactividad pueden vivir bien y tener vidas productivas. En algunas profesiones es muy útil tener mucha energía.

¿Mantienen "alterado" al niño los estimulantes?
Los estimulantes *no alteran* al niño. Tampoco lo mantienen con sueño, ni lo ponen "bobo". Pero es importante que su niño reciba el tipo apropiado y la cantidad correcta de medicina. Por esta razón, es importante tener citas regulares con el doctor.

¿Las escuelas pueden recetar las medicinas para niños con el déficit de atención con hiperactividad?
A veces los maestros son los primeros en darse cuenta de los síntomas de hiperactividad. Pero sólo el doctor puede indicar si su niño padece de ADHD. Sólo el doctor puede recetarle la medicina.

American Academy of Pediatrics

DEDICATED TO THE HEALTH OF ALL CHILDREN™

What to Do for ADHD

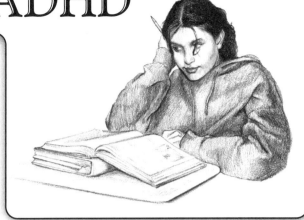

ADHD is short for **attention-deficit/hyperactivity disorder** (uh-TEN-shun DEF-uh-sit HYE-pur-ak-TIV-uh-tee dis-ORD-ur). There is no cure for ADHD yet. But there are many good treatments to help your child. As a parent, you play a big role in your child's treatment.

Making a Plan

Your child's doctor will help you make a plan for managing your child's ADHD. Most plans include:

Medicine. For most children, drugs called stimulants (STIM-yuh-lints) are safe and work well. They speed up the signals in your child's brain. This helps your child focus and can help other symptoms too.

Behavior therapy. This focuses on changing things *around* your child to help your child behave better. See "Behavior Therapy" on the second page of this handout.

Working with the school. Treatment works best when everyone works as a team. The team should include doctors, parents, teachers, caregivers, and children themselves. By law, public schools have to pay for testing and give extra help for children with ADHD or learning problems.

Medicine

Stimulant medicines are safe and help ADHD symptoms for most children. Stimulants help children focus their thoughts, like glasses help people focus their eyes. This helps children pay attention and control their behavior.

There are a few different types of stimulants. Some brand names are Adderall, Concerta, and Ritalin. Short-acting forms work quickly and are usually taken 2 to 3 times during the day. Long-acting medicines are usually taken once in the morning. There are also patches with these medicines to put on your child's skin. Your child's doctor will help you find what works best for your child.

There is a new medicine that is not a stimulant. It's brand name is Strattera. It may not work as well as stimulants. But if stimulants are not helping or are causing bad side effects, the doctor may want your child to try it.

Which Medicine Is Best for My Child?

Your child may need to try different types and doses of stimulants. Some children do well with one kind, but not another. If one stimulant doesn't work, your child's doctor may switch to a different one.

It is important for your child to have regular checkups when taking medicine. Your child's doctor needs to track how well the medicine is working. The doctor will also check for side effects and change the dose of the medicine, if needed.

What Side Effects Can Stimulants Cause?

Not all children get side effects. If they do, these are the most common:

- Not feeling hungry; losing weight
- Sleep problems
- Not wanting to be with or play with others
- Being even more active or in a bad mood as the medicine wears off (rebound effect)
- Headaches or stomachaches

Rare side effects include:

- Small, jerky movements that come and go (tics)
- Slower growth

Continued on back

continuedfrom front

Behavior Therapy

Behavior therapy helps parents, teachers, and other caregivers learn better ways to relate to the child with ADHD. You will learn how to set and enforce rules. And your child will learn better ways to control his or her behavior.

Making It Work

- **Set goals.** Set clear, small goals that your child can reach. Example: Stay focused on homework for 15 minutes at a time.
- Look for **slow progress, not instant success.** Be sure your child knows it's OK to take small steps to learn self-control.
- **Find things your child can do well.** Children need to succeed to feel good about themselves.
- **Help your child stay "on task."** Use charts and checklists to track homework or chores. Keep instructions short. Offer friendly reminders.
- **Give rewards.** Give your child something nice when he or she does the right thing. (This is positive reinforcement.) It could be something simple, like 10 extra minutes of playtime.
- **Give consequences** (KAHN-suh-kwent-siz). Give your child a consequence when he or she fails to meet a goal. A consequence might be losing a privilege or not getting something he or she wants. For example, the child loses playtime for not getting homework done. (*Never* hit your child. It doesn't help.)
- **Stick with your system and watch it work!** Find rewards and consequences that work for you and your child. Then use them the same way every day.

Warning

If your child has a serious heart problem, he or she should probably not take stimulants. Check with your child's doctor.

Working With the School

Your child's school can help your child with ADHD. The school should work with you and your child's doctor.

Two federal laws say what schools must do to help:

- The Individuals with Disabilities Education Act, Part B (IDEA)
- Section 504 of the Rehabilitation Act of 1973

These laws say public schools *must*:

- Pay for testing for a child with learning problems.
- Use teaching methods that meet children's learning needs.
- Give extra help when needed.

This extra help might be a classroom aide, private tutoring, special classroom settings, or even a special school. Talk with the teacher or principal if you think your child needs more help.

You may want to share the ideas below with people who work with your child at school:

- Keep assignments short or break them into sections.
- Keep an eye on the child and help him or her stay on task.
- Use clear rewards and consequences.
- Send parents daily or weekly "report cards" on the child's behavior in school.

Children with ADHD *can* do well in school when they get the help and support they need.

To learn more, visit the American Academy of Pediatrics (AAP) Web site at www.aap.org.

Your child's doctor will tell you to do what's best for your child.
This information should not take the place of talking with your child's doctor.

Note: Brand names are for your information only. The AAP does not recommend any specific brand of drugs or products.

Adaptation of the AAP information in this handout into plain language was supported in part by McNeil Consumer Healthcare.

© 2008 American Academy of Pediatrics

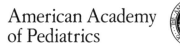

American Academy of Pediatrics
DEDICATED TO THE HEALTH OF ALL CHILDREN™

¿Cómo se trata el déficit de atención con hiperactividad? (What to Do for ADHD)

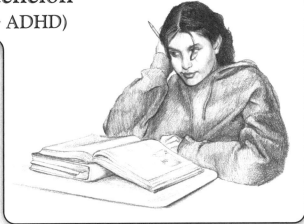

El déficit de atención con hiperactividad se conoce en inglés como ADHD. Todavía no existe cura para este problema. Pero hay muchos tratamientos buenos para ayudar a su niño. Como padre, usted juega una parte importante en el tratamiento de su niño.

Cómo hacer un plan de tratamiento

El doctor de su niño le ayudará a hacer un plan para controlar la hiperactividad de su niño. La mayoría de los planes incluyen:

La medicina: Para la mayoría de los niños, las medicinas que se conocen como estimulantes son seguras y funcionan bien. Éstas aceleran las señales químicas en el cerebro de su niño. Además, le ayudan a concentrarse y a aliviar otros síntomas.

La terapia de la conducta. Se enfoca en cambiar cosas en el ambiente de su niño para ayudarlo a comportarse mejor. Lea "terapia de la conducta" en la segunda página de este folleto.

Trabajo en equipo con el personal de la escuela. El tratamiento funciona mejor cuando se trabaja en conjunto. Este equipo debe incluir a los doctores, los padres, los maestros, los cuidadores y a los mismos niños. Por ley, las escuelas públicas deben pagar las pruebas para diagnosticar este problema o problemas de aprendizaje en el niño y darles más ayuda.

La medicina

Las medicinas estimulantes son seguras y ayudan a controlar los síntomas en la mayoría de los niños con déficit de atención con hiperactividad. Los estimulantes hacen que los niños se enfoquen en lo que piensan. Esto es igual a como los anteojos ayudan a que las personas enfoquen sus ojos. De esta forma, los niños ponen atención y controlan su conducta.

Existen diferentes tipos de estimulantes. Algunos nombres comerciales son, Adderall, Concerta y Ritalin. Las medicinas de acción corta actúan rápidamente y hay que tomarlas entre 2 y 3 veces al día. Las medicinas de acción larga generalmente se toman una vez por la mañana. También existen los parches para la piel de su niño. Estos liberan las medicinas en la piel. El doctor le ayudará a encontrar el tratamiento que mejor se adapte a las necesidades de su niño.

Existe una nueva medicina que no es un estimulante. Su nombre comercial es Strattera. Probablemente no funcione tan bien como los estimulantes. Pero si los estimulantes no están ayudando o están provocando malos efectos secundarios, el doctor puede recomendarle esta medicina para su niño.

¿Cuál medicina es mejor para mi niño?

Puede ser que su niño tenga que probar diferentes tipos y dosis de estimulantes. A algunos niños les funciona una medicina, pero a otros no. Si un estimulante no funciona, puede ser que el doctor de su niño decida cambiarlo.

Es importante que su niño vaya a sus chequeos regulares cuando está tomando la medicina. El doctor de su niño debe controlar cómo está funcionando la medicina. También, chequeará si hay efectos secundarios y cambiará la dosis de la medicina, si fuera necesario.

¿Qué efectos secundarios pueden provocar los estimulantes?

No todos los niños tienen efectos secundarios. Si su niño los sintiera, estos son los más comunes:

- Falta de hambre; pérdida de peso
- Problemas para dormir
- No desean estar o jugar con otros niños
- Se ponen más activos o de mal humor mientras desaparece el efecto de la medicina. (Esto se llama efecto de rebote).
- Dolores de cabeza o de estómago

Efectos secundarios poco comunes:

- Movimientos pequeños e irregulares que aparecen y desaparecen (tics).
- Crecimiento más lento.

Continúa atrás

Terapia de la conducta

La terapia de la conducta ayuda a que los padres, los maestros y otros cuidadores aprendan mejores formas de relacionarse con el niño. Usted aprenderá como establecer las reglas y mantenerlas. Su niño aprenderá mejores formas de controlar su conducta.

Para lograr que funcione

- **Defina metas.** Establezca metas pequeñas y claras que su niño pueda lograr. Ejemplo: Concentrarse en sus tareas escolares por períodos de 15 minutos.
- **Observe los pequeños avances, no el éxito instantáneo.** Asegúrese de que su niño sepa que es bueno dar pequeños pasos para aprender el autocontrol.
- **Descubra las cosas que su niño puede hacer bien.** Los niños necesitan tener éxito para sentirse bien con sí mismos.
- **Ayude a que su niño se concentre "en la tarea".** Use gráficas y listas para llevar un control de los trabajos. Use instrucciones cortas. Recuérdele de una manera agradable.
- **Dele premios.** Cuando su niño haga bien las cosas, regálele algo (refuerzo positivo). Puede ser algo sencillo como 10 minutos más de juego.
- **Establezca consecuencias.** Cuando su niño no cumpla una meta, imponga una consecuencia. Podría ser la pérdida de un privilegio o no recibir algo que desea. Por ejemplo, el niño pierde tiempo de juego por no haber terminado las tareas. (Nunca le pegue al niño. Esto no ayuda en nada).
- **¡Cumpla con las reglas y verá que funcionan!** Busque premios y consecuencias que funcionen para usted y su niño. Luego, úselos todos los días de la misma forma.

Advertencia

Si su niño tiene un problema serio en el corazón, probablemente no debería tomar estimulantes. Consulte con el doctor de su niño.

Trabajo en equipo con el personal de la escuela

La escuela puede ayudar a su niño con ADHD. La escuela debe colaborar con usted y con el doctor de su niño.

Hay dos leyes federales que indican lo que las escuelas deben hacer para ayudar.

- La "Ley de educación para personas con discapacidades, parte B (IDEA siglas en inglés)"
- Sección 504 de la "Ley de rehabilitación de 1973".

Estas leyes establecen que las escuelas públicas deben:

- Pagar por las pruebas para evaluar los problemas de aprendizaje.
- Usar métodos de enseñanza que apoyen las necesidades de aprendizaje de los niños.
- Brindar más ayuda cuando sea necesario.

Esta ayuda extra puede darse en forma de un auxiliar en la clase, una tutoría privada, clases especiales en grupo o hasta una escuela especial. Hable con el maestro o el director si cree que su niño necesita más ayuda de la escuela.

Puede compartir las ideas que aparecen a continuación con las personas que trabajan con su niño en la escuela:

- Asignar tareas cortas o divididas en secciones.
- Vigilar al niño y ayúdarlo a concentrarse en la tarea.
- Usar premios y explicar bien las consecuencias.
- Enviar a los padres, todos los días o semanalmente, "tarjetas de reporte" sobre la conducta del niño en la escuela.

A los niños con hiperactividad les puede ir bien en la escuela cuando reciben la ayuda y el apoyo que necesitan.

Para aprender más, visite el sitio de la Academia Americana de Pediatría (AAP) en www.aap.org.
Su pediatra le dirá qué es lo mejor para la salud de su hijo.
Esta información no debe usarse en lugar de consultar con su doctor.
Nota: Los nombres de marca son para su información solamente.
La AAP no recomienda ninguna marca o producto de medicina específicamente.
La adaptación de la información de este folleto de la AAP a lenguaje sencillo se hizo con el apoyo de McNeil Consumer Healthcare. La traducción al español fue patrocinada por Leyendo Juntos (Reach Out and Read), un programa pediátrico de alfabetización.

American Academy of Pediatrics

DEDICATED TO THE HEALTH OF ALL CHILDREN™

Bedwetting

Bedwetting, or nocturnal enuresis, affects 5 to 7 million children in the United States. While most children learn bladder control between 2 to 4 years of age, 15% of 5-year-olds still wet their beds at night and 1% of 15-year-olds do too. Most children who wet the bed have no underlying medical or psychological problem.

Bedwetting usually goes away as the child gets older, with 15% of children who wet their beds stopping each year without any treatment. Bedwetting runs in families; more than two-thirds of children with enuresis have a parent who had the problem as a child.[1,2]

Areas of potential confusion and miscommunication include

- Causes and risk factors
- Evaluation and diagnosis
- Management and treatment

Ask Me 3

During your patient encounter, you should communicate using plain language and health literacy principles so that by the end of the visit, the parent or child will know the answers to the *Ask Me 3* questions.

A Patient Story . . .

Maria is 6 years old and still wets her bed 3 or 4 times each week. Her mom asks the pediatrician, Dr Garcia, what she should do about it.

Dr Garcia finds out that Maria's father wet his bed as a child, and that Maria does not wet her pants during the day and has normal urination and bowel movements. Maria has always wet her bed, but now that she is going to school, her mom is concerned that she hasn't stopped.

Maria's urinalysis was normal.

Dr Garcia advises Maria's mother to decrease fluids before bedtime, have Maria help in the cleanup in the morning, and use a chart to reward Maria for each night she is dry.

Maria and her mom return 3 weeks later with no improvement. Maria's mom reports that they have been fighting each night about not drinking any fluids, and Maria says she is very thirsty and can't fall asleep.

Maria has also become very upset about having to clean up in the morning, and feels that her mother is angry with her when she wets her bed. Her mother reports that Maria says there is something wrong with her.

· ·

Dr Garcia could have told Maria's mother that Maria should agree to any fluid restriction, rather than have it imposed on her.

He also could have made it clear that if Maria were going to help clean up on mornings after she wet her bed, her participation should be natural and positive, not punitive.

Dr Garcia could also have focused the discussion on the possible damage to Maria's self-esteem if parents or siblings are critical or make fun of her inability to stay dry during the night.

Patient: Michael, a 6-year-old who wets his bed at night	
Ask Me 3 questions	**What the parent should understand at the end of the visit**
What is my child's main problem?	Michael wets his bed on many nights, which concerns him because he feels different from other children and is embarrassed.
What do I need to do?	• I need to make sure Michael doesn't drink much more than one glass of fluid in the 2 hours before bedtime, especially drinks that contain caffeine, including many sodas, coffee, and tea. I will make sure he agrees with this. • We will keep track of Michael's dry nights on a chart that will let him earn rewards, and also show us if he's doing better. (See the sample reward chart on page 107.) • I will not punish Michael or make him feel that it is his fault. I'll make sure his brothers and sisters don't tease him about it. • I will have Michael use the toilet just before bedtime, and wake him up 1 to 2 hours after going to sleep to use the toilet.
Why is it important for me to do this?	If I follow these steps, Michael should wet his bed less frequently, or even stop wetting it altogether over the next several months. He will also feel better about himself and not blame himself for bedwetting or think he is bad.

Patient: Angelica, a 10-year-old who wets her bed	
Ask Me 3 questions	**What the parent and patient should understand at the end of the visit**
What is my child's main problem?	Angelica wets her bed on many nights, which concerns her because she feels different from other children and is embarrassed.
What do I need to do?	• We'll attach the alarm to Angelica's underwear and pajamas like you showed us. (See the diagram in the "Bedwetting" handout on page 108.) The alarm will go off when Angelica wets herself during the night, and I will help Angelica change her pajamas and sheets. • We understand that the alarm may take several months to really work, so we'll be patient and we won't stop using it. • We'll agree that Angelica won't drink much more than one glass of fluid in the 2 hours before bedtime, especially drinks that contain caffeine, including many sodas, coffee, and tea. • We will keep track of Angelica's dry nights on a chart that will let her earn rewards and also show us if she's doing better. • I will not punish Angelica or make her feel that it is her fault, and I'll make sure her brothers and sisters don't tease her about it. • I will have Angelica use the toilet just before bedtime, and wake her up 1 to 2 hours after going to sleep to use the toilet. • I'll put a plastic cover under the sheets to protect Angelica's bed.
Why is it important for me to do this?	If we follow these steps, Angelica should wet her bed less frequently, or even stop wetting it altogether over the next several months. She will also feel better about herself and not blame herself for bedwetting or think something is wrong with her.

Medical Terms and Plain Language Alternatives

Many of the medical terms we use every day don't mean much to many parents. Below is a list of medical terms that may be confusing or difficult to explain and suggestions for plain language alternatives.

Medical Terms	Plain Language Alternatives
Bedwetting alarm	An alarm that attaches to your child's pajamas or underwear and goes off when it gets wet, which happens when the child wets the bed
Bladder	A hollow place—like a balloon—that holds urine in the body until you go to the toilet
DDAVP	A medicine that can be taken as a pill or sprayed in the nose. It works by helping the child make less urine during the night and can be helpful for older children when they have a sleepover or go away to camp.
Low self-esteem	When a child feels bad about himself or herself and thinks he or she is not as good as other children
Motivational therapy	Using reward charts and letting the child earn points or tokens for dry nights toward getting something they want or doing something special
Nocturnal enuresis	Wetting the bed at night (peeing in the bed during sleep)
Reward chart	A calendar that the parent uses with the child, marking each success with a star or other sticker, and allowing the child to trade in a certain number of earned stars or stickers for rewards. (See page 107 for more on reward charts.)
Urine	Pee, pee-pee, number 1

Confusing Terms and Concepts

With any condition, there are likely to be terms or concepts for which patients and families have a different understanding than a health care professional. These may include preventive strategies, complex disease processes, medication or treatment regimens, abstract laboratory results or measurements, technical terms, or words that have a different meaning in the health care arena than in everyday use. Cultural issues and misconceptions can also contribute to lack of understanding.

Consider the following when talking with parents about bedwetting:

Causes and Risk Factors

Parents may not understand what causes bedwetting, so start with the basics.

- We don't know what causes enuresis, but we know it seems to run in families. It is probably caused by a number of different factors. Mostly we view it as a normal lag or delay in development or maturing. Some children take longer to be able to hold their urine, or pee, in during the night than others.

- We think that some children are deep sleepers and don't wake up when they have to pee. Some children may have a bladder that is still too small to hold the urine all night. Some children have trouble passing stool (poop). The extra stool can put pressure on the bladder.
- The child isn't purposely wetting the bed.

Explain that bedwetting is rarely caused by some medical or physical problem but that you will be checking for medical problems by asking questions, doing a physical examination, and sending a sample of urine to the laboratory. Sometimes when a child gets sick with a cold or other illness they may wet the bed for a short while.

Parents should understand that psychological (emotional) problems rarely cause bedwetting, but occasionally stress or change may cause the child to wet the bed again after being dry at night. Also, children may get emotional problems and feel bad about themselves (called "low self-esteem") because other people criticize them or tease or make fun of them for bedwetting.

Diagnosis

Parents may want their children to have tests or be sent to subspecialists to make sure there is nothing wrong with them physically. Explain that bedwetting is rarely caused by some medical or physical problem; fewer than 1 in every 20 children who wets the bed has any physical cause.[1,2]

Explain what you will be doing to look into the child's bedwetting.

- I will be asking questions about the bedwetting and other medical problems that will help me decide if I need to do tests or refer to a subspecialist doctor.
- I will be doing a careful physical examination that will also help me decide if we need to do tests or refer to a subspecialist doctor.
- I will be sending a sample of the child's urine (pee) for tests that will make sure the child doesn't have an infection in the urine or a problem, such as diabetes, that may cause the child to be making too much urine (pee) at night.
- If I find any problems during the history, physical examination, and urine tests, I will tell you about them and follow up with more tests or referrals to subspecialist doctors.

Management and Treatment

The most important messages you can deliver with regard to managing and treating bedwetting are as follows.

Natural history of bedwetting: Most children who wet the bed get better on their own.

- Before the age of 5, parents should take a wait and see attitude.

- After age 5 about 1 out of every 6 (15%) children with enuresis gets better with each year.

- After age 5, some management may be needed. But first steps are doing the simple things, like trying to decrease the amount of fluids before bedtime and using reward charts to reward the child for dry nights.

Cultural Spotlight

Traditional Chinese Remedies for Bedwetting

In traditional Chinese medicine, the body and mind are inseparable and express themselves through the functions of various body organs and their vital substances or Qi (pronounced "chee").

Enuresis (bedwetting) may be due to lung, kidney, or spleen Qi deficiency. These may be differentiated by the amount and color of the urine, as well as other symptoms such as cold limbs, fatigue, hyperactivity, and lack of concentration. Different herbs may be used depending on which deficiency is suspected.

Sometimes moxibustion or acupuncture is also used to treat bedwetting. Moxibustion is the burning of "moxa" made from the mugwort herb on the skin or in conjunction with acupuncture.

It is worthwhile exploring these health beliefs with a family that practices traditional Chinese medicine. Generally these treatments will not interfere with your treatments, but incorporating them into your treatment or management, if the family is using them, will make it more likely the family will adhere to your suggestions.

Behavioral and conditioning therapies for bedwetting: For older children, bedwetting alarms work well and are the best treatment, but they need a big commitment from parents to be involved and keep going (because they may take several months to work).

- Bedwetting alarms only work if the parent is involved each night in helping the child wake up, clean up, and finish peeing in the toilet.

- Bedwetting alarms may take several months to work. Explain this to the parent so that they don't give up and stop using it after several weeks. Make sure to say this at the beginning and do a teach-back about how long it may take to work.

- Bedwetting alarms usually work better if combined with other treatments, such as rewards and reward charts, or even medications.

Medication: Medications are sometimes used, but usually in older children.

- Desmopressin acetate (DDAVP), either as a pill by mouth or as a nose spray, is helpful for children going away on sleepovers or to summer camp. It does not cure the bedwetting, but helps the child stay dry for a small number of nights. Once the medicine is stopped, the bedwetting is likely to return.

- Explain to parents that DDAVP can cause low salt in the blood by keeping too much water in the body. So they should only give the child the amount you tell them and no more. And they should make sure not to give the child too much fluid in the evening before bedtime.

Low self-esteem: Children may develop low self-esteem if parents are not clear that they should never punish the child or criticize the child for failure to stay dry during the night.

- Explain to parents that children do not purposely wet the bed. Specifically discuss the problem of self-esteem of children with bedwetting.

- Make sure parents take responsibility for ensuring that siblings do not tease or make fun of the child who is wetting the bed.

Cultural Beliefs

Families from different cultures may have their own ideas of what causes bedwetting. Extended family members may play an important role in decision-making and management, which can contribute to confusion or lack of adherence to suggested management.

Explore this by asking the parent what they think is causing bedwetting, and what they think will make it better. This will increase your understanding of their culture while uncovering possible roadblocks or cultural issues with treatment before they arise. Usually the parents' or families' beliefs will pose no harm to the child. Try to incorporate their beliefs into your treatment plan, if possible.

Behavior Change

Behavior change is a key element in preventing and managing many pediatric conditions. Shifting from paternalistic advice that is either too vague or too complicated to a patient- or family-centered approach that incorporates elements of motivational interviewing and goal-setting, and that makes use of plain language, can be an effective way to empower patients and families to make changes and improve their health.

Families with a child who is wetting the bed will need to be familiar with reward charts and the use of tokens and rewards for dry nights. The following are issues that are worth discussing:

Motivational therapy: Reward charts are useful for tracking dry nights and rewarding the child for success.

- Use stickers or stars for each dry night.

- Celebrate progress.

- For older children, decide on other rewards such as activities they want to do and how many dry nights or tokens lead to different rewards.

Bedwetting alarms are used to slowly "condition" the child to wake up before wetting the bed.

- The alarm wakes the child and parent from sleep. Initially this occurs after the child has already wet the bed. Unless the child is able to wake up himself or herself, the parent will have to wake up the child and take him or her to the toilet.
- Over time, weeks to months, the child will wake more quickly and perhaps stop peeing and be able to complete the urination in the toilet.
- Eventually, the child will wake up to pee before the alarm goes off, or prevent wetting the bed and hold the urine until morning.
- Parents need to be actively involved in the response to the alarm as well as know how to put it on the child. They need to have patience and wait for the effect, which may take several months.
- Parents may want to leave a light on, or give the child a flashlight, so that children who are afraid of the dark may be able to walk to the toilet.

Hypnotherapy and dry-bed training may also be part of the treatment of enuresis.

Hypnotherapy involves taking the mystery out of what is happening by explaining how the brain communicates to the bladder, as well as

- Teaching relaxation techniques
- Having the child practice imagery of awakening to urinate in the toilet or staying dry prior to bedtime
- Pluses and minuses
    + May be combined with bedwetting alarm
    – Requires frequent visits until the pediatrician is sure the child can practice the imagery by himself or herself prior to bedtime

Dry-bed training involves waking the child each night on a schedule of decreasing time starting about the time the child usually wets the bed. As with bedwetting alarms, the goal is for the child to eventually wake himself or herself up to go to the toilet.

Child Involvement

Including the child, to the extent possible, is respectful and patient-centered and can contribute to developing health literacy skills as the child moves toward managing his or her own health as an adolescent and an adult. It can include direct, age-appropriate statements to the child, and also ways for the child to be involved in his or her health.

Most children treated for bedwetting will be school-aged. They should participate actively in the behavioral management of bedwetting, including choosing rewards for dry nights, progressively taking responsibility for the bedwetting alarm intervention, and direct involvement in guided imagery if that is part of the management.

It is important that children understand that bedwetting is not due to their being inferior or bad or unworthy. All communications with the child should be positive, encouraging and, when appropriate, congratulatory. Conversations with the child should explore their self-esteem and their views on how the therapies are working. Children should be directly told that bedwetting is a common and routine problem. Children should be asked if anyone teases them or criticizes them because of bedwetting.

Teach-back

The concept of teaching back entails asking parents or patients to demonstrate understanding *using their own words*, not simply asking whether they have questions or whether they understand, because that may not elicit lack of understanding. Having patients explain in their own words not only assesses their understanding, but it reinforces the information by repeating it and internalizes it for the patient. When there is a lot of information, go over each concept and elicit a teach-back before moving to the next idea.

When using teach-back, it's important to keep the burden on yourself. Avoid the perception that you are quizzing the parent or patient— emphasize that you want to be sure you've explained things clearly.

The practice of using teach-back can be especially important over the phone, because it may be the only way to gauge whether the parent or patient understands.

Here are some approaches to using teach-back when talking with a parent of a child who is bedwetting.

- To make sure this plan works for you, what will you do tomorrow morning if Yvonne wakes up and has wet her bed?
- What will you do if, tomorrow morning, Holly has had a dry night?
- Show me how you will put the bedwetting alarm on José.
- What will you tell your wife to do if the bedwetting alarm goes off some night?

Key Messages for Use by All Members of the Health Care Team

It is important to reinforce key messages for parents and children so they hear them more than once and recognize them as priorities in managing their health. In addition, families should not receive conflicting advice about their health and what to do.

Key concepts for bedwetting are

- Bedwetting is a common problem. Children are not purposely wetting their beds at night. Children should never be criticized or made fun of because of bedwetting.
- Most children stop wetting the bed as they get older. Some children take longer than others, and we can help them by using reward charts and rewards, bedwetting alarms, and sometimes medication.
- Bedwetting alarms take weeks to months to work. Parents should not give up on them after a few weeks. Parents need to be actively involved, especially at first, in waking up the child when the alarm goes off.

Some routine actions parents can take to help are

- Protect the child's bed by placing a plastic cover under the sheets.
- Limit fluids, especially those containing caffeine, 1 to 2 hours before bedtime. Make sure to agree on with the child.
- Make sure the child goes to the toilet before bedtime.
- Don't make bedwetting a big issue so the child won't feel that it is.

Some health information is complicated but important. You can always explain more to parents if they ask questions, or you can ask them if there are other questions that they have. But it is essential that all parents leave the office with the basic key concepts as noted above.

Miscellaneous

Communicating Reassurance Versus Concern to Parents

Most children who wet the bed have what is called "monosymptomatic nocturnal enuresis" (MNE). A few will have what is called "polysymptomatic nocturnal enuresis" (PNE). Those children will also have daytime wetting or other bladder symptoms, such as frequency, urgency, or voiding difficulties. Parents of children with PNE should not be reassured as we have suggested with children with MNE, and may require further evaluations with tests such as renal ultrasound, voiding cystourethrogram, urodynamics, and pediatric neurologic and urologic evaluations.

Primary Versus Secondary Enuresis

Most children have primary enuresis; that is, they have never had consistently dry nights. Some children have secondary enuresis; that is, they start after a period of 6 months or more of being dry. These children may have medical causes of enuresis, such as urinary tract infections, diabetes, and constipation. History, physical examination, and a simple urinalysis will rule out common medical causes of secondary enuresis in most cases. The pediatrician should communicate to parents about the difference between primary and secondary enuresis, if indicated.

References

1. Lawless MR, McEdlerry DH. Nocturnal enuresis: current concepts. *Pediatr Rev.* 2001;22:399–406

2. Medline Plus Medical Encyclopedia. Bedwetting. http://www.nlm.nih.gov/medlineplus/ency/article/001556.htm

Bedwetting

Most children learn to use the toilet between 2 and 4 years of age. Even after children are toilet-trained, they may wet the bed until they are older. It's even common for 6-year-olds to wet the bed once in a while. Some children still wet the bed at age 12.

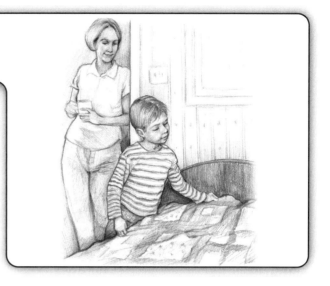

What to Do About Bedwetting

Bedwetting usually goes away as your child gets older. Talk with the doctor if you or your child are worried about bedwetting. These tips can help in the meantime.

Try These Tips

- **Protect the bed.** Put a plastic cover under the sheets.
- **Have your child use the toilet just before bedtime.**
- **Don't give your child soda pop (especially cola) before bed.**
- **Wake your child up to use the toilet** 1 or 2 hours after going to sleep. This will help him or her stay dry through the night.
- **Reward your child for dry nights.** Try a star chart. (See "Using a Star Chart" on the right.) Do not punish your child for wet nights.
- **Let your child help change wet sheets and covers.** But don't force your child to do this. If you do, your child will think he or she is being punished.
- **Set a no-teasing rule in your family.** Let others know that it's not the child's fault.
- **Don't make bedwetting a big issue** so your child won't either.

Tell Your Child

- Wetting the bed is not his or her fault.
- It won't last forever.
- Lots of kids go through this, but no one talks about it at school.

I Can Keep Dry!

Week	S	M	T	W	T	F	S
1		★		★		★	★
2		★		★	★		★
3	★	★	★		★	★	★
4		★	★	★	★		★

Using a Star Chart

Try using a calendar and star-shaped stickers to keep track of your child's "dry" nights. Each morning, check your child's bed. If it stayed dry all night, praise your child. Let him or her put a sticker on the calendar for that day. (You can also make a chart that shows the days of the week. See the chart above.)

For many children, just seeing the stars add up is enough. Other children may need a reward. For example, do something special with your child after a whole week of dry nights.

Continued on back

If You Need More Help...

Try the tips on the first page of this handout for 1 to 3 months. Then, talk with your child's doctor if bedwetting is still a problem. The doctor may suggest one of the following:

A Bedwetting Alarm

You can use a bedwetting alarm. The alarm goes off when it gets wet. Then the child learns to wake up to use the toilet. Over time, this helps a child stay dry at night. But don't give up. It can take weeks or months to work.

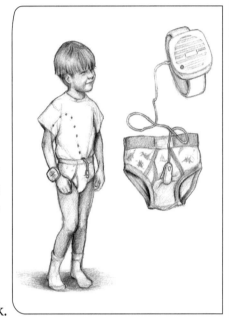

Bedwetting alarms tend to work best for children who have some dry nights. Ask your child's doctor what kind of alarm would be best for your child.

Medicine

There are some medicines for treating bedwetting in older children. They almost *never cure* bedwetting. But they can help your child go to a sleepover or camp. Ask your child's doctor about them.

Reasons for Bedwetting

We don't always know what causes bedwetting. Here are some possible reasons:

- There is a family history of bedwetting. (Most children who wet the bed have at least one parent who did it as a child.)
- Your child is a deep sleeper and doesn't wake up when he or she has to pee.
- Your child's **bladder*** is still too small to hold urine all night.
- Your child has trouble passing stool (poop). This can put pressure on the bladder.
- Your child has a minor illness, is very tired, or is going through changes or stress at home.

Signs of a Health Problem

Talk with your child's doctor if:

- Your child has been completely toilet-trained for more than 6 months AND
- Your child starts wetting the bed again.

These 2 things together *may* mean that your child has a health problem.

✳ **Word to Know**

bladder—a hollow organ that holds urine in the body until you go to the toilet.

To learn more, visit the American Academy of Pediatrics (AAP) Web site at www.aap.org.

Your child's doctor will tell you to do what's best for your child.
This information should not take the place of talking with your child's doctor.

Adaptation of the AAP information in this handout into plain language was supported in part by McNeil Consumer Healthcare.

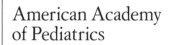

American Academy
of Pediatrics

DEDICATED TO THE HEALTH OF ALL CHILDREN™

Orinar o mojar la cama
(Bedwetting)

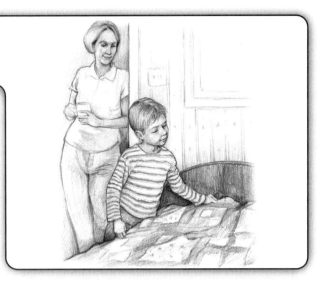

La mayoría de los niños aprenden a ir al baño entre los dos y cuatro años. Incluso después de que aprenden a ir al baño, pueden seguir mojando la cama. Es común que los niños de seis años se orinen de noche de vez en cuando. Algunos niños todavía la mojan a los 12 años.

Qué hacer si el niño moja la cama

A medida que crecen, los niños dejan de mojar la cama. Hable con el doctor si usted o el niño están preocupados porque el niño sigue teniendo ese problema. Estos consejos pueden ayudarle mientras tanto.

Pruebe estos consejos

- **Proteja la cama.** Coloque una cubierta plástica bajo las sábanas.
- **Haga que su niño vaya al baño antes de acostarse.**
- **No le dé refrescos (especialmente soda de cola, té o café) antes de acostarse.**
- **Levante a su niño para que vaya al baño una o dos horas después de acostarse.** Esto le ayudará a mantenerse seco toda la noche.
- **Dele una recompensa cuando esté seco toda la noche.** Trate de usar una gráfica para poner estrellas. (Vea el cuadro a la derecha "Cómo usar la gráfica de las estrellas"). No castigue a su niño por mojar la cama de noche.
- **Pídale ayuda a su niño para cambiar las sábanas y cobijas mojadas.** Pero, no lo obligue a que lo haga. Si lo obliga, su niño pensará que lo está castigando.
- **Imponga una regla en la familia de no burlarse.** Dígales a los otros niños que no es culpa del niño.
- **No le dé mucha importancia al asunto de mojar la cama** para que su niño tampoco lo haga.

Dígale a su niño

- Que mojar la cama no es su culpa.
- Que esto no va a durar para siempre.
- Que muchos niños pasan por esto, pero nadie lo comenta en la escuela.

¡Puedo mantenerme seco!

Semana	D	L	M	M	J	V	S
1		★		★		★	★
2		★		★	★		★
3	★	★	★		★	★	★
4		★	★	★	★		★

Cómo usar la gráfica de las estrellitas

Trate de utilizar un calendario y estrellitas adhesivas para llevar la cuenta de las noches que su niño pasa "seco". Revise la cama cada mañana. Si estuvo seco toda la noche, felicite a su niño. Dígale que pegue una estrellita en el calendario por ese día. (También puede hacer una gráfica que muestre los días de la semana. Vea la gráfica de arriba).

Para muchos niños, el ver que se acumulan las estrellas es suficiente. Otros niños tal vez necesiten una recompensa más. Por ejemplo, haga algo especial con su niño después de lograr una semana completa de noches en seco.

Continúa atrás

Si necesita más ayuda…

Pruebe los consejos en la página anterior por un período de uno a tres meses. Consulte con el doctor si su hijo tiene problemas de mojar la cama después de ese tiempo. El doctor puede sugerir una de las siguientes opciones:

Alarma para la cama mojada

Puede usar una alarma que se activa cuando se moja la cama. Entonces, el niño aprende a levantarse para ir al baño. Con el tiempo, la alarma ayuda al niño a mantenerse seco toda la noche. Puede llevar semanas o meses para que esto funcione.

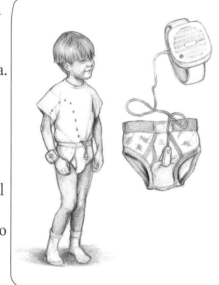

No se dé por vencida. Las alarmas para las camas mojadas tienden a funcionar mejor en niños que pasan algunas noches secos. Pregunte al doctor de su niño qué tipo de alarma sería la mejor para su caso.

Medicina

Hay algunas medicinas para tratar a los niños mayores que mojan la cama. Éstas casi nunca curan el problema. Pero pueden ayudar al niño cuando vaya a dormir a la casa de un amigo o a un campamento. Pregunte al doctor de su niño sobre estas medicinas.

Razones por las que moja la cama

No siempre sabemos por qué los niños mojan la cama. Estas son algunas de las posibles razones:

- Han habido personas en la familia que mojaban la cama. (La mayoría de niños que mojan la cama tienen al menos un padre que también lo hizo de niño).
- Su niño duerme profundamente y no se despierta cuando tiene que orinar.
- La **vejiga*** de su niño es aún muy pequeña para retener la orina por toda la noche.
- Su niño tiene problemas para defecar (hacer pupú). Esto puede presionar la vejiga.
- Su niño tiene alguna enfermedad leve, está muy cansado o está pasando por cambios o estrés en la casa.

Señales de un problema de salud

Hable con el doctor de su niño si:

- Ya sabía ir al baño por más de seis meses y de nuevo comienza a mojar la cama.

✳ *Palabra que debe conocer*

vejiga: Donde el cuerpo sostiene la orina dentro de su cuerpo hasta que va al baño.

Para aprender más, visite el sitio de la Academia Americana de Pediatría (AAP) en www.aap.org.
Su pediatra le dirá qué es lo mejor para la salud de su hijo.
Esta información no debe usarse en lugar de consultar con su doctor.
La adaptación de la información de este folleto de la AAP a lenguaje sencillo se hizo con el apoyo de McNeil Consumer Healthcare. La traducción al español fue patrocinada por Leyendo Juntos (Reach Out and Read), un programa pediátrico de alfabetización.

American Academy
of Pediatrics

DEDICATED TO THE HEALTH OF ALL CHILDREN™

Bronchiolitis/Respiratory Syncytial Virus (RSV)

Recurrent upper respiratory infections caused by respiratory syncytial virus (RSV) and other viruses occur throughout life. But lower respiratory tract infections from RSV—including bronchiolitis—are the most common cause of hospitalization among infants younger than 1 year. Hospitalization rates for this population due to RSV, bronchiolitis, and pneumonia increased 25% between 1997 and 2002.

The most vulnerable population—infants from birth to 1 year of age, particularly those with prematurity, chronic lung disease, neuromuscular disease, or congenital heart disease—are at highest risk for hospitalization. Because there are no treatment options other than supportive care, prevention is critically important in this vulnerable population.

Areas of potential confusion and miscommunication include

- Causes and risk factors
- Prevention and health promotion
- Diagnosis
- Treatment

Ask Me 3

During your patient encounter, you should communicate using plain language and health literacy principles so that by the end of the visit, the parent or child will know the answers to the *Ask Me 3* questions.

A Patient Story. . .

It is October in Houston and Dr Paulson is seeing Joey, a 4-month-old former 35-week gestation infant, for a routine health supervision visit.

She inquires about the home environment and learns that Joey has a 5-year-old sister, that they live in a trailer, and that no one smokes cigarettes.

She tells the parents to keep Joey away from cigarette smoke and crowds.

Two months later, Joey is hospitalized with RSV pneumonia. At the hospital, Dr Paulson notices 2 cigars in Joey's father's shirt pocket.

. . . .

The parents did not understand that environmental pollution in the home is not only due to cigarettes, but also from pipes and cigars. Vapors from a number of cleaning solvents and formaldehyde (which may be found in trailers) may also contribute.

Dr Paulsen could have stressed the importance of making everyone in the family wash their hands before touching Joey, or given them tips to encourage his young sister to wash her hands. It wasn't explained that simple hand-washing could prevent the transmission of many infective agents, including RSV.

Patient: Sajada, 16-month-old girl with RSV bronchiolitis	
Ask Me 3 questions	**What the parent should understand at the end of the visit**
What is my child's main problem?	• My baby has a cold and an infection of her breathing tubes. • Her cough and stuffy nose will probably get better over the next 7 to 14 days.

What do I need to do?	• I need to use the saltwater nose drops and bulb syringe to help her breathe easier. [Demonstrate use, and give handout.]
	• Everyone in our family must wash their hands often with soap and water.
	• I need to watch her breathing closely. ***If one of the following things happens, I must get her to the hospital fast:***
	  • She breathes very hard and fast, with the spaces between her ribs sucking in.
	  • She turns blue around the mouth.
	  • She breathes so hard she can't drink.

Why is it important for me to do this?	• Breathing hard can keep her from feeding well and dry her out or make her very weak. • Checking how she breathes will help her get more care if she needs it.

Patient: Julia, 3-month-old girl (former 31-week gestation premature baby), at her well-baby examination. She is 1 of 3 children; all attend child care.	
Ask Me 3 questions	**What the parent should understand at the end of the visit**
What is my child's main problem?	• Julia was born early and can get very sick if she gets an infection in her lungs from a germ called RSV. • Adults and children with RSV infection can spread it to Julia and make her sick too. • There is a shot she can get once a month that will help keep her from getting a bad infection from the RSV germ.
What do I need to do?	• I need to bring Julia to the doctor for the RSV shot every month for 5 months, starting today. • Everyone in our family must wash their hands often with soap and water. • I need to keep Julia away from sick children, crowds, and smokers as much as I can.
Why is it important for me to do this?	Getting the shots for Julia, washing our hands, and keeping her away from sick people will help protect her from the dangerous RSV germ.

Medical Terms and Plain Language Alternatives

Many of the medical terms we use every day don't mean much to many parents. Below is a list of medical terms that may be confusing or difficult to explain and suggestions for plain language alternatives.

Communication Tip

Remember to give parents backup information in plain language that they can take home. That way, they can read and refer to it later.

Medical Terms	Plain Language Alternatives
Apnea	Stop breathing
Bronchiolitis	An infection of the tubes that carry air into the lungs
Cyanosis	Blue color of the tongue, lips, or body
Dehydrated	Dry; dried out. The body needs water and other liquids to stay healthy; when it doesn't have enough, it dries out, or gets "dehydrated," which can be dangerous.
Hand hygiene	Keeping hands clean by washing them with soap and water
Lethargic	Tired, sleepy, weak
Nasal congestion	Stuffy, runny nose
Retractions	When the spaces between the ribs suck in from hard breathing
Rhinorrhoea	Runny nose
RSV	Germ that can cause infections ranging from a cold to bronchiolitis and pneumonia
Tachypnea	Breathing a lot faster than usual
Tachycardia	When the heart is beating a lot faster than usual
Temperature; fever	The temperature is how warm or cold your body is. If the temperature is higher (hotter) than usual, you have a "fever."
Upper respiratory infection (URI)	Cold; the common sickness that gives you a cough, runny nose, and sometimes a fever or other symptoms.
Worsening respiratory symptoms	Breathing harder, faster, or when the spaces between the ribs start to suck in

Confusing Terms and Concepts

With any condition, there are likely to be terms or concepts for which patients and families have a different understanding than a health care professional. These may include preventive strategies, complex disease processes, medication or treatment regimens, abstract laboratory results or measurements, technical terms, or words that have a different meaning in the health care arena than in everyday use. Cultural issues and misconceptions can also contribute to lack of understanding.

Consider the following when talking with parents about RSV and bronchiolitis:

Prevention and Health Promotion

Parents may not understand how viruses are transmitted. Be sure to incorporate a discussion of how severe viruses can be and how important it is to guard against them. Explain the important infection-preventing role played by keeping the family's hands clean, and be very precise in your instructions. For example, tell parents to wash their hands with soap and water for as long as it takes them to sing "Happy Birthday" or "Mary Had a Little Lamb." Also, have the parents teach their children how to wash their hands.

Parents aren't likely to know what makes one child more susceptible than others to RSV. Siblings, child care, and crowding make it more likely that a child will get RSV. But being born prematurely or having chronic lung or heart disease make it more likely that a child who gets RSV will be severely affected. Smoking probably increases both frequency and severity.

Parents may not know that babies who were born early may need special medicine (palivizumab prophylaxis) throughout the RSV season.

Diagnosis

Parents may not know what viruses are or that you do not treat a viral infection with antibiotics. You may need to explain that a virus is a germ that makes you sick and that antibiotics don't usually work for viruses.

Visual aids and handouts can help caregivers understand the condition. The 2 or 3 most important concepts can be printed on a piece of paper and given to the caregiver. For example, pictures of the airways of a term infant versus those of an infant born preterm may enhance parental understanding.

Symptoms

Parents may not know the symptoms associated with bronchiolitis. The following are easily recognizable and understood terms that indicate a child may have bronchiolitis.

- She breathes fast and the spaces between her ribs are sucking in.
- He may have a blue color around his lips.
- A wheezing—or whistling sound—is heard when she breathes.
- He coughs a lot.

Management and Treatment

Parents want their child to feel better and may not realize that using saline nose drops with a bulb syringe can decrease a child's congestion, making it easier to breathe, feed, and sleep. Demonstrate how to use saline nose drops with a bulb syringe. Give parents a handout to take home.

Parents may not understand how the work of breathing can cause a baby to dehydrate. Advise parents that they can continue to breastfeed, or offer the child small frequent feedings of formula or other liquids.

Parents may not understand how long the symptoms will last and that the symptoms may get worse before they start to improve. Explain the usual duration and natural course of RSV infection so they know what to watch for and when to call or have their infant rechecked for worsening symptoms.

Cultural Beliefs

Families from different cultures may have their own ideas of what causes the symptoms of bronchiolitis and how to treat it. Their beliefs can result in confusion and lack of adherence to suggested management if they are not understood.

Ask parents what they think is causing the cold or the breathing symptoms and what they think will make it better. This will increase your understanding of their culture while uncovering possible road-blocks or cultural issues with treatment before they arise.

Try to incorporate their beliefs into your treatment plan. Usually parents' or families' beliefs will pose no harm to the child.

Worsening Condition

Parents may think that because they saw the doctor earlier in the day or yesterday there is no need to check in again, even if the child seems worse.

Parents may not know what to look for when determining whether their child's condition is worsening.

Be clear and tell them when they should call you or go to the emergency department.

Cultural Spotlight

Upper Respiratory Infection for Some Latino Cultures

Some Latinos may treat upper respiratory infections with a variety of teas for each symptom.

For example, the yerbero or curandero would recommend salvia (sage) tea as a tonic; gordolobo (mullein) tea as an antispasmodic; eucalipto (eucalyptus) tea for bronchodilation, and oregano de la sierra (oregano) tea for its antitussive and sore throat effects.

Even if the parent doesn't mention teas to help relieve symptoms, it is helpful to address this treatment concept.

Source: Hispanic Center of Excellence (a partnership of the Baylor College of Medicine and University of Texas-Pan American). http://www.rice.edu/projects/HispanicHealth/Courses/mod7/mod7.html. Accessed March 19, 2008.

- The child gets very tired or limp.
- The child stops eating or has trouble feeding.
- The child starts to turn blue.

In particular, explain clearly what they should look for as signs of a more severe problem (eg, turning blue, breathing very hard). Give them a handout to take home so they have something to refer to later. Point out and mark the most important information.

Behavior Change

Behavior change is a key element in preventing and managing many pediatric conditions. Shifting from paternalistic advice that is either too vague or too complicated to a patient- and family-centered approach that incorporates elements of motivational interviewing and goal-setting, and that makes use of plain language, can be an effective way to empower patients and families to make changes and improve their health.

Explain how important it is for everyone in the family to keep their hands clean, especially before and after diaper changing or going to the bathroom, and before preparing food or eating. Stress the importance of hand-washing in terms of making sure the rest of the family doesn't get sick too—not just with bronchiolitis or RSV, but with many common and potentially serious illnesses.

Explain that smoking increases the risk of getting RSV and its seriousness, and that no one should smoke around the child. There should be absolutely no smoking in the home or car.

Child Involvement

Including the child, to the extent possible, is respectful and patient-centered and can contribute to developing health literacy skills as the child moves toward managing his or her own health as an adolescent and an adult. Involve the child by directing age-appropriate statements to the child, and introducing ways the child can keep himself or herself healthy.

For example, even children younger than 2 years can be taught how to wash their hands with help. And older children can easily be given the responsibility of washing their hands too.

Teach-back

The concept of teaching back entails asking parents or patients to demonstrate understanding *using their own words*, not simply asking whether they have questions or whether they understand, because that may not elicit lack of understanding. Having patients explain in their own words not only assesses their understanding, but reinforces the information by repeating and internalizing it for the patient. When there is a lot of information, go over each concept and elicit a teach-back before moving to the next idea.

When using teach-back, it's important to put the burden on yourself. Avoid the perception that you are quizzing the parent or patient—emphasize that you want to be sure you've explained things clearly and thoroughly.

The practice of using teach-back is especially important over the phone, because it may be the only way to gauge whether the parent or patient understands.

Here are some approaches to using teach-back when preventing or managing bronchiolitis.

- To make sure your baby stays as healthy as possible this winter, what will you do to prevent colds and bronchiolitis?
- What will you tell your husband needs to be done to help Logan through this sickness?
- I want to make sure I was clear when I explained this to you. To check, can you tell me which symptoms of John's will make you call me back? What things might mean that he is getting worse?

Key Messages for Use by All Members of the Health Care Team

It is important to reinforce key messages for parents and children so they hear them more than once and recognize them as priorities in managing their health. At a well-baby visit, you and your staff can introduce and reinforce ideas regarding risk reduction for both RSV and other viruses, particularly those involving hand-washing and avoiding tobacco smoke. At subsequent visits, your staff can reemphasize the importance of core concepts. Sick visits also provide a chance to reinforce key prevention measures.

By developing some key concepts and reviewing them with your staff, you can ensure that families don't receive conflicting advice about their health and what to do.

Remember: Don't try to teach parents the pathophysiology of RSV or bronchiolitis, but explain the basic key concepts thoroughly and consistently.

Information in a simple handout can be given to the parents on how the caregiver can recognize severe breathing problems and when to call the doctor.

- Explain the differences between symptoms associated with mild upper respiratory infection (a stuffy or runny nose and a mild cough) and those of severe lower respiratory tract illness (turning blue, fast heartbeat, fast breathing, difficulty breathing or feeding, a bad cough).
- Having a fever and being unable to sleep or eat sometimes accompany the increasing respiratory symptoms.

Bronchiolitis and colds are caused by viruses and will not be helped by antibiotics. (For some patients, palivizumab may be used to reduce the risk of severe disease due to RSV.)

- Palivizumab requires monthly injections during the RSV season; one injection is not enough.
- Palivizumab does not prevent illness from other respiratory viruses.

Important factors that can increase the risk of infection

- Child care
- Environmental air pollution, including smoke
- School-aged siblings

Important factors that can increase the severity of infection

- Premature birth
- Chronic lung disease
- Hemodynamically significant congenital heart disease
- Environmental air pollution, including smoke
- HIV or other diseases or conditions that compromise the immune system

Bronchiolitis and many other illnesses can often be prevented by regular hand-washing.

Miscellaneous

It is essential that all parents leave the office with the basic concepts on RSV or bronchiolitis, as noted above, but some parents will want to know more about their child's condition. You can explain more to parents who have questions, or ask if they have other questions.

You may also send them to reliable Internet sites for more in-depth discussion on the child's condition. Consider giving them a list of reliable sites. Below are several sites that present information on RSV and bronchiolitis at various reading levels (some are in Spanish).

Medical Encyclopedia

- Entry on **bronchiolitis**:
  http://www.nlm.nih.gov/medlineplus/ency/article/000975.htm

- Entry on **RSV:**
  http://www.nlm.nih.gov/medlineplus/ency/article/001564.htm
- Information also available in Spanish
- US National Library of Medicine, National Institutes of Health

Kids' Health for Parents

- http://www.kidshealth.org/parent/infections/bacterial_viral/
  bronchiolitis.html
- Information also available in Spanish
- Nemours Foundation

"Bronchiolitis and Your Child"

- http://familydoctor.org/020.xml
- Information also available in Spanish
- American Academy of Family Physicians

"RSV: When It's More Than Just a Cold" (PDF)

- http://www.aap.org/healthychildren/08winter/HC-winter08-
  rsv.pdf
- American Academy of Pediatrics
- *Healthy Children*, Winter 2008

NLM Easy-to-Read Resources and Services

- http://www.nlm.nih.gov
- The MedlinePlus tutorials with pictures, sound, and text make
  health information especially easy to understand for people
  with different learning needs
  http://www.nlm.nih.gov/medlineplus/tutorial.html.
- Includes MedlinePlus http://medlineplus.gov;
  http://medlineplus.gov/spanish/; NIHSeniorHealth
  http://nihseniorhealth.gov/;
  http://nihseniorhealth.gov/toolkit/toolkit.html; MedlinePlus
  Magazine
  http://www.nlm.nih.gov/medlineplus/magazine.html

RSV, Bronchiolitis, and Your Baby

RSV is the short name for respiratory syncytial virus (RES-pruh-tor-ee sin-SISH-ul VYE-ris). Almost all children get RSV at least once before they are 2 years old. For most healthy children, RSV is like a cold. But some children get very sick with RSV.

Symptoms may include:

- Runny nose.
- Coughing.
- Low fever.

These symptoms should go away in 5 to 7 days. And you can treat them the same way you would treat a cold.

But RSV can be dangerous for some children. It is the main cause of **pneumonia*** and **bronchiolitis*** in children younger than 2 years.

Bronchiolitis is an infection that is common in babies. One symptom of bronchiolitis is trouble breathing. This can be scary for both parents and children.

Call the Doctor Right Away If…

…your baby shows any of these signs:

- Trouble breathing or breathing faster than usual
- **Wheezing***
- Acting fussy and restless
- Not wanting to eat

Call 911 or an Ambulance If…

- Your baby's lips and fingertips start to turn blue.
- Your baby stops breathing.

What Will the Doctor Do?

The doctor will check to see what the infection is. Then the doctor will talk with you about the best way to care for your baby. If your baby is very sick, the doctor may need to keep him or her in the hospital for a few days.

Home Treatment

You can't cure a virus. But you can help your baby's symptoms.

To Help a Stuffy Nose

Thin the mucus (MYOO-kus). Only use saline (saltwater) nose drops. *Never* use any other kind of nose drops unless your baby's doctor prescribes them.

Clear your baby's nose with a suction bulb. (This is also called an ear bulb.) Squeeze the bulb first and hold it in. Gently put the rubber tip into one **nostril***, and slowly release the bulb. This will suck the clogged mucus out of the nose. It works best when your baby is younger than 6 months.

✳ Words to Know

acetaminophen (uh-see-tuh-MIN-uh-fin)— a medicine for pain and fever. Tylenol is one brand of acetaminophen.

bronchiolitis (brahn-kee-yoh-LYE-tis)—an infection that makes the lining of small breathing tubes of the lungs swell. The swelling blocks airflow, making it hard to breathe.

ibuprofen (eye-byoo-PROH-fin)— a medicine for pain and fever. Advil and Motrin are brands of ibuprofen.

nostril (NAH-strul)—1 of 2 holes in the bottom of the nose, where air goes in and out.

pneumonia (nuh-MOH-nyuh)— an infection of the lungs. Many different germs can cause pneumonia.

wheezing (weez-ing)—high-pitched whistling sounds when breathing.

Continued on back

Continued from front

Put a cool-mist humidifier in your child's room. A humidifier (hyoo-MID-uh-fye-ur) puts water into the air to help clear your child's stuffy nose. Be sure to clean the humidifier often.

Don't give your baby any cold medicines without asking the doctor.

To Help Fever

Give your baby acetaminophen* or ibuprofen* (for a baby older than 6 months). Be sure to get the right kind for your child's age. Ask the doctor how much to give your baby.

Don't give aspirin to your baby. It's dangerous for children younger than 18 years.

Make Sure Your Baby Drinks Lots of Liquids

Your baby needs to drink plenty of liquids if he or she has a fever or has trouble sucking or nursing.

Your baby may want clear liquids instead of milk or formula. Good choices are water and juice mixed with water. Offer a little bit at a time. Your baby may feed more slowly or not feel like eating because it's hard to breathe.

Who Can Get Very Sick?

RSV can be serious for babies whose lungs are not strong. These include:

- Babies younger than 6 weeks.
- Babies who were born more than 8 weeks early (before 32 weeks of pregnancy).
- Babies who were born with severe heart or lung disease.

RSV also can be serious for young children with health problems like:

- Chronic (long-term) lung disease.
- Serious heart problems.
- Problems fighting infections because their immune system does not work well.

When and How Does RSV Spread?

RSV and other viruses are very easy to catch. Children can pick up germs from:

- Countertops, tables, and playpens.
- Unwashed hands.
- Touching or kissing someone with a cold.

Can You Prevent RSV?

It's important to try to protect your child from RSV and other viruses. This is especially true when your child is younger than 6 months. Here are some things you can do:

- Make sure everyone washes their hands before touching your baby.
- Keep your baby away from anyone who has a cold, fever, or runny nose.
- Don't take your baby to crowded places like shopping malls.
- Don't smoke around your baby.
- Keep your baby away from cigarette and other tobacco smoke.

For Babies Who Can Get Very Sick…

Ask your child's doctor if your baby is at high risk for getting very sick from RSV. If so, follow the tips above and ask the doctor if your baby should get special shots that can help prevent RSV.

> ### Remember Flu Shots
> All babies older than 6 months should get a flu shot. And make sure the whole family gets the flu vaccine too!

To learn more, visit the American Academy of Pediatrics (AAP) Web site at www.aap.org.

Your child's doctor will tell you to do what's best for your child. This information should not take the place of talking with your child's doctor.

Note: Brand names are for your information only. The AAP does not recommend any specific brand of drugs or products.

Adaptation of the AAP information in this handout into plain language was supported in part by McNeil Consumer Healthcare.

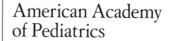

American Academy of Pediatrics

DEDICATED TO THE HEALTH OF ALL CHILDREN™

VSR, bronquiolitis y su bebé
(RSV, Bronchiolitis and Your Baby)

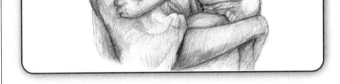

VSR son las siglas del virus sincitial respiratorio. En inglés lo llaman "RSV". Casi todos los niños padecen de este virus por lo menos una vez antes de cumplir los 2 años. Para la mayoría de los niños saludables, el VSR es como un resfriado. Pero algunos niños se enferman mucho con este virus.

Los síntomas pueden incluir:

- Secreción nasal (mocos).
- Tos.
- Fiebre leve.

Estos síntomas casi siempre mejoran después de 5 a 7 días. Usted puede tratarlos de la misma forma como trataría un resfriado.

Aún así, el virus VSR puede ser peligroso para algunos niños. Este virus es la causa principal de **neumonía*** y **bronquiolitis*** en los niños menores de 2 años.

La bronquiolitis es una infección que es común en los bebés. Uno de los síntomas de la bronquiolitis es dificultad para respirar. Esto puede asustar tanto a los padres como a los niños.

Llame al doctor de inmediato si...

…su bebé tiene cualquiera de estos síntomas:

- Dificultad para respirar o respira más rápido que lo normal
- Silbido al respirar* (wheezing)
- Está irritable e intranquilo
- No quiere comer

Llame al 911 ó una ambulancia si...

- Los labios y las puntas de los dedos de su bebé comienzan a ponerse azules.
- Su bebé no respira.

¿Qué hará el doctor de su niño?

El doctor evaluará que tipo de infección tiene el bebé. Si su bebé está muy enfermo, puede ser que el doctor decida que se quede unos días en el hospital.

Tratamiento en casa

No hay medicina para curar este virus. Aún así, usted puede aliviar los síntomas de su bebé.

Para aliviar la nariz tapada

Reduzca la mucosidad. Puede utilizar las gotas nasales salinas (agua con sal). Nunca utilice ninguna otra clase de gotas nasales a menos que el doctor de su bebé las prescriba.

Limpie la nariz de su bebé con una bomba de succión (Éstas son las mismas bombas que se usan para los oídos). Primero apriete la bomba y sosténgala de esta forma. Suavemente coloque la punta de hule dentro de la **fosa nasal*** del bebé, lentamente afloje su mano de la bomba. Esto aspirará la mucosidad de la nariz. Este método funciona mejor en bebés menores de 6 meses.

✱ Palabras que debe conocer

acetaminofén: Es una medicina para el dolor y la fiebre. Tylenol es una marca de acetaminofén.

bronquiolitis: Es una infección de los pequeños tubos respiratorios de los pulmones. Ésta bloquea el flujo de aire, dificultando la respiración.

ibuprofeno: Es una medicina para el dolor y la fiebre. Advil y Motrin son marcas de ibuprofeno.

fosa nasal: 1 de los 2 orificios en la nariz, donde entra y sale el aire.

neumonía: Es una infección de los pulmones. Muchos gérmenes diferentes pueden causar la neumonía.

silbido al respirar: Sonidos de pito producidos al respirar. En inglés se le llama "wheezing".

Continúa atrás

Coloque un humidificador en el dormitorio de su niño. El aire húmedo ayuda a destapar la nariz de su niño. Asegúrese de limpiar con frecuencia el humidificador.

No le dé a su bebé ningún medicamento para el resfriado sin preguntarle al doctor.

Para aliviar la fiebre

Dele a su bebé acetaminofén* (para bebés de más de 6 meses) o ibuprofeno*. Pregúntele al doctor cuánto debe darle.

No le dé aspirina. Es peligroso para niños menores de 18 años.

Asegúrese de que su bebé tome bastante líquido.

Necesita tomar más líquidos si tiene fiebre o dificultad para comer.

Puede ser que su bebé quiera otros líquidos en lugar de leche o fórmula. Los mejores son agua y jugo mezclado con agua o pedialyte. Ofrézcale un poco a la vez. Puede ser que su bebé coma menos o no sienta ganas de comer porque se le dificulta respirar.

¿Quién puede enfermarse seriamente con este virus?

El VSR puede ser serio en los bebés cuyos pulmones no son fuertes. Como:

- Bebés de menos de 6 semanas.
- Bebés que nacieron prematuros por más de 8 semanas (antes de las 32 semanas de embarazo).
- Bebés que nacieron con enfermedad severa del corazón o enfermedad de los pulmones.

El VSR también puede ser serio en niños pequeños con problemas de salud como:

- Enfermedad crónica (de largo plazo) de los pulmones.
- Problemas serios del corazón.
- Problemas del sistema inmunológico.
  (el cuerpo no puede combatir infecciones).

¿Cuándo y cómo se propaga el VSR?

Es muy fácil contagiarse de VSR y de otros virus. Los niños pueden agarrar los gérmenes de:

- Mostradores, mesas y parques.
- Manos sucias.
- Otros niños o adultos que esten resfriados.

¿Se puede prevenir el VSR?

Es importante tratar de proteger a su hijo del VSR y de otros virus. Esto es especialmente importante cuando su niño es menor de 6 meses.

- Asegúrese de que todos se laven las manos antes de tocar a su bebé.
- Mantenga a su bebé alejado de cualquier persona que tenga resfrío, fiebre o mucosidad.
- No lleve a su bebé a lugares con mucha gente como a los centros comerciales.
- No fume cerca de su bebé.
- Mantenga a su bebé alejado del humo del tabaco de otras personas.

Para los bebés que corren el riesgo de enfermarse seriamente...

Pregúntele a su doctor si su bebé corre alto riesgo de enfermarse de este virus. Si es así, siga los consejos anteriores. También pregúntele al doctor si su bebé necesita la vacuna contra el VSR.

Recuerde las vacunas contra la gripe

Todos los bebés de más de 6 meses deben tener una vacuna contra la gripe. ¡Asegúrese de que toda su familia también se vacune contra la gripe!

Para aprender más, visite el sitio de la Academia Americana de Pediatría (AAP) en www.aap.org.
Su pediatra le dirá qué es lo mejor para la salud de su hijo.
Esta información no debe usarse en lugar de consultar con su doctor.
Nota: Los nombres de marca son para su información solamente. La AAP no recomienda ninguna marca o producto de medicina específicamente.
La adaptación de la información de este folleto de la AAP a lenguaje sencillo se hizo con el apoyo de McNeil Consumer Healthcare. La traducción al español fue patrocinada por Leyendo Juntos (Reach Out and Read), un programa pediátrico de alfabetización.

American Academy of Pediatrics

DEDICATED TO THE HEALTH OF ALL CHILDREN™

Calcium

Most children older than 8 years in the United States fail to achieve the recommended intake of calcium. Maintaining adequate calcium intake during childhood and adolescence is necessary to attain peak bone mass, which may be important in reducing the risk of fractures and osteoporosis later in life.

Good bone health requires satisfactory intake of both calcium and vitamin D. While calcium requirements vary by age, current recommended adequate vitamin D intake for all infants, children, and adolescents is 200 IU per day.

Optimizing calcium intake is particularly important during adolescence. Peak calcium-accretion rate is attained at an average of 12½ years in girls and 14 years in boys. During the 3- to 4-year period of increased bone mass acquisition that occurs during adolescence, 40% of total lifetime bone mass is accumulated. Yet only 10% of adolescent girls achieve the recommended daily intake of calcium.[1]

Prevention of future osteoporosis and possibility of a decreased risk of fractures in childhood and adolescence should be discussed with patients and families as potential benefits for achieving the goal of adequate calcium intake.

Common areas for miscommunication may include

- Prevention and health promotion
- Management and treatment
- Nutrition and physical activities
- Peak bone mass accrual

A Patient Story. . .

Dr Tremont is seeing Sarah—who is 13 years old, an excellent student, and a very good athlete—for a follow-up appointment related to a sports injury.

Sarah never eats breakfast because she gets up too late and is in a hurry to get to school. She is starting to worry about her appearance and doesn't want to get fat. Sarah cares about her participation in sports, hopes to play on the high school team, and intellectually knows that eating healthy is important, but everything seems to be fine right now. Her mother and older sister each drink 2 to 4 diet sodas every day.

Sarah recently heard her grandmother telling her mother that she has to start taking some kind of medicine because she has weak bones.

Sarah was evaluated for a sports injury that turned out to be a severe bruise, although there was concern it might have been a fracture. She is eager to get back to softball. Dr Tremont said the injury was healing properly and sent Sarah home with instructions to call if anything more happens.

. . . .

The sports injury could have provided a hook to engage Sarah in a conversation about the critical window of opportunity she has to build strong bones now and for the future.

Motivational interviewing techniques might have spurred Sarah to take action to get more calcium in her diet. Dr Tremont could also have talked Sarah through some of the difficulties she may have in making changes in her diet, considering the diets of others in her home.

Dr Tremont could also have pointed out that teens who don't get enough calcium can be at increased risk for fractures. The potential seriousness of Sarah's recent injury—and how it could have hurt her chances to stay active in sports—might have been the catalyst Sarah needed to engage in some healthier behaviors.

Ask Me 3

During your patient encounter, you should communicate using plain language and health literacy principles so that by the end of the visit, the parent or child will know the answers to the *Ask Me 3* questions.

Patient: Illiana, a 13-year-old with a calcium deficiency	
Ask Me 3 questions	**What the patient should understand at the end of the visit**
What is my main problem?	I'm not getting enough calcium through what I usually eat and drink.
What do I need to do?	• I'm going to work on drinking 3 glasses of milk a day. • I'm going to start by mixing 2% and skim milk until I get used to the flavor. Or I might try the flavored milk at school. • I'll also eat a carton of yogurt for a snack and drink a glass of calcium-fortified orange juice at breakfast.
Why is it important for me to do this?	I need to get enough calcium to keep me from breaking a bone now and when I'm older. This is the only chance I have to get really strong bones; and once I turn 21 it's practically too late.

Patient: Ella, a 10-year-old at risk for suboptimal calcium intake	
Ask Me 3 questions	**What the parent and patient should understand at the end of the visit**
What is my child's main problem?	She isn't getting enough calcium through what she usually eats and drinks, which could make her bones weak.
What do I need to do?	• I'm going to start buying chocolate skim milk, and she and I will both drink a glass at breakfast and dinner. • I'll get string cheese and yogurt cups for her after-school snack. • And, at least 3 times a week, we'll take a walk together right after dinner to help keep her bones strong.
Why is it important for me to do this?	• I know it's important for her to start building lifelong healthy habits now. • I need to make some healthy changes too. • Doing this will help both of us get more calcium and help keep us from breaking bones later. And it will also give us some time together!

Medical Terms and Plain Language Alternatives

Many of the medical terms we use every day don't mean much to many parents. Below is a list of medical terms that may be confusing or difficult to explain and suggestions for plain language alternatives.

Medical Terms	Plain Language Alternatives
Adequate calcium intake	Getting enough calcium through food and drinks
Bone density test	The way we measure how strong a person's bones are
Bone mass accrual	How bones store calcium for the rest of the body, like a bank keeps money for when you need it
Calcium	A mineral that the body needs to build strong bones and teeth
Dairy products	Foods and drinks that come from milk and have a lot of calcium in them
Diet	A general word for what a person usually eats. It can also be used to describe special ways to eat that help you be healthy (like a high-calcium diet or a low-salt diet). "Diet" doesn't always mean limiting what you eat to help you lose weight.
Fracture	Broken bone
Lactose intolerance	When a person gets a stomachache or a lot of gas from eating or drinking things that have milk in them
Osteoporosis	When bones get so weak or fragile they can break from just bending over
Peak bone mass	The time when bones have the most calcium they will ever have—usually in your early teens and before age 21
Weight-bearing exercise	Activities that you do on your feet—like walking, running, dancing, tennis, or soccer—and other activities like weight lifting help your bones get strong (Activities like swimming and biking are healthy and make your heart beat faster, but they aren't weight-bearing exercises.)

Confusing Terms and Concepts

With any condition, there are likely to be terms or concepts for which patients and families have a different understanding than a health care professional. These may include preventive strategies, complex disease processes, medication or treatment regimens, abstract laboratory results or measurements, technical terms, or words that have a different meaning in the health care arena than in everyday use. Cultural issues and misconceptions can also contribute to lack of understanding.

Consider the following when talking with families about calcium:

Prevention and Health Promotion

Because the amount of calcium needed changes by age, it may be hard for children, teens, and parents to know how much calcium they need. Parents and teens may not understand that in addition to getting enough calcium, they need vitamin D and weight-bearing exercise to build strong bones.

Many things affect calcium requirements, including gender, physical activity, and race or ethnicity, so it can be hard to determine the optimal amount of intake. Other dietary factors are important to maximize retention of dietary calcium, including alcohol, caffeine, oxalates, phytates (eg, in soy), and protein.

People may not know how to read and use food nutrition labels to see how much calcium is in a food or drink.

Show them how to read food labels to find the amount of calcium in a serving. Explain the amount of calcium in a serving is listed as "% Daily Value" not as milligrams, and that 100% of the daily value is 1,000 mg of calcium per day for an adult and 1,300 mg a day for people between 9 and 18 years old.

Show them an easy way to find out how many milligrams of calcium are in a serving; then they can add them up. Put a "0" at the end of the number listed for the daily value to get the number of milligrams.

Use the AAP handout on calcium or a laminated copy of a food label to demonstrate.

Diagnosis

Teens and parents may not make the connection between a fracture or a family history of osteoporosis and the need for ensuring adequate calcium intake during adolescence.

Instead of trying to explain genetics to the family, put the potential condition into real-world examples that will help the parent and patients visualize the effects of not getting enough calcium. When asking about family history, ask if grandma has a hunched back, or if she has gotten shorter as she has aged. You can use that later to talk about how grandma probably didn't have enough calcium as a child.

It can be hard to explain the concept of peak bone mass accrual and bone density, especially when an adolescent looks and feels healthy. Consider using the "bone bank" metaphor.

- Calcium is stored in the bones now for the rest of your body as if it were in a savings account at the bank. You can only put money into this account until you're 21, then you have to live the rest of your life on what's in there. From then on, your body mainly takes calcium out of your bones.

- Do you think you can start saving more calcium up in your bone bank? Can you think of ways you can save up more calcium?

- When you get older, your bones will still need calcium, but if you don't have any to withdraw, your bones will get weak and may start to break—even when you do simple things like bend

---

✓ **Communication Tip**

Remember to explain to patients and parents that getting enough calcium isn't the only way to strong bones!

✓ Everyone needs vitamin D to make strong bones too. Vitamin D comes from fortified milk and from sunlight, and it helps calcium work.

✓ Weight-bearing exercise is also important in achieving maximal peak bone mass.

over. Even now, if you don't have enough calcium you can break a bone when you run or dance.

Symptoms

Because few symptoms of low bone-mineral density are apparent until a fracture occurs, it is often difficult to explain to a teenager how important bone density is. Discovering the potential problem may come through gathering the family history or exploring the patient's interest in sports.

Management and Treatment

Parents may not recognize the critical role they play in influencing their children's lifelong eating habits. Emphasize the importance of establishing dietary practices in childhood that promote adequate calcium intake throughout life, and point out that a mother's consumption of milk predicts how much milk young female children will consume.

Help them recognize that it helps the teen to eat healthy foods and good sources of calcium when the whole family has healthy eating habits too.

It can be difficult to get some patients—especially teenaged girls—to consume more dairy products because they erroneously think all dairy products are "fattening."

- There are skim milks and fat-free and low-fat yogurts and cheeses.
- You can look on the food labels to see how many calories and how much fat foods contain.

Some patients may ask about the calcium in nondairy foods. (See the list on page 130 under Cultural Beliefs for suggestions on calcium-rich, nondairy foods.)

- Even though there are nondairy foods that are high in calcium, you have to eat a lot more of them to get enough calcium every day.
- Plus, if you rely on calcium-fortified foods or nondairy foods for calcium, you will still need another source of vitamin D, because both are critical to optimal bone health.

Some may ask if they can take calcium supplements instead. Explain to parents and patients that supplements are a good alternative source of calcium for some people, but getting calcium from foods is preferred—that's because supplements don't offer the added nutritional benefits that calcium-rich foods do. Adherence can also be a problem because supplements have to be taken every day.

The Problem of Lactose Intolerance

Primary lactose intolerance may be a problem for some populations. It is more common in children of African, Mexican, Native American, and Asian descent than it is among white children.

Many children with lactose intolerance can drink small amounts of milk without discomfort, especially when accompanied by other foods.

Alternative ways for lactose-intolerant children to get calcium is through fermented dairy products, such as hard cheese and yogurt, which they may tolerate better than milk.

In addition, lactose-free and low-lactose milks are now widely available.

Cultural Beliefs

Nondairy food products (such as calcium-fortified soy milk) may be used as other calcium sources, especially for vegetarians who do not consume dairy products, although the calcium in soy products has low bioavailability.

Alternative sources of calcium are important for children and adolescents who do not drink milk. Most vegetables contain calcium, although at relatively low density. Thus large servings are needed to equal the total intake achieved with typical servings of dairy products. (Note: If a patient relies on calcium-fortified foods or nondairy foods that are low in vitamin D, then they must also have another source of vitamin D to provide the adequate intake of 200 IU per day.)

Good vegetable sources of calcium include cabbage; bok choy; dark, leafy greens, such as mustard, collard, dandelion, or turnip greens; spinach; kale; broccoli; and okra.

Drinking orange juice fortified with calcium is a good alternative to dairy products for getting enough calcium.

Other good alternatives include canned salmon, canned sardines, tofu, soybeans, blackstrap molasses, white beans and navy beans, chickpeas (garbanzo beans), instant oats, almonds, sesame seeds, and sesame butter (tahini).

Worsening Condition

It may not be possible to know that an adolescent has osteopenia or even osteoporosis without testing bone mineral density, so efforts must focus on assessing calcium intake and risk factors for suboptimal bone health at least 3 times during well-child visits: at 2 to 3 years of age, during preadolescence, and during early adolescence.

Some questions that are helpful to ask to find out about bone health are

- How many times a day do you (does your child) drink milk?
- How often do you (does your child) eat cheese, yogurt, or other dairy foods?
- Do you (does your child) drink juice with added calcium or cereals with added calcium?
- Do you (does your child) eat any of the following vegetables: broccoli, beans, collard greens? How often? How much at a time?

- How often do you (does your child) do activities like walking, running, soccer, tennis, dancing, or lifting weights?
- Have you (has your child) ever had a broken bone?[1]

Note: Children need 3 servings (4 for adolescents) of dairy foods per day to get enough calcium.

Behavior Change

Behavior change is a key element in preventing and managing many pediatric conditions. Shifting from paternalistic advice that is either too vague or too complicated to a patient- or family-centered approach that incorporates elements of motivational interviewing and goal-setting, and that makes use of plain language, can be an effective way to empower patients and families to make changes and improve their health.

Inadequate calcium intake in a child or adolescent is a family problem. Parental intakes and practices influence their children's intakes. If the parent is not achieving the recommended calcium intake, it is unlikely the child will. Thus family dietary behavior should be considered when encouraging children and adolescents to drink milk.

Because some children, teens, and families may have long-term habits that contribute to suboptimal calcium intake and bone health, it may be hard to make changes in their behavior. Providers may want to use principles from the stages of change model to help motivate changes in behavior, moving patients from pre-contemplation to contemplation to action.[2]

Also, when dealing with behavior change it's important to have the patient and/or parent identify what they think will work best for them, set small goals that they believe are achievable, and identify ways to help them succeed. Motivational interviewing techniques can be used to help them build conviction (the belief that "this is important" so they know why they should change) and confidence (the belief that they can actually carry it out successfully)[3] to make sustained behavior changes to increase calcium intake and promote physical activity.

Parent

- On a scale of 1 to 10, with 1 being "not at all" and 10 being "completely," how convinced are you that helping Tina get more calcium is important?
  - You say "8"—that's great.
- On a scale of 1 to 10, with 1 being "not at all" and 10 being "completely," how confident are you that you will be able to change Gina's afternoon snack to yogurt instead of chips?

- You say "3"—why is that, and what would it take to move that to a "4"?

Parent and Young School-Aged Child
- How confident are you that you can get rid of the juice and pop, and switch over to water or low-fat milk?

Teen

- How confident are you that you will never drink pop again? Is it more realistic to say you will only have pop on special occasions or when you go out with your friends?
- You say you would only give yourself a 4 in how confident you are that you can stop drinking so much soda. What would it take to move that to a 5?
- Anna, you say you aren't convinced that you need to drink more milk. You say you feel healthy even though you don't drink milk and skip breakfast every day, you have your whole life to get more calcium, and by the time you're old they'll have pills to keep you from getting osteoporosis. Is there anything you can think of that might make you want to start getting more calcium now instead of waiting?

Child Involvement

Including the child, to the extent possible, is respectful and patient-centered and can contribute to developing health literacy skills as the child moves toward managing his or her own health as an adolescent and an adult. It can include direct, age-appropriate statements to the child, and also ways for the child to be involved in his or her health.

Young school-aged children can keep track of their own and family members' dairy servings daily, and keep a chart on the refrigerator.

Older school-aged children can read nutrition labels and chart not only dairy servings, but also the daily intake amounts of calcium and vitamin D.

Children and teens can track exercise too.

- They can count reps (for weight-bearing exercises) and steps (for walking and running).
- They can use a pedometer to track their number of steps and set goals.
- They can mark milestones, family and personal records, achievements, and goals and monitor frequency and other statistics.
- The family can have healthy competitions, among themselves or with neighbors and friends.

- Children can earn rewards for achievement of health goals.

Teach-back

The concept of teaching back entails asking parents or patients to demonstrate understanding *using their own words*, not simply asking whether they have questions or whether they understand, because that may not elicit lack of understanding. Having patients explain in their own words not only assesses their understanding, but it reinforces the information by repeating it and internalizes it for the patient. When there is a lot of information, go over each concept and elicit a teach-back before moving to the next idea.

When using teach-back, it's important to keep the burden on yourself. Avoid the perception that you are quizzing the parent or patient—emphasize you want to be sure you've explained things clearly.

The practice of using teach-back can be especially important over the phone, because it may be the only way to gauge whether the parent or patient understands.

Here are some approaches to using teach-back when talking about calcium.

Teens

- Now that we've discussed why calcium is good for you and some ways you can eat and drink more things that have calcium in them, tell me where you're going to start.
- To make sure this plan works for you, what will you tell your friends when you get together and go out to eat?
- Because your grandmother and aunt both have osteoporosis, I really want to be sure I've done a good job going over everything that you can do to stay healthy and not have the same problem when you're older. It can be kind of complicated, so can you tell me in your own words, so I can make sure I was clear?

Preteens

- Payton, now that we've gone over everything, what will you tell your dad tonight about some good ways to get more calcium into your diet so you can build strong bones?

Parents of Younger Children

- What will you tell Kristin's father and your after-school child care provider about the changes you want to make to help her get more calcium?

Key Messages for Use by All Members of the Health Care Team

It is important to reinforce key messages for parents and children so they hear them more than once and recognize them as priorities in managing their health. In addition, families should not receive conflicting advice about their health and what to do.

Key concepts for calcium are

- The easiest way to achieve adequate calcium intake is to consume 3 servings of dairy products per day and 4 servings per day for adolescents.

- Low-fat dairy products, including skim milk and low-fat yogurts, are good sources of calcium, and there is hardly any difference in their calcium content compared with whole milk products.

- Calcium intakes on food labels are indicated as a percentage of the daily value in each serving. This daily value is currently set at 1,000 mg per day, which is the adult requirement. There's an easy way to find out how many milligrams of calcium are in a serving; then you can add them up. (Use the How to Read Food Labels section of the handout on page 138.)

- If you rely on calcium-fortified foods or nondairy foods that are low in vitamin D, you need another source of vitamin D to get adequate daily intake.

- If you don't consume dairy products, alternative nondairy sources of calcium include most vegetables and calcium-fortified juices, breakfast cereals, and soy beverages.

- Calcium supplements can help, but they don't have all the other nutrients that are important for good health, and it can be hard to take them regularly.

- Physical activity—mainly weight-bearing exercise—is an important part of an overall healthy bone program.

- Early adolescence, the time for peak bone mass accrual, is a critical window of opportunity to build strong bones for a lifetime.

- Establishing healthy eating habits as a child is important to lifelong health, so the whole family needs to be involved.

Miscellaneous

There are many resources online that have good information on nutrition. Print out appropriate sections for patients, or write down Web addresses for them.

The US Department of Agriculture food pyramid Web site (http://www.mypyramid.gov/) has a variety of resources, including printable posters and materials—for children and adults—to help keep track of daily intake and to see what international foods fall into which category. To help families make sure they're eating the proper amount of each food group every day, consider giving parents and older children a chart they can take home, such as a printout of the food pyramid: http://www.mypyramid.gov/downloads/MiniPoster.pdf.

The US Food and Drug Administration has a complete plain language explanation of how to read a nutrition label: http://www.cfsan.fda.gov/~dms/foodlab.html#ca.

The Mayo Clinic has a very helpful interactive guide to the nutrition label at http://www.mayoclinic.com/health/nutrition-facts/NU00293. And the Nemours Foundation has a similar explanation for children at http://kidshealth.org/kid/stay_healthy/food/labels.html.

Doctors and other health professionals can learn more about this topic by reading the American Academy of Pediatrics clinical report, "Optimizing Bone Health and Calcium Intakes of Infants, Children, and Adolescents" (*Pediatrics*. 2006;117(2):578–585). The report is available online at http://aappolicy.aappublications.org/cgi/content/full/pediatrics;117/2/578.

References

1. Greer FR, Krebs NF, American Academy of Pediatrics Committee on Nutrition. Optimizing bone health and calcium intakes of infants, children, and adolescents. *Pediatrics*. 2006;117:578–585

2. DiClemente CC, Prochaska J. Toward a comprehensive, transtheoretical model of change: stages of change and addictive behaviors. In: Miller WR, Heath N, eds. *Treating Addictive Behaviors*. 2nd ed. New York, NY: Plenum; 1998

3. Rollnick S, Mason P, Butler C. *Health Behavior Change: A Guide for Practitioners*. London, UK: Churchill Livingstone; 1999

Calcium

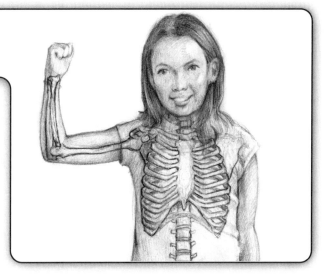

What Calcium Is and Why You Need It

Calcium is a mineral that your body needs. Its main job is to build strong bones and teeth. Your bones store calcium for the rest of your body, like a bank keeps money for when you need it.

You need the most calcium when you are between 9 and 18 years old. By the time you are 21 years old, your bones are as strong as they will ever be. From then on, your body mainly takes calcium out of your bones.

If you don't get enough calcium, your body will take the calcium it needs *from your bones.* They will get weak. They can break when you run or dance.

When you get older, you could have a disease called osteoporosis (ah-stee-yoh-puh-ROH-sis). It makes bones so fragile, they can break from just bending over. By then, it is usually too late to rebuild your bones.

How to Get Calcium

The best way to get calcium is by eating foods with lots of calcium. Here are some of the best ones:

- Low-fat milk, yogurt, and other milk products (These have the most calcium.)
- Flavored milks, like chocolate or strawberry (These can have more calories than plain milk.)
- Kale, collard greens, and other dark green, leafy vegetables (but *not* spinach)
- Chickpeas, lentils, split peas
- Canned salmon and sardines (and other fish with bones)
- Cereals and juices *with added calcium* (No more than 1 cup of juice a day, or you'll get too much sugar.)
- Tofu, soy milk with calcium added (Check the label.)

Ask the doctor if you think you need to take extra calcium or if you have trouble digesting milk.

How Much Calcium Do You Need?

This depends on your age. Here's what is recommended:

Daily Calcium Needs

Age	You Need This Much Calcium (mg per day)
4–8 years	800 mg
9–18 years	1,300 mg
19–50 years	1,000 mg

Calcium is measured in milligrams. The short way to write milligrams is *mg*.

Source: National Academy of Sciences

Tips for Getting More Calcium

- Choose milk or smoothies instead of soda pop.
- Add calcium to salads with low-fat cheese, tofu, or beans.
- Choose low-fat yogurt as a snack. Add it to pancakes, waffles, shakes, salad dressings, dips, and sauces.
- Look for foods with added calcium.

Continued on back

How to Read Food Labels

Food labels list the amount of calcium in a serving as "% Daily Value," not as milligrams (mg). **100% of the Daily Value = 1,000 mg of calcium per day for an adult.**

But, if you're between 9 and 18 years old, you need 1,300 mg a day (not 1,000 mg).

Here's an easy way to find out how many milligrams of calcium are in a serving. Then you can add them up.

Put a "0" at the end of the number listed for the daily value to get the number of milligrams.

For example, a serving of orange juice with added calcium might list the amount of calcium as 30% of the daily value.

30% Daily Value = 300 mg calcium

Usually, foods with at least 20% daily value (200 mg) are high in calcium. Foods with less than 5% of the daily value are low in calcium.

This food has 30% of the calcium an adult needs each day or 300 mg.

Nutrition Facts

Serving Size 1 cup (236ml)
Servings Per Container 1

Amount Per Serving

Calories 80	Calories from Fat 0

	% Daily Value*
Total Fat 0g	**0%**
Saturated Fat 0g	**0%**
Trans Fat 0g	**0%**
Cholesterol Less than 5mg	**0%**
Sodium 120mg	**5%**
Total Carbohydrate 11g	**4%**
Dietary Fiber 0g	**0%**
Sugars 11g	
Protein 3g	**17%**

Vitamin A 10%	•	Vitamin C 4%
Calcium 30%	•	Iron 0% • Vitamin D 25%

*Percent Daily Values are based on a 2,000 calorie diet. Your daily values may be higher or lower depending on your calorie needs.

Source: US Food and Drug Administration

Amounts of Calcium in Some Foods

Check food labels for the exact amounts. (See "How to Read Food Labels" on the left.)

Milk Group	Calcium (mg)
Milk, regular or low-fat, 1 cup	245–265
Yogurt, nonfat, fruit, 1 cup	260
Cheese, 1-oz slice	200
Frozen yogurt, 1/2 cup	105
Soy milk, with added calcium, 1 cup	200–500

Protein Group	Calcium (mg)
White beans, cooked, boiled, 1 cup	160
Salmon, canned with bones, 3 oz	205
Tofu, firm, with added calcium, 1/2 cup	205

Vegetables/Fruits	Calcium (mg)
Collards, cooked, 1 cup	265
Orange juice, with added calcium, 1 cup	300

Source: US Department of Agriculture

Health Tip: Choose low-fat or nonfat foods. Make trade-offs. For example, if you drink a milk shake, skip the fries. Low-fat milk has as much calcium as whole milk. (Taking fat out of food does not take out calcium.)

Other Tips for Strong Bones

Calcium doesn't work alone. You need 3 more things:

1. **A healthy diet**—Eat lots of fruits, vegetables, and whole grain foods.
2. **Exercise**—Get lots of weight-bearing exercise. This is any exercise you do on your feet, like walking, running, dancing, tennis, or soccer. You can also lift weights to help your bones.
3. **Vitamin D**—This can come from:
   • Sunlight. (Your body makes vitamin D when the sun shines on your skin.)
   • Milk, other dairy products, drinks, and foods, like cereals, with added vitamin D. (Check the label.)
   • Multivitamins (mull-tee-VYE-tuh-minz).

To learn more, visit the American Academy of Pediatrics (AAP) Web site at www.aap.org.

Your doctor will tell you to do what's best for you.

This information should not take the place of talking with your doctor.

Adaptation of the AAP information in this handout into plain language was supported in part by McNeil Consumer Healthcare.

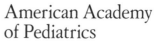American Academy of Pediatrics

DEDICATED TO THE HEALTH OF ALL CHILDREN™

Calcio (Calcium)

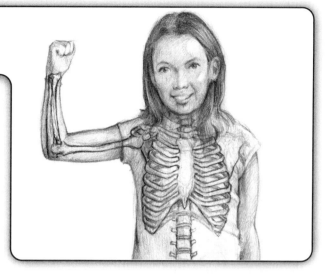

Qué es el calcio y por qué lo necesita

El calcio es un mineral que el cuerpo necesita. Su función principal es hacer que los huesos y dientes sean fuertes. Los huesos almacenan calcio para el resto de su cuerpo, así como un banco guarda el dinero para cuando usted lo necesita.

Los niños entre los 9 y 18 años necesitan tomar mucho calcio. Cuando llegan a los 21 años sus huesos son tan fuertes como lo serán de allí en adelante.

Cuando uno no toma suficiente calcio, el cuerpo obtiene el calcio que necesita de los huesos. Los huesos se ponen débiles y se pueden quebrar más fácilmente.

Cuando uno envejece, puede padecer de una enfermedad llamada osteoporosis. Esta hace que los huesos sean muy frágiles y se puedan quebrar con tan sólo una torcerdura. Para entonces, ya es demasiado tarde para reconstruir los huesos.

Cómo obtener el calcio

La mejor forma de obtener el calcio es comiendo alimentos que contengan mucho calcio. Estos son algunos de los mejores alimentos:

- Leche baja en grasa, yogurt y otros productos lácteos. (Estos son los que tienen más calcio).
- Leche con sabor (chocolate o fresa). (Estas pueden tener más calorías que la leche común).
- Col, variedades de acelgas y otros vegetales de hojas verdes (pero *no* la espinaca).
- Garbanzos, lentejas y guisantes.
- Salmón y sardinas enlatados (y otros tipos de pescado con espinas).
- Cereales y jugos con *calcio agregado*. (No más de una taza de jugo al día o tomará demasiada azúcar).
- Tofu, leche de soya (soja) con calcio agregado. (Revise la etiqueta).

Pregúntele al doctor si su niño debe tomar calcio extra. Cuéntele al doctor si su niño tiene problemas para digerir la leche.

¿Qué cantidad de calcio se necesita?

Esto depende de la edad. A continuación están las cantidades recomendadas:

Cantidades necesarias diarias de calcio

Edad	Necesita esta cantidad de calcio (mg por día)
4–8 años	800 mg
9–18 años	1,300 mg
19–50 años	1,000 mg

El calcio se mide en miligramos. La abreviatura de miligramos es mg.

Fuente: National Academy of Sciences

Consejos para obtener más calcio

- Elija leche o batidos de leche en lugar de bebidas gaseosas.
- Agréguele calcio a las ensaladas poniéndoles quesos bajos en grasa, tofu o frijoles (habichuelas).
- Agréguele yogurt bajo en grasa a los panqueques, wafles, batidos, aderezo para ensaladas, dips y salsas.
- Escoja alimentos que contengan calcio agregado.

Continúa atrás

Cómo leer las etiquetas de los alimentos

La etiqueta de los alimentos indica la cantidad de calcio en una porción como un "% de la cantidad diaria," y no como miligramos (mg). El **100% de la cantidad diaria es 1,000 mg de calcio al día para un adulto.**

Recuerde que los niños entre los 9 y 18 años de edad necesitan 1,300 mg al día (no 1,000 mg).

Para saber cuantos miligramos de calcio hay en una porción de comida:

Coloque un "0" al final del número mencionado en la cantidad diaria.

Por ejemplo, una porción de jugo de naranja con calcio agregado podría indicar la cantidad de calcio como 30% de la cantidad diaria.

El 30% de la cantidad diaria equivale a 300 mg.

Escoja alimentos con más de 20% de la cantidad diaria (200 mg). Los alimentos con menos del 5% tienen un bajo contenido de calcio.

Estos alimentos contienen 30% del calcio que un adulto necesita cada día ó 300 mg.

Nutrition Facts

Serving Size 1 cup (236ml)
Servings Per Container 1

Amount Per Serving

Calories 80	Calories from Fat 0

% Daily Value*

Total Fat 0g	**0%**
Saturated Fat 0g	**0%**
Trans Fat 0g	**0%**
Cholesterol Less than 5mg	**0%**
Sodium 120mg	**5%**
Total Carbohydrate 11g	**4%**
Dietary Fiber 0g	**0%**
Sugars 11g	
Protein 3g	**17%**

Vitamin A 10%	•	Vitamin C 4%
Calcium 30%	• Iron 0% •	Vitamin D 25%

*Percent Daily Values are based on a 2,000 calorie diet. Your daily values may be higher or lower depending on your calorie needs.

Fuente: US Food and Drug Administration

Cantidades de calcio en algunos alimentos

Revise las etiquetas de los alimentos para conocer las cantidades exactas de calcio. (Vea "Cómo leer las etiquetas de los alimentos" a la izquierda).

	Calcio (mg)
Leche, regular o baja en grasa, 1 taza	245–265
Yogurt, sin grasa, 1 taza	260
Queso, una rodaja de 1 onza	200
Helado/mantecado de yogurt, ½ taza	105
Leche de soya, con calcio agregado, 1 taza	200–500

	Calcio (mg)
Frijoles blancos, cocidos o hervidos, 1 taza	160
Salmón, enlatado con espinas, 3 onzas	205
Tofu, sólido, con calcio agregado, ½ taza	205

	Calcio (mg)
Acelgas cocidas, 1 taza	265
Jugo de naranja, con calcio agregado, 1 taza	300

Fuente: US Department of Agriculture

Consejo de salud: Elija alimentos con poca grasa. Haga un intercambio. Por ejemplo si se toma un batido de leche, no se coma las papitas fritas.
La leche con poca grasa contiene tanto calcio como la leche entera. (El quitarle la grasa a los alimentos no le quita el calcio).

Otros consejos para tener huesos fuertes

El calcio no trabaja por sí solo. Se necesitan 3 cosas más:

1. **Una dieta saludable**—Ofréscale a su hijo muchas frutas, muchos vegetales y alimentos de grano entero.

2. **Hagan ejercicio**—Especialmente ejercicios levantando los pies. Por ejemplo: caminar, correr, bailar o jugar fútbol. También puede hacer ejercicio con pesas para mantener los huesos fuertes.

3. **Obtengan vitamina D**—La vitamina D se encuentra en:
   - La luz del sol. (El cuerpo produce vitamina D cuando se expone la piel al sol).
   - La leche, otros productos lácteos, bebidas y alimentos con vitamina D agregada, como los cereales. (Revise la etiqueta).
   - Multivitaminas.

Para aprender más, visite el sitio de la Academia Americana de Pediatría (AAP) en www.aap.org.
Su pediatra le dirá qué es lo mejor para la salud de su hijo.
Esta información no debe usarse en lugar de consultar con su doctor.
La adaptación de la información de este folleto de la AAP a lenguaje sencillo se hizo con el apoyo de McNeil Consumer Healthcare. La traducción al español fue patrocinada por Leyendo Juntos (Reach Out and Read), un programa pediátrico de alfabetización.

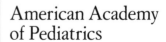
American Academy of Pediatrics
DEDICATED TO THE HEALTH OF ALL CHILDREN™

Colds and Flu
Upper Respiratory Infection

Studies have demonstrated pediatricians are more likely to give a parent a prescription if he or she feels the parent is expecting one. However, in the current era of antibiotic resistance, health care providers are being called on to use antibiotics less frequently. Educating staff and providing consistent messages that illnesses such as the common cold do not require antibiotics can help alleviate the strain on the pediatric health care system during the peak winter months. Equally important is managing parents' expectations and educating them about the natural course of illness, and symptoms that mean a child needs further evaluation.

Clear communication around the nature of a viral illness—as well as supportive care at home, expectations for improvement, and instructions about when parents should seek medical care—may improve parent and provider satisfaction.

Common areas for miscommunication may include

- Diagnosis
- Management and treatment expectations
- Expected course of illness
- Indicators that a child is getting worse and needs attention

Ask Me 3

During your patient encounter, you should communicate using plain language and health literacy principles so that by the end of the visit, the parent or child will know the answers to the *Ask Me 3* questions.

A Patient Story. . .

It is mid-winter and this is the tenth patient Dr Roosevelt has seen this morning for fever, cough, and aches.

As she finishes examining Jayden, she informs his mother: "Mrs Johnson, your son has the flu. Give him plenty to drink and have him rest and he will be better soon."

As Dr Roosevelt prepares to leave the room, Mrs Johnson asks that familiar question: "But, he's sick. Aren't you going to give him an antibiotic?"

. . . .

Mrs Johnson is the exception, because she spoke up when she had a question—many parents don't; they just leave unsatisfied, and do whatever they would have done had they not brought the child to see the doctor.

This illustration points out the need for health care providers to take the time to clarify their instructions with the patients and their parents.

Dr Roosevelt could have told Mrs Johnson what signs would indicate a worsening condition, how much "plenty" of fluids means, when Jayden should start feeling better, and even what she means by "rest."

And she should have been prepared for the question and had a direct discussion about antibiotics with Mrs Johnson. Or, if antiviral medications are given, the doctor should have been ready to explain how they are used.

Providing this information at the outset would allow the parent to take comfort in the doctor's counsel, and might lead to improved adherence for Jayden.

Patient: Arden, 6-year-old girl with influenza	
Ask Me 3 questions	**What the parent should understand at the end of the visit**
What is my child's main problem?	Arden has the flu, which is caused by a virus. It's not the stomach flu, but the kind that causes fever and cough.
What do I need to do?	• I need to keep Arden comfortable. I can give her a medicine like acetaminophen for fever or body aches and to help her rest easier. The doctor will tell me the right dose and how often I can give it. • I must give Arden the medicine you prescribed to help get rid of the flu virus. • I should give her small amounts of healthy fluids often so her body doesn't dry out. • *I will call the doctor if...*Arden has trouble breathing, ear pain, a fever after 3 or 4 days, if cough is still there after 1 week, or if she doesn't start feeling better after a few days.
Why is it important for me to do this?	• The virus medicine should shorten how long Arden is sick. • Most children get better from the flu within a week, but sometimes the flu might lead to something else. • I can help Arden feel comfortable and watch for signs that something else might be going on.

Patient: Andrew, 18-month-old boy with a viral upper respiratory infection (a cold)	
Ask Me 3 questions	**What the parent should understand at the end of the visit**
What is my child's main problem?	Andrew has a cold, which is caused by a virus. There is no medicine for it, but there are some things I can do to make him rest easier until he starts feeling better.

What do I need to do?	• I need to make sure Andrew gets rest and doesn't get dried out, so I'll keep him calm and give him water and other healthy fluids to drink.
	
	• I will NOT buy over-the-counter cold and cough medicines to give Andrew. These medicines
	
	  • May be dangerous to young children like Andrew
	
	  • Won't make him get better
	
	• *I will call the doctor if*...Andrew's fever lasts more than 2 or 3 days, if he gets worse instead of better after a week, if he has trouble breathing or drinking, if he has ear pain, or if he is very cranky or very sleepy.

Why is it important for me to do this?	This will help Andrew feel better while his body gets rid of the infection on its own and keep him from drying out.

Medical Terms and Plain Language Alternatives

Many of the medical terms we use every day don't mean much to many parents. Below is a list of medical terms that may be confusing or difficult to explain and suggestions for plain language alternatives.

Medical Terms	Plain Language Alternatives
Antibiotics	Medicine to get rid of the germs, called "bacteria," that cause infections. Antibiotics don't work against viruses.
Antiviral medicine	Medicine that can treat the flu if the child is seen in the first 2 days and is older than 1 year
Dehydrated	Dry; dried out. The body needs water and other liquids to stay healthy; when it doesn't have enough, it dries out, or gets "dehydrated," which can be dangerous.
Diarrhea	Watery poop (stool)
Fluids	Liquids or things to drink or swallow without chewing (like soup)
Gastroenteritis	Stomach infection, or stomach flu, that causes you to throw up and have diarrhea (This is different from influenza.)
Influenza	Flu. A virus that causes high fever, aches, cough, runny nose, and sometimes other symptoms; it's different from the stomach flu that makes you throw up and have diarrhea.
Lethargic	Tired, sleepy, weak
Nasal spray	Medicine that you squirt up the nose to help you breathe easier
Nauseous/ nauseated	Feeling sick to your stomach
Temperature; fever	The temperature is how warm or cold your body is. If the temperature is higher (hotter) than usual, you have a "fever."
Upper respiratory infection (URI)	Cold; the common sickness that gives you a cough, runny nose, and sometimes a fever or other symptoms.
Vaccine	A shot or nose spray to keep people from getting sick with illnesses like the flu. In this case, it's commonly called the "flu shot."
Viral illness	Consider using terms such as "cold" or "flu."
Virus	A germ that makes you sick. Antibiotics don't usually work for viruses.
Vomiting	Throwing up

Confusing Terms and Concepts

With any condition, there are likely to be terms or concepts for which patients and families have a different understanding than a health care professional. These may include preventive strategies, complex disease processes, medication or treatment regimens, abstract laboratory results or measurements, technical terms, or words that have a different meaning in the health care arena than in everyday use. Cultural issues and misconceptions can also contribute to lack of understanding.

Consider the following when talking with families about influenza:

Prevention and Health Promotion

Parents may not be aware of evolving recommendations for influenza vaccine. Explain the specifics of influenza vaccination, and any other details they need to know, including

- Who should be vaccinated?
  Among those who should get the vaccine are
    - All children aged 6 to 59 months, or 6 months to 4 years
    - Children and adolescents receiving long-term aspirin treatment
    - Children and adults with high-risk conditions, such as certain chronic or immunosuppressive conditions, or other illnesses that compromise respiratory function
    - Healthy household members and others who care for children or for people with high-risk conditions
    - All well children and adolescents aged 5 to 18 years (new 2008 recommendation)
    - Residents of nursing homes and other chronic care facilities
    - Women who will be pregnant during the flu season
    - People aged 50 years and older
    - Health care workers
    - Travelers
    - Anyone who wants to decrease his or her chance of getting ill from influenza
- What is a flu vaccine?
  There are 2 types of vaccines
    - Live attenuated nasal vaccine, in which a vaccine with weakened flu virus is gently sprayed into the nose
    - Inactivated injected vaccine, a vaccine that contains flu virus that has been killed; it is given as a shot
- What are the side effects?
  People often say they got the flu vaccine and then they got the flu, or even that they caught the flu *from* the vaccine. Because of this kind of confusion about the side effects of the vaccine, it's important to clear up misperceptions right away.

  Communicate clearly what side effects can really accompany the flu vaccine (eg, soreness, low-grade fever, muscle aches) versus symptoms of the stomach flu (eg, vomiting and diarrhea) or actual influenza.
- When is the best time to get vaccinated?

Explain that ideal timing of flu vaccination depends on several factors, and offer some guidelines about timing the vaccine.

- Influenza season usually peaks in the United States between December and March.[1]
- It takes about 2 weeks for the vaccine to work.
- You can still get the vaccine even after the flu season has started.
- Children aged 6 months to 8 years who are getting the vaccine the first time need 2 doses 1 month apart.

- How well does the vaccine work?
  The effectiveness of the vaccine depends on the match between the flu viruses in the vaccine and the ones that are causing illness during the current year's flu season.

  Flu vaccine developers have to predict which flu virus types are going to be active almost a year ahead of time; sometimes the virus types change after they start manufacturing the vaccine. Then the vaccine is not as good a match and may not work as well.

- Why should I have my child vaccinated against the flu?

  Even when the vaccine doesn't work 100%, it can still provide protection against more severe illness and having to be in the hospital.

  The Centers for Disease Control and Prevention estimates that an average of 36,000 people die from influenza-related complications each year in the United States.[1]

Diagnosis

You may need to explain the difference between viral and bacterial illness.

- The flu virus is different from most viruses because antibiotics don't usually work for viruses, but there are some drugs that may help cure the flu. These drugs are different from the usual antibiotics that help treat other infections, like strep throat and urinary tract infection.
- If a child is older than 1 year and it's within 2 days of the start of symptoms, there is a treatment for the child.

If you are using a rapid test for flu, explain how these tests are like tests looking for strep throat.

There is sometimes confusion because viral gastroenteritis is called the "stomach flu." Ask parents to describe what the child's stool looks like. Reinforce to parents that although a child with the flu can also have vomiting or diarrhea, this is different from the stomach flu, which is caused by different viruses.

Symptoms

Parents often are concerned that fevers may pose risk to a child. Make sure that parents are aware of what constitutes a fever for infants older than 2 months and children. And reassure them that fevers are an important part of the body's response to the cold/flu and won't hurt the child.

Management and Treatment

Avoid generalities such as "a few days" when you can. Tell parents how many days the symptoms should last—even if it's a range (2 or 3 days). Also explain that as long as the child isn't getting worse and there are no signs of dehydration, the child is probably getting better.

> • With a cold, most children will start to get better after 2 to 3 days, but that it will take 7 to 10 days before they are back to normal.

Be clear about when parents need to bring children back for reevaluation (eg, if fever continues past 3 days or the child develops new symptoms, such as ear pain or signs of increased trouble breathing).

Many parents feel the need to provide medications to alleviate symptoms of the cold and flu. Explain that treatments that may alleviate symptoms include the use of acetaminophen (or ibuprofen for infants older than 6 months), rest, and encouraging fluids.

Tell parents that treatment may be available if the flu is diagnosed in the first 2 days of symptoms, and explain that over-the-counter (OTC) cold medications are not indicated for children younger than 2 years (see box on the left). They don't work to cure the illness and can have dangerous side effects. Emphasize that aspirin should never be given to a child.

Cultural Beliefs

Explore a family's cultural beliefs by asking the parent what they think is causing the condition and what they think will make it better. This will increase your understanding of their culture while uncovering possible roadblocks or cultural issues with treatment before they arise.

If you find that the family subscribes to such common health theories as "hot-cold" beliefs, you may need to tailor your advice to what is consistent with their beliefs. For example, if the family believes that milk is "cold" and should not be used to treat a cold or flu, explore with them what fluids they would feel to be appropriate (eg, "hot").

Usually the parents' or families' beliefs will pose no harm to the child. Try to incorporate their beliefs into your treatment plan.

Did You Know...?

In January 2008 the US Food and Drug Administration issued a public health advisory stating that children younger than 2 years should not be given cold medications because of serious and life-threatening side effects. The American Academy of Pediatrics (AAP) position is as follows:

• Over-the-counter cough and cold medicines do not work for children younger than 6 years and in some cases may pose a health risk.

• The efficacy and risk of such medications needs to be studied in children. As the AAP has testified: "If a medicine will be used in children, it should be studied in children. Cough and cold medications should not be exceptions to this rule."

• The labeling needs to reflect what we know—the medications are not effective for children younger than 6 years and their use, and misuse, could cause serious, adverse side effects.

Worsening Condition

It is important to emphasize to parents when they need to either call the doctor or bring their child back in to be reassessed. Be clear about when fevers should improve and what temperature constitutes a fever so parents know what to expect and when to call.

When these points are emphasized, it is helpful to provide the handout and point to the information as it is explained to parents. Underlining or circling the section can help parents to quickly locate the information at home if needed. Try to limit this to 3 main points, and avoid medical jargon.

Providing anticipatory guidance on these points can help to alleviate parental concerns, as well as decrease unnecessary phone calls.

Behavior Change

Behavior change is a key element in preventing and managing many pediatric conditions. Shifting from paternalistic advice that is either too vague or too complicated to a patient- or family-centered approach that incorporates elements of motivational interviewing and goal-setting, and that makes use of plain language, can be an effective way to empower patients and families to make changes and improve their health.

To avoid colds, families can be encouraged to wash their hands often, avoid touching their faces, and not to smoke or expose each other to smoke. Explain that smoking increases the risk of getting a respiratory infection, and its seriousness, and that no one should smoke around the child. There should be absolutely no smoking in the home or car.

Explain how important it is for everyone in the family to keep their hands clean, especially before and after diaper changing or going to the bathroom, and before preparing food or eating. Stress the importance of hand-washing in terms of making sure the rest of the family doesn't

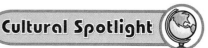

Cultural Spotlight

Shared Misperceptions About Colds

Many cultures share misperceptions about upper respiratory infections (URIs). For example, studies have found that a great many cultures believe exposure to drafts causes URIs. Similarly, there is the shared misperception that exposure to extreme temperatures causes URIs.

In Latin American cultures, exposure to extreme temperatures is believed to upset the body's self-regulatory system, causing illness. Generally, the remedy for a "cold" is something hot. Urban Guatemalans classified "flu" as needing hot remedies, and most rural Guatemalans in the study classified both "cold" and "flu" as needing "hot" remedies.

"However, the classification of foods, medicines, and diseases as either hot or cold is not necessarily dependent on their temperature, but rather on an innate quality of "hotness" or "coldness."

A study of Puerto Ricans in Connecticut uncovered the belief that a hot-cold balance must be maintained for good health. Specifically, the study found that a child who has a cold should not have milk, which is classified as "cold."

For the Mestizos in Sonora, Mexico, fresh homemade cheese is considered to be muy fresca (very cool) and therefore shouldn't be eaten by someone who has a cold. Another example of these relationships was seen among Tarascan Indians; eating "cold" foods was believed to be a cause of gripa (cold or flu). It was also believed that to cure this illness, "hot" foods should be consumed.

Source: Baer RD, Weller SC, Pachter L, et al. Cross-cultural perspectives on the common cold: data from five populations. *Hum Organ*. 1999. http://findarticles.com/p/articles/mi_qa3800/is_199910/ai_n8873496/pg_1. Accessed April 30, 2008.

get sick too—not just with a cold or the flu, but with many common and potentially serious illnesses.

Recommend that patients and their families get the flu vaccine. Motivational interviewing can help with this behavior change.

- How convinced are you that getting the flu vaccine for J.J. is important?
- Do you think you could write a reminder on your calendar to bring Toni for her flu vaccine in October?

Child Involvement

Including the child, to the extent possible, is respectful and patient-centered and can contribute to developing health literacy skills as the child moves toward managing his or her own health as an adolescent and an adult. Involve the child by directing age-appropriate statements to the child, and introducing ways the child can keep himself or herself healthy.

It is important to engage children in assisting with their care as they are able. For example, even children younger than 2 years can be taught how to wash their hands with help. Older children can easily be given the responsibility of washing their hands too. As children become preschool age, they may be encouraged to wash their hands often and, when they're sick, to rest or drink fluids as they are able.

Teach-back

The concept of teaching back entails asking parents or patients to demonstrate understanding *using their own words,* not simply asking whether they have questions or whether they understand, because that may not elicit lack of understanding. Having patients explain in their own words not only assesses their understanding, but it reinforces the information by repeating it and internalizes it for the patient. When there is a lot of information, go over each concept and elicit a teach-back before moving to the next idea.

When using teach-back it's important to keep the burden on yourself. Avoid the perception that you are quizzing the parent or patient—emphasize that you want to be sure you've explained things clearly.

The practice of using teach-back can be especially important over the phone, because it may be the only way to gauge whether the parent or patient understands.

Potential teach-back concepts for cold and flu are

- How will you explain to your babysitter how to give the acetaminophen to the baby? How much and how often?

- Pretend I am grandma. Can you teach me how to use the bulb syringe and what I use it for?

- I want to be sure I explained this to you clearly. Can you tell me the symptoms that will make you call me?

- Because the flu medicine has some side effects, what will you tell your wife to watch for?

Key Messages for Use by All Members of the Health Care Team

It is important to reinforce key messages for parents and children so they hear them more than once and recognize them as priorities in managing their health. In addition, families should not receive conflicting advice about their health and what to do.

Key concepts for colds

- There is no treatment to cure colds.
- The illness can last for up to 10 days.
- Mucus in your child's nose may turn yellow or green after 3 or 4 days.
- Children can get one cold after another.
- Fever should only last for the first 2 to 3 days of the cold.
- Do NOT give the child aspirin. It is dangerous.
- If your child is younger than 2 years, do NOT give her OTC cold and cough medicines.
- Treatment
  - Cool mist humidifier
  - Bulb suction
  - Fluids
  - Acetaminophen (or ibuprofen for children older than 6 months), if needed

Key concepts for the flu

- We can only give antiviral medicines that can cure the flu if the child is within 2 days of starting the illness and older than 1 year.
- The worst of the illness should be the first 2 to 3 days.
- If child has problems breathing, pain in the ear, the fever doesn't get better after 3 days, or the child doesn't start to feel better after 2 or 3 days, call the doctor.

Did You Know...?

In one study, 4 Latino groups were asked for the differences between the common cold (*catarro*), *resfriado*, and *gripe*. Mexicans tended to define *gripe* the same as *catarro*. Some Texas respondents classified *gripe* as "a cold" and others as "the flu."

At all study sites except Texas, the symptoms offered for gripe focused on upper respiratory complaints. The Texas respondents included fever as a symptom of *gripe*.

Resfriado showed a somewhat different pattern, with a focus on symptoms of coldness (as seen in responses such as "cold sweats," "chills," "cold hands and feet," "feel cold"), particularly in Guatemala, Mexico, and Texas.

Source: Baer RD, Weller SC, Patcher L, et al. Cross-cultural perspectives on the common cold: data from five populations. *Hum Organ*. 1999. http://findarticles.com/p/articles/mi_qa3800/is_199910/ai_n8873496/pg_1. Accessed April 30, 2008.

- The child needs a lot of rest and to drink plenty of fluids.
- The child can be given acetaminophen (or ibuprofen for children older than 6 months) to lower the fever and help aches. Do *not* give the child aspirin. It is dangerous.
- The flu vaccine can prevent the flu. Your child will need it each year in the fall.

Miscellaneous

Because the US Food and Drug Administration has withdrawn pediatric cold remedies for infants and toddlers younger than 2 years, this may be a shift in thinking for some parents, who may be used to giving their children a cold medicine. This can give a parent the sense that he has actively done something to alleviate or cure the child's condition.

Addressing this expectation may avoid conflict later on, and lead to improved parental expectations and satisfaction. In addition, providing other suggestions for supportive care—such as the use of a bulb syringe or a cool mist humidifier—may provide an active alternative for caregivers.

Reference

1. Centers for Disease Control and Prevention. CDC finds annual flu deaths higher than previously estimated [press release]. http://www.cdc.gov/od/oc/Media/pressrel/r030107.htm. Accessed June 3, 2008

Colds

Most children get 8 to 10 colds before they are 2 years old. Most colds come and go without any big problems.

There is *no* cure for the common cold since colds are caused by viruses. Antibiotics don't kill viruses so they will not make your child's cold better. But you can help your child *feel* better until the cold goes away.

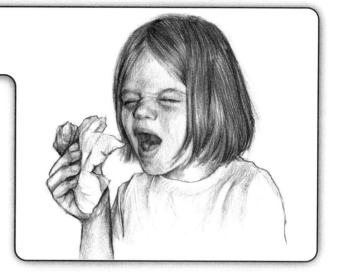

Signs of a Cold

A child with a cold may show these signs:

- Stuffy, runny nose
- Sneezing
- Coughing
- Watery eyes
- Eating more slowly, not feeling hungry
- Sore throat

There may also be a mild fever (under 102°F or 38.9°C) or headache. All this can make your child fussy too.

Colds usually last about a week but can even last for 10 days. If there is fever, it should come at the start of the cold and then go away. Mucus (MYOO-kus) in your child's nose may turn yellow or green after 3 or 4 days. Children can get one cold right after another. So it may seem like your child is sick for a long time.

Call the Doctor If...

...your child has any of these signs:

- Fever lasting more than 2 or 3 days
- Cold symptoms that get worse, instead of better, after a week.
- Trouble breathing or drinking
- Ear pain
- Acting very sleepy or fussy
- Coughing more than 10 days

What to Do for a Cold

To Help a Stuffy Nose

Put a cool-mist humidifier in your child's room. A humidifier (hyoo-MID-uh-fye-ur) puts water into the air to help clear your child's stuffy nose. Be sure to clean the humidifier often.

Thin the mucus. Use saline (saltwater) nose drops. Never use any other kind of nose drops unless your child's doctor prescribes them.

Clear your baby's nose with a suction bulb. (This is also called an ear bulb.) Squeeze the bulb first and hold it in. Gently put the rubber tip into one **nostril***, and slowly release the bulb. This will suck the clogged mucus out of the nose. It works best for babies younger than 6 months.

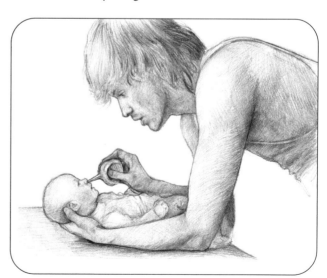

Continued on back

Continued from front

To Help Fever and Aches

- For a baby 6 months or younger, give **acetaminophen***.
- For a baby or child older than 6 months, give *either* acetaminophen or **ibuprofen***.

Both of these drugs help with fever. But they are not the same. Be sure to get the right kind of medicine for your child's age and weight. Follow what the label says, or ask your child's doctor how much to give.

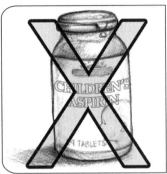

Note: *Never* give your child aspirin. It's dangerous for children younger than 18 years.

Don't give any other medicines without asking your child's doctor.

Make Sure Your Child Drinks Lots of Liquids

Make sure your child drinks plenty of liquids to avoid getting dehydrated (dee-HIGH-dray-ded). Being dehydrated means your child's body loses water and gets very dry inside. Clear liquids like juice mixed with water may work better than milk or formula if your child's nose is very stuffy.

Can You Prevent Colds?

There is no special way to prevent colds. But you can help keep viruses and other infections from spreading:

- Make sure everyone washes their hands often. Hand-washing helps keep germs from spreading.
- Cough and sneeze into a tissue. If you don't have time to get a tissue, bend your arm and sneeze into it.
- Keep your child away from anyone who has a cold, fever, or runny nose.
- Don't share spoons, forks, or drinking cups with anyone who has a cold, fever, or runny nose.
- Wash dishes in hot, soapy water.
- Don't smoke around your child. Keep your child away from cigarette and other tobacco smoke.

A Warning About Cold and Cough Medicines

The American Academy of Pediatrics strongly recommends that over-the-counter cough and cold medications not be given to infants and children younger than 2 years because of the risk of life-threatening side effects. Also, several studies show that cold and cough products don't work in children younger than 6 years and can have potentially serious side effects.

✳ *Words to Know*

acetaminophen (uh-set-uh-MIN-uh-fin) —a medicine for pain and fever. Tylenol is one brand of acetaminophen.

ibuprofen (eye-byoo-PROH-fin)— a medicine for pain and fever. Advil and Motrin are brands of ibuprofen.

nostril (NAH-strul)—1 of 2 holes in the bottom of the nose, where air goes in and out.

To learn more, visit the American Academy of Pediatrics (AAP) Web site at www.aap.org.

Your child's doctor will tell you to do what's best for your child.
This information should not take the place of talking with your child's doctor.

Note: Brand names are for your information only. The AAP does not recommend any specific brand of drugs or products.

Adaptation of the AAP information in this handout into plain language was supported in part by McNeil Consumer Healthcare.

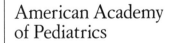

American Academy of Pediatrics

DEDICATED TO THE HEALTH OF ALL CHILDREN™

Resfriados (Colds)

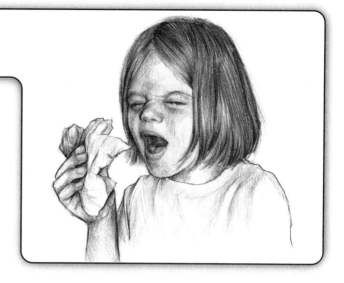

La mayoría de los niños sufren entre 8 y 10 resfriados antes de los 2 años. Casi todos los resfriados aparecen y desaparecen sin grandes problemas.

No hay cura para el resfriado común, ya que los virus son la causa. Los antibióticos no matan los virus, así que no mejorarán el resfriado de su niño. Pero usted puede ayudar a que su niño se sienta mejor hasta que el resfriado desaparezca.

Signos de un resfriado

Un niño con resfriado puede mostrar estos signos:

- Nariz tapada o con secreción
- Estornudos
- Tos
- Ojos llorosos
- Falta de apetito o comer más despacio
- Dolor de garganta

También puede tener una fiebre leve (más baja que 102°F ó 38.9°) o dolor de cabeza. Estos malestares pueden inquietar a su niño.

Normalmente, los resfriados tardan casi una semana, pero pueden durar hasta 10 días. Si hay fiebre, sucede al principio del resfriado. Luego desaparecerá. Después de 3 ó 4 días, los mocos de su niño tal vez cambien a color amarillo o verde. Los niños pueden padecer un resfriado tras otro. Puede ser que sienta como que su niño ha estado enfermo por mucho tiempo.

Consulte con el doctor si...

...su niño tiene alguno de estos signos:

- Fiebre que dura más de 2 ó 3 días.
- Síntomas de resfriado que empeoran, en lugar de mejorar, después de una semana.
- Dificultad para respirar o tragar.
- Dolor del oído.
- Mucho sueño o está inquieto.
- Tose por más de 10 días.

Qué hacer con un resfriado

Para aliviar la nariz tapada

Coloque un humidificador en la habitación de su niño. El humidificador hace que el vapor del agua se una con el aire y ayuda a que se le destape la nariz tapada de su niño. Asegúrese de limpiar con frecuencia el humidificador.

Para suavizar los mocos. Use gotas salinas para la nariz (agua con sal). Nunca use otro tipo de gotas nasales, a menos que el doctor se las recete.

Limpie la nariz de su bebé con un aspirador nasal. (También se conoce como aspirador para los oídos). Primero, presione el aspirador y manténgalo así. Con suavidad coloque la punta dentro de la **fosa nasal***, y suelte lentamente el aspirador. Así succionará los mocos que tapan la nariz. Esto funciona muy bien en bebés menores de 6 meses.

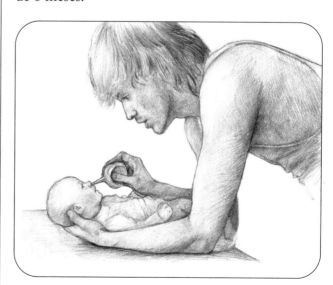

Continúa atrás

Viene de la página anterior

Para controlar la fiebre y los dolores

- Déle **acetaminofén*** al bebé de 6 meses o menos.
- Déle **ibuprofeno*** o acetaminofén al bebé o niño mayor de 6 meses.

Estas dos medicinas ayudan a controlar la fiebre. Pero no son iguales. Sólo dé a su niño el tipo correcto de medicina, de acuerdo a su edad y peso. Siga las instrucciones de la etiqueta o pregunte al doctor de su niño la cantidad que debe darle.

Nota: *Nunca* le dé aspirina a su niño. Es peligroso para niños menores de 18 años.

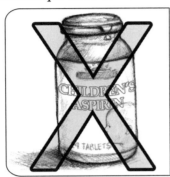

No le dé otras medicinas a su niño sin preguntarle a su doctor.

Déle bastantes líquidos a su niño

Asegúrese de que su niño tome una buena cantidad de líquidos. Esto evitará que se deshidrate. Estar deshidratado significa que el cuerpo de su niño pierde agua y se reseca mucho por dentro. Tomar líquidos claros como el jugo mezclado con agua son mejores que la leche o la leche de fórmula cuando la nariz de su niño está muy tapada.

¿Se pueden prevenir los resfriados?

No existe una forma especial de prevenir los resfriados. Pero puede evitar que los virus y otras infecciones se propaguen:

- Asegúrese de que todos se laven las manos con frecuencia. Lavarse las manos ayuda a evitar que los microbios se propaguen.
- Tosa y estornude en un pañuelo de papel. Si no tiene tiempo de alcanzarlo, doble el brazo y estornude en él.
- Aleje a su niño de cualquier persona con resfriado, fiebre o secreción nasal.
- No comparta cucharas, tenedores o vasos con alguien que tenga resfriado, fiebre o secreción nasal.
- Lave los platos en agua caliente con jabón.
- No fume cerca de su niño. Aléjelo del humo de cigarrillos y de otros productos de tabaco.

Una advertencia sobre medicinas para la tos y el resfriado

La Academia Americana de Pediatría recomienda enfáticamente que las medicinas de venta libre para la tos y el resfriado no se administren a bebés y niños menores de dos años de edad, debido al riesgo de efectos secundarios que pueden ser letales. Asimismo, varios estudios indican que los productos para los resfriados y la tos no son efectivos en niños menores de seis años y pueden tener efectos adversos potencialmente graves.

✳ *Palabras que debe conocer*

acetaminofén: Una medicina para el dolor y la fiebre. Tylenol es una marca de acetaminofén.

ibuprofeno: Una medicina para el dolor y la fiebre. Advil y Motrin son marcas de ibuprofeno.

fosa nasal: 1 de los 2 hoyos en la nariz por donde el aire entra y sale.

Para aprender más, visite el sitio de la Academia Americana de Pediatría (AAP) en www.aap.org.
Su pediatra le dirá qué es lo mejor para la salud de su hijo.
Esta información no debe usarse en lugar de consultar con su doctor.
Nota: Los nombres de marca son para su información solamente. La AAP no recomienda ninguna marca o producto de medicina específicamente.
La adaptación de la información de este folleto de la AAP a lenguaje sencillo se hizo con el apoyo de McNeil Consumer Healthcare. La traducción al español fue patrocinada por Leyendo Juntos (Reach Out and Read), un programa pediátrico de alfabetización.

American Academy of Pediatrics

DEDICATED TO THE HEALTH OF ALL CHILDREN™

The Flu

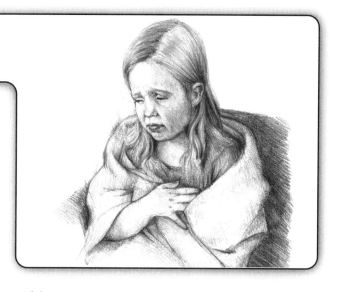

The flu (influenza) is an illness caused by a virus. It affects the whole body. This is not the same as what we often call the "stomach flu."

Flu season is mostly in the winter. Each year the flu is a little different because there are different types of flu viruses and they change over time. So, people can get the flu many times in their life.

Signs of the Flu

The flu can last a week or more. Your child usually will feel the worst during the first 2 or 3 days. Flu symptoms include:

- A sudden fever (usually over 101°F or 38.3°C).
- Chills and shakes with the fever.
- Headache, body aches, and extreme tiredness.
- Sore throat and/or dry, hacking cough.
- Stuffy, runny nose.
- Throwing up (vomiting) and loose, runny stools (diarrhea).

Is It the Flu or a Cold?

Both the flu and colds are caused by viruses. They can have some of the same symptoms. But there are differences:

Flu

- Children get sick quickly, often within 1 day.
- Children usually feel very sick and achy.
- Most children will need to stay in bed for a few days.
- Flu is more common in the winter.

Cold

- Children usually have low fever or none at all.
- Coughing is mild.
- Children with colds usually have the energy to play and keep up with their routines.
- Colds can happen any time of year.

What to Do for the Flu

Call the Doctor…

Right away—if your baby is 2 months or younger and has a fever.

Within 24 hours—if your child is older than 1 year and shows signs of flu. The doctor may be able to treat the flu with an **antiviral drug***. But this only works if your child gets the drug in the first day or two of illness.

Usually there are no serious problems with the flu. But sometimes your child can get an ear infection, a **sinus infection***, or **pneumonia***.

✳ Words to Know

acetaminophen (uh-see-tuh-MIN-uh-fin)—a medicine for pain and fever. Tylenol is one brand of acetaminophen.

antiviral (ant-ee-VYE-rul) **drug**— a medicine that can kill some flu viruses.

disinfectant (dis-in-FEK-tint)— a cleaner that kills germs.

ibuprofen (eye-byoo-PROH-fin)— a medicine for pain and fever. Advil and Motrin are brands of ibuprofen.

pneumonia (nuh-MOH-nyuh)— an infection of the lungs.

sinus infection (SYE-nis in-FEK-shun)— an infection of the spaces inside your head, behind your nose (sinuses).

wheeze (weez) or **wheezing** (weez-ing)— high-pitched whistling sound when breathing.

Continued on back

At *any* age, call the doctor if your child has one of these signs with the flu:

- Trouble breathing
- A cough that won't go away after a week
- Pain in the ear
- Fever that continues or comes back after 3 to 4 days
- Does not start to feel better after a few days

Other Tips

Extra rest and lots of fluids can help your child feel better. You can also give your child medicine to bring down the fever:

- For a baby 6 months or younger, give **acetaminophen***.
- For a child older than 6 months, give *either* acetaminophen or **ibuprofen***.

Both of these drugs help with fever. They are not the same. Be sure to get the right kind of medicine for your child's age. Follow what the label says.

Never give your child aspirin. Aspirin puts your child at risk for Reye syndrome, a serious illness that affects the liver and brain.

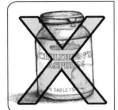

Check with your child's doctor before giving your child any *other* medicines. This includes over-the-counter cold and cough medicines. Antibiotics *don't* help the flu.

Don't smoke around your child. Smoke makes children cough and **wheeze*** more. And it makes it harder for them to get over the flu.

How to Prevent the Flu

The flu spreads very easily, especially to children and adults who spend time with children. It usually spreads during the first several days of the illness.

There are 3 ways to prevent the flu:

Good Hygiene (HYE-jeen)

Keeping germs from spreading is the best way to avoid spreading the flu. These tips will help protect your family from getting sick:

1. Teach your child to cover his or her mouth and nose when coughing or sneezing. Show your child how to use a tissue or a sleeve, not a hand.
2. Use tissues for runny noses. Throw them in the trash right away.
3. Avoid kissing a sick child on the mouth or face.
4. Make sure everyone washes their hands often.
5. Wash dishes, spoons, and forks in hot, soapy water or the dishwasher.
6. Don't let children share pacifiers, cups, spoons, forks, washcloths, or towels. *Never* share toothbrushes.
7. Use paper cups in the bathroom and kitchen. Throw them away after each use.
8. Wash doorknobs, toilet handles, countertops, and even toys. Use a **disinfectant*** or soap and hot water.

Flu Vaccines

There are safe **vaccines** to protect against the flu. They come as shots and a nose spray. Ask your child's doctor what is best for your child. Most healthy children need a flu vaccine every fall. All their family members should get the vaccine too. Call the doctor in September to find out more.

Antiviral Drugs

These drugs are taken before the child is exposed to the flu. These are very important for children with serious health problems who have not had a flu vaccine.

To learn more, visit the American Academy of Pediatrics (AAP) Web site at www.aap.org.

Your child's doctor will tell you to do what's best for your child.
This information should not take the place of talking with your child's doctor.

Note: Brand names are for your information only. The AAP does not recommend any specific brand of drugs or products.

Adaptation of the AAP information in this handout into plain language was supported in part by McNeil Consumer Healthcare.

American Academy of Pediatrics

DEDICATED TO THE HEALTH OF ALL CHILDREN™

La gripe (The Flu)

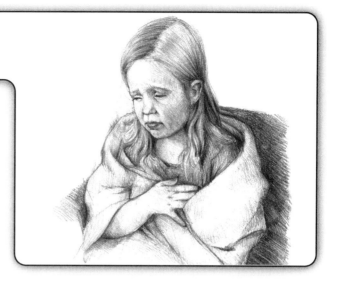

La gripe (influenza) es una enfermedad causada por un virus. La gripe afecta todo el cuerpo. No es lo mismo que la "gripe intestinal".

La época de gripe es más común en el invierno. Cada año la gripe es diferente. Esto sucede porque hay diferentes tipos de virus de la gripe y estos cambian con el tiempo. Las personas pueden sufrir de gripe muchas veces en su vida.

Señales de la gripe

La gripe puede durar una semana o más. Su niño se sentirá muy mal los primeros 2 ó 3 días. Los síntomas de la gripe incluyen:

- Fiebre que aparece de repente (arriba de 101°F ó 38.3°C).
- Escalofríos y temblores junto con la fiebre.
- Dolor de cabeza, dolor de cuerpo y mucho cansancio.
- Dolor de garganta y tos cortada o seca.
- Congestión y mucosidad nasal.
- Vómitos y heces aguadas (diarrea).

¿Cómo sé si es gripe o resfriado?

Tanto la gripe como los resfriados son causados por un virus. Los dos pueden tener algunos de los mismos síntomas. Pero son diferentes:

La gripe

- Los niños se enferman muy rápido, a veces en un día.
- Casi todos los niños se sienten muy enfermos y sienten dolor.
- Muchos niños tienen que quedarse en cama durante algunos días.
- La gripe es más común en el invierno.

El resfriado

- Casi todos los niños tienen fiebre baja o no les da fiebre.
- A los niños les da una tos ligera.
- Casi todo los niños con resfriado tienen energía para jugar y continuar con sus rutinas.
- Los resfriados se pueden dar en cualquier época del año.

Qué debe hacer contra la gripe

Llame al Doctor…

De inmediato—si su bebé tiene 2 meses o menos y tiene fiebre.

Dentro de las primeras 24 horas—si su niño es mayor de 1 año y muestra señales de tener gripe.

Puede ser que el doctor le recete una **medicina antiviral*** para la gripe. Pero esta sólo funciona si su niño toma la medicina en el primer o segundo día de la enfermedad.

En la mayoría de los casos no hay problemas serios con la gripe. Pero algunas veces su niño puede tener una infección de oídos, **sinusitis*** o **neumonía***.

✳ *Palabras que debe conocer*

acetaminofén: Es una medicina para el dolor y la fiebre. Tylenol es una marca de acetaminofén.

medicina antiviral: Es una medicina que puede combatir algunos virus de la gripe.

desinfectante: Es un limpiador que mata los gérmenes.

ibuprofeno: Es una medicina para el dolor y la fiebre. Advil y Motrin son marcas de ibuprofeno.

neumonía: Es una infección de los pulmones.

sinusitis: Es una infección en las cavidades dentro de la cabeza, detrás de la nariz.

sibilancias: Sonidos que se parecen a un silbido producido al respirar.

Continúa atrás

Llame al doctor si usted ve una de estas señales de gripe, sin importar que edad tenga el niño:

- Dificultad para respirar
- Tos que no desaparece después de una semana
- Dolor de oído
- Fiebre continua o que vuelve después de 3 ó 4 días
- Falta de mejoría después de algunos días

Otros consejos

Haga que su niño repose y tome bastantes líquidos para aliviarlo a sentirse mejor. También puede darle medicina para bajar la fiebre:

- Para un bebé de 6 meses o menos, dele **acetaminofén***.
- Para un niño de más de 6 meses, dele acetaminofén o **ibuprofeno***.

Ambas medicinas alivian la fiebre. Pero no son lo mismo. Asegúrese de tener el tipo de medicina correcto para la edad de su niño. Siga lo que indica la etiqueta.

Nunca le dé a su niño aspirina. La aspirina pone a su niño en riesgo de tener el síndrome de Reye. Esta es una enfermedad seria que afecta el hígado y el cerebro.

Pregunte al doctor de su niño antes de darle cualquier otra medicina. Esto incluye las medicinas para la tos y el resfriado de venta sin receta médica. Los antibióticos no ayudan contra la gripe.

No fume cerca de su niño. El humo causa más tos y **sibilancias*** en los niños. Y les dificulta que combatan la gripe.

Cómo prevenir la gripe

La gripe se contagia muy fácilmente, especialmente a los niños y adultos que pasan tiempo con niños. En la mayoría de casos la gripe se contagia durante los primeros días de la enfermedad.

Existen 3 formas de prevenir la gripe:

Tener buena higiene

Evitar que los gérmenes se rieguen es la mejor manera de evitar que la gripe se propague. Estos consejos le ayudarán a proteger a su familia contra la gripe:

1. Enséñele a su niño a cubrirse la boca y la nariz al toser o estornudar. También enséñele a utilizar un pañuelo o su manga, no la mano.
2. Use pañuelos de papel para limpiarse la nariz. Tírelos en la basura después de usarlos.
3. Evite besar a un niño enfermo en la boca o la cara.
4. Asegúrese de que todos se laven las manos con frecuencia.
5. Lave los platos, cucharas y tenedores en agua caliente con jabón o en la máquina de lavar platos.
6. No permita que los niños compartan chupetes, tazas, cucharas, tenedores, paños para lavarse o toallas. *Nunca* comparta el cepillo de dientes.
7. Utilice vasitos desechables en el baño y en la cocina. Tírelos después de usarlos.
8. Limpie los jaladores de las puertas, del inodoro, las superficies y hasta los juguetes. Use un **desinfectante*** o jabón y agua caliente.

Vacunas contra la gripe

Hay vacunas **seguras** para protegerse contra la gripe. Vienen en forma de inyecciones y rociadores nasales. Pregúntele al doctor qué es lo mejor para su niño. La mayoría de los niños sanos necesitan una vacuna contra la gripe cada otoño. Todos sus familiares deberían vacunarse también. Llame al doctor en septiembre para preguntarle.

Medicinas antivirales

Estos medicamentos se toman antes de que el niño esté expuesto a la gripe. Estas medicinas son muy importantes para los niños con problemas serios de salud cuando no se les puso una vacuna contra la gripe.

Para aprender más, visite el sitio de la Academia Americana de Pediatría (AAP) en www.aap.org.
Su pediatra le dirá qué es lo mejor para la salud de su hijo.
Esta información no debe usarse en lugar de consultar con su doctor.
Nota: Los nombres de marca son para su información solamente.
La AAP no recomienda ninguna marca o producto de medicina específicamente.
La adaptación de la información de este folleto de la AAP a lenguaje sencillo se hizo con el apoyo de McNeil Consumer Healthcare. La traducción al español fue patrocinada por Leyendo Juntos (Reach Out and Read), un programa pediátrico de alfabetización.

© 2008 Academia Americana de Pediatría

American Academy of Pediatrics

DEDICATED TO THE HEALTH OF ALL CHILDREN™

Constipation

Age Group: 1–18 years
Preventive: ✓
Acute:
Chronic: ✓

This section focuses on constipation, which is a common underlying reason children (particularly those who are toilet training) and teens visit the doctor. Parents might bring their children in for abdominal pain or petechiae only to learn that the child is suffering from constipation.

In fact, at least 3% of visits to pediatricians and 25% of visits to pediatric gastroenterologists are due to problems with constipation, according to the North American Society for Pediatric Gastroenterology, Hepatology and Nutrition.

Taking the time to make sure that parents understand the details of treatment for constipation, and the fact that constipation is typically a chronic condition, may improve adherence and increase parent and patient satisfaction. Early treatment of constipation may prevent long-term complications like encopresis, and may help stave off related self-esteem problems.

Common areas for miscommunication may include

- Diagnosis
- Symptoms
- Prevention and health promotion
- Management and treatment

Ask Me 3

During your patient encounter, you should communicate using plain language and health literacy principles so that by the end of the visit, the parent or child will know the answers to the *Ask Me 3* questions.

A Patient Story. . .

Sara is a 6-year-old who has hard, painful bowel movements every 3 to 4 days. Sara's mother states that Sara sometimes complains of abdominal pain but has not had any other symptoms.

The workup shows there is no underlying pathology with Sara, who is healthy and developing normally. She is a picky eater and refuses to eat vegetables. Her physical examination is normal except for palpable stool in the left lower quadrant of the abdomen.

Dr Clymer determines from the workup that Sara is suffering from chronic constipation. The doctor advises that Sara needs to eat more fiber, drink more water, and engage in more physical activity to clear up the constipation in a few weeks.

A month later, Sara is taken back to Dr Clymer because her abdominal pains have gotten worse.

. . . .

Sara's mother wasn't told which foods—aside from vegetables—contain fiber, and how to determine how much fiber a given food contains. She also didn't know how much fiber Sara needed. Additionally, she wasn't given any guidance on the amount of fluid Sara needed, and she wasn't given a definite timeline about when to expect Sara's constipation to clear up.

Patient: Tina, 7-year-old girl with constipation of several months' duration	
Ask Me 3 questions	What the parent should understand at the end of the visit
What is my child's main problem?	Tina has constipation, and it is going to take time for it to get better.
What do I need to do?	I need to give her more water to drink and at least 12 g of fiber in her food every day—like it says on the sheet the doctor gave me. I can feed her high-fiber foods, like the ones on the sheet the doctor gave me, or I can see how much fiber is in a food by looking at the label, like the doctor taught me.
Why is it important for me to do this?	More water and fiber will make her poop softer over time. That will make it easier to go to the bathroom, and she won't say it hurts.

Patient: Robert, 15-year-old boy	
Ask Me 3 questions	What the parent and patient should understand at the end of the visit
What is my child's main problem?	I have constipation, and it is going to take time for it to improve.
What do I need to do?	I need to take Miralax. Miralax is a powder, and I can use the cap of the bottle to measure how much to take. I also need to drink a lot of water and eat at least 20 g of fiber in my food every day—like the sheet says. I can eat high-fiber foods, like the ones on the sheet the doctor gave me, or I can see how much fiber is in a food by looking at the label, like the doctor taught me.
Why is it important for me to do this?	Eating more fiber and taking this medicine will help me have softer stools. It may not work right away, so I won't stop taking it until the doctor and I know the constipation has cleared up. Even after I stop taking the medicine, I need to keep eating a lot of fiber and drinking water. This will help make my stomach hurt less, and I won't be embarrassed when I go to the bathroom.

Medical Terms and Plain Language Alternatives

Many of the medical terms we use every day don't mean much to many parents. Below is a list of medical terms that may be confusing or difficult to explain and suggestions for plain language alternatives.

Medical Terms	Plain Language Alternatives
Anus	Bottom, butt, rear; where the poop comes out
Bowel movement	Stool, poop, BM, number 2, caca, poo-poo
Constipation	Stopped up; can't poop; poop that is so hard it causes pain in your belly or hurts when you go to the bathroom
Encopresis	When poop gets so hard and big that it can barely come out, and some watery poop leaks out around the hard parts

Fiber	Fiber comes from certain foods, including vegetables, fruits, and grains. It helps absorb water like a sponge, so your stool gets softer and easier to pass.
Intestine	Gut; the part of your body that food goes through after you eat it; the healthy parts of the food get absorbed into your body and the leftover parts get made into poop
Peristalsis	The way muscles squeeze to move food through your gut, like the way you squeeze toothpaste out of its tube
Rectum	Where your poop is before it comes out when you go to the bathroom

Confusing Terms and Concepts

In any condition, there are likely to be terms or concepts for which patients and families have a different understanding than a health care professional. These may include preventive strategies, complex disease processes, medication or treatment regimens, abstract laboratory results or measurements, technical terms, or words that have a different meaning in the health care arena than in everyday use. Cultural issues and misconceptions can also contribute to lack of understanding.

Consider the following when talking with parents about constipation:

Prevention and Health Promotion

Parents may not understand how bad experiences during toilet-training can lead to stool withholding. Advise parents to understand the problem the child is facing, and be patient while trying to help the child work through it and get back on track with toilet-training.

After a child has a bad experience with going to the bathroom—for example, the last time he went, it hurt when the poop came out—he may not want to go again, which may make him hold it in. But after he holds it in, the poop gets even bigger and more difficult to pass, and the problem starts all over again. This can also lead to setbacks in toilet-training.

Parents may not understand how establishing healthy dietary practices early can avoid problems with constipation.

- What the child eats and drinks (or doesn't eat and drink) is usually the cause of constipation.
- Eating too much of some foods and not enough of other foods can make the stool hard, and painful to pass.

Diagnosis

Parents might not know what causes constipation.

- What the child eats and drinks (or doesn't eat and drink) is usually the cause of constipation. Eating too much of some foods and not enough of other foods can make the stool hard, and painful to pass.

Tell the parent or patient what kinds of foods are best for the constipated child, including ethnic and cultural examples when you can. Give specific examples of high-fiber foods and a handout to take home.

Explain how to read food labels and give them the patient handout that tells how to calculate the amount of fiber a child needs every day.

Symptoms

Parents might not know what to look for when it comes to constipation.

- Sometimes it may look like the child is pushing and straining to poop, but he may really be holding it in because he is afraid that it will hurt.

- Standing on their toes, often in a corner, and rocking can be a sign that the child is trying to hold it in, which can lead to continued constipation.

Often when a parent is asked the number of times a child has had a bowel movement in a day, the parent's answer is based only on daylight hours. To make sure you're getting an accurate count, ask them for specific times when the child has pooped.

Parents may not recognize some symptoms of constipation. Ask about bowel movements that stop up the toilet, and their shape and consistency (eg, little, hard balls).

Patients and parents may be embarrassed to talk about bowel movements. Put them at ease by acknowledging that it can be difficult to talk about, but that they can't tell you much you haven't already heard. You might point out to the children (patients) that to help keep them from being embarrassed when they're with their friends, you have to know what's going on.

Management and Treatment

It is good for parents to understand constipation, and how foods and liquids work to prevent or manage the condition.

- Encopresis—while it may look like diarrhea, is a sign of bad constipation.

- Drinking water and eating high-fiber foods make stools (poop, BMs, bowel movements) softer and easier to pass.

- There is a cycle that comes from withholding: Hard stools can cause pain, which can lead to withholding the stool or "holding it in." Holding the stool in can cause constipation. It can also make the stool harder and larger and hurt more to pass, which can cause the child to keep holding it in. The big hard stools stretch the gut and that's what causes the pain.

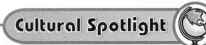

Constipation Among Latinos

Empacho is the belief among many Latino families that there is something "stuck" in the child's stomach or intestine. It may be gum, food, or paper (or any of the many things children put in their mouths).

The treatment for *Empacho* is giving oil to the child or taking him to a *Sobador* who will give him deep massages to help pass whatever is stuck.

When Latino children present with symptoms of constipation, it is possible that their parents think that they have *Empacho*, and the etiology and treatment of constipation and *Empacho* are basically the same: getting rid of the impacted fecal material.

Thus explaining that the poop "is stuck" in the intestines, and that we need to give the child a medicine that will help it come out, resonates with parents' existing beliefs, and it can help to increase understanding of the problem and adherence with therapy.

Mazanilla (Chamomile) tea is also commonly used by Latinos for abdominal pain, and may be what grandma has already told them to do. Mentioning tea as a possible liquid to give the child can be reassuring for the parents.

Parents and doctors may not have a shared understanding of what types of foods to give a child who is constipated. The usual food for a family might not be food that the physician would recommend. Explain what kinds of foods are best for the constipated child, and give specific examples and a handout to take home.

Be specific about how much fiber the child needs every day and how to find out how much fiber is in a food using the food label. Kids and parents may be surprised about how much fiber is needed to make a difference.

Allay parents' fears about using medication for this condition. These fears need to be addressed up front if the parents are to continue to give medications for long periods.

Explain that it took a long time for the child to get constipated and it will often take that long for them to get back to normal, which may mean taking medicine for a few weeks or even months. But, even if they have to take it for a long time, Miralax and some of the gentle, modern medications aren't ones the child can get "hooked on." And finally, explain that it can come back if they don't keep eating foods with a lot of fiber.

Cultural Beliefs

Families from different cultures may have their own ideas of what causes constipation and how to treat it. Their beliefs can result in confusion and lack of adherence to suggested management if they are not understood.

Ask parents what they think is causing the constipation, and what they think will make it better. This will increase your understanding of their culture while uncovering possible roadblocks or cultural issues with treatment before they arise.

Usually parents' or families' beliefs will pose no harm to the child, but some remedies are potentially toxic. Try to incorporate their beliefs into your treatment plan when they won't be harmful to the child.

Worsening Condition

Explain clearly how long it could take the constipation to improve, and when they should contact you if it doesn't get better. Avoid generalities such as "a few days," in favor of more specific time frames, even if they are a range (2 or 3 days).

Explain that if the child develops diarrhea or if the constipation hasn't eased in a definite number of days, they need to call you to have their medicine adjusted. If there is a possibility that a serious problem exists, be sure to give them 2 or 3 specific parameters that should make them call you back. Writing the parameters down for them would be wise.

Consider sending them home with a checklist or a chart they can use to keep track of the child's illness and progress—or lack of progress—noting how many times the child pees, how much the child is eating and drinking, what the child is eating and drinking, whether the child has produced any stool at all, what it looked like, and whether it was painful.

Be sure they know that encopresis—while it may look like diarrhea—is another sign of constipation, and that it may come back if they don't eat foods with a lot of fiber.

Behavior Change

Behavior change is a key element in preventing and managing many pediatric conditions, including constipation.

Shifting from paternalistic advice that is either too vague or too complicated to a patient- or family-centered approach that incorporates elements of motivational interviewing and goal-setting, and that makes use of plain language, may be an effective way to empower patients and families to make changes and improve their health.

The treatment of constipation, especially in older children, primarily requires changes in habits and routines, as well as dietary changes that may affect the whole family. The following are examples of motivational interviewing questions that can help you gauge how likely the parent and patient are to make the recommended changes.

- On a scale of 1 to 10, how convinced are you that you can give Adam more high-fiber foods?

- How confident are you that Caleb will take his medicine every morning when he gets up?
- How convinced are you that you can get Maggie to sit on the toilet each morning?

These can be applied for older children to involve them in making changes by asking them directly and including them in goal-setting.

- How confident are you that you can eat 2 bowls of bran-containing cereal every day?
- How will you get more fiber in the foods you eat every day?

Child Involvement

Including the child, to the extent possible, is respectful and patient-centered and can contribute to developing health literacy skills as the child moves toward managing his or her own health as an adolescent and an adult. It can include direct, age-appropriate statements to the child, and also ways for the child to be involved in his or her health.

Young Children

Between 4 and 6 years of age, children's language and cognitive skills are developed enough to begin to involve them in the discussion about constipation and the treatment plan. This includes discussions about diet changes, toilet habits, and incentive systems.

Simple messages for the child can include

- You need to eat more fruit so your poop won't be hard and it won't hurt so much when it comes out.
- Sit on the toilet every morning and try to poop. The more you do it, the easier it gets!
- This medicine helps so you don't have to push so hard to poop and it won't hurt.

School-aged Children

Schoolchildren should be able to take more responsibility for their dietary choices (especially when they are at school), and for remembering to take their medication. School-aged children can also learn to count and add up grams of fiber on food labels. However, constipation in older children is more often associated with behavior issues and encopresis.

Finding high-fiber foods that the child likes to eat will increase the chances that your recommendation will be followed. A handout for your patients, like the one shown on page 168, can be very helpful in demonstrating how many high-fiber foods they can choose from. More information on a wide variety of foods can be found online at http://www.nal.usda.gov/fnic/foodcomp/Data/SR20/nutrlist/sr20a291.pdf.

One effective way to encourage children to get involved in the process is through reward charts. Suggestions on developing reward charts can be found on page 107.

Adolescents

Reward calendars also work for older children, for whom ownership comes with being involved in designing the system: from setting the goals to determining the incentives or rewards.

Teach-back

The concept of teaching back entails asking parents or patients to demonstrate understanding *using their own words*, not simply asking whether they have questions or whether they understand, because that may not elicit lack of understanding. Having patients explain in their own words not only assesses their understanding, but it reinforces the information by repeating it and internalizes it for the patient. When there is a lot of information, go over each concept and elicit a teach-back before moving to the next idea.

When using teach-back, it's important to keep the burden on yourself. Avoid the perception that you are quizzing the parent or patient—emphasize that you want to be sure you've explained things clearly.

The practice of using teach-back can be especially important over the phone, because it may be the only way to gauge whether the parent or patient understands.

Here are some approaches to using teach-back when managing constipation.

- To make sure I explained things clearly, what are you going to do at home for Andrew's constipation?
- What will you tell Alicia's babysitter about the changes you need to make in what Alicia eats?
- How much and how often are you going to give the Miralax to Blakeley?

Key Messages for Use by All Members of the Health Care Team

It is important to reinforce key messages for parents and children so they hear them more than once and recognize them as priorities in managing their health. In addition, families should not receive conflicting advice about their health and what to do. For constipation, staff should reinforce these basic concepts.

- Constipation can take a long time to get better.
- The longer your child has had constipation, the longer it will take for him/her to get better. It's something that can come back, so you will probably need to do some of these things for a long time.
- Keep giving your child the medicine until your doctor tells you to stop, even if he/she is better.
- Fruits and vegetables are healthy for you. Keep eating them, even if you are not constipated anymore.
- Drink a lot of water every day to keep stools soft.
- We may need to make changes to the plan, so be sure to come back or call the office like we discussed.
- Remember, your child needs a certain amount of fiber every day. You can figure out how much by taking your child's age and adding 5 to it. Age + 5 = the grams of fiber the child needs every day. Use food labels to find out how much fiber is in foods.
- Use the nutrition facts label to find foods that have 3 or more grams of fiber per serving. Because people often use 2 slices of bread to make a sandwich, it may take 2 slices to get 3 grams of fiber.

Miscellaneous

Make sure that you talk with parents thoroughly enough to determine whether the child has encopresis. Like other toileting issues, not all parents will bring it up on their own, so you must put them at ease and draw accurate information from them. It's imperative for your diagnosis and treatment.

Find plain language about encopresis in the "Constipation" handout on page 169.

Sample handout

Have fun with fiber!

The following are a few examples of high-fiber foods from different areas of the world. Have fun discovering more!

Mexican/Mexican-American

beans	burritos
corn tortillas	chili
jicama	guava
mango	

Chinese/Asian

stir-fried vegetables

Puerto Rican

yucca	rice and beans
tostones	

Middle Eastern

figs	tabouli
chick peas	babaganouche

Eastern European

sauerkraut	rye bread
potatoes	pirogues

Other high-fiber foods that can be part of or added to any cuisine

artichokes	oatmeal	raisin bran	
oatmeal-raisin cookies			
peanuts	bran muffins	fig cookies	brown rice
celery	broccoli	barley	almonds
pears	apples	green peas	split peas
soy	lentils	prunes	uncooked vegetables
hazelnuts	raisins	potatoes and sweet potatoes (with skin)	
dried fruits	popcorn	kidney, black, navy, and pinto beans	
oranges	berries	whole-grain cereals and breads	

Use food labels to find out how much fiber is in each food item. Or, for fiber information on hundreds of foods, visit http://www.nal.usda.gov/fnic/foodcomp/Data/SR20/nutrlist/sr20a291.pdf.

Formula for success

Every child needs to eat a certain amount of fiber every day. You can figure out how much your child needs by taking the child's age and adding 5 to it.

Age + 5 = the grams of fiber your child needs every day

Constipation

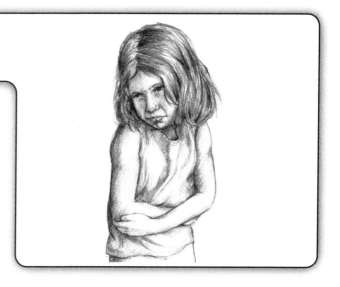

Constipation (kahn-sti-PAY-shun) is common. Children with constipation have stools (poops) that are hard, dry, and difficult or painful to get out. Constipation can be treated.

You may worry your child is constipated if he or she doesn't have a **bowel movement*** (BM) every day. But every child is different. Most children have BMs 1 or 2 times a day. Others may go 2 to 3 days or longer between BMs.

Signs of Constipation

- Hard or painful stools
- Many days between bowel movements
- Bleeding from the child's bottom where stool comes out
- Stomachaches, cramping, **nausea***
- Brownish wet spots in the underwear (See "What Is Encopresis?" on the second page of this handout.)

Your Child May Also:

- Have BMs that stop up the toilet.
- Make faces like he or she is in pain.
- Clench his or her bottom. It may look like your child is trying to push the stool out. But he or she is really trying to hold it in, because it hurts to come out.

Call the Doctor If...

- Your child doesn't have a BM at least every 2 to 3 days.
- Passing a stool hurts your child.

What to Do for Constipation

Treatment is based on your child's age and how bad the problem is. Usually no special tests are needed.

Constipation can get worse if it isn't treated. The longer stool stays inside the body, the larger and drier it gets. Then it hurts to pass it. This starts a cycle. The child becomes afraid to have a BM, and holds it in even more.

For Babies

Constipation is rarely a problem in babies. It may become a problem when starting solid foods. Your child's doctor may suggest you give more water or juice. Pear juice and prune juice work well. Talk with the doctor before giving extra water to your baby.

For Children and Teens

Children and teens who are constipated often aren't getting enough high-fiber foods and water. Your child's doctor may suggest adding more high-fiber foods to your child's diet and drinking more water.

For Very Bad Constipation

Your child's doctor may prescribe medicine to soften or remove the stool. Never give your child **laxatives*** or **enemas*** unless you check with the doctor. These drugs can be dangerous to children if used wrong.

❋ Words to Know

bowel movement—when stool passes out of your child's body. Also called a "BM."

diarrhea (dye-uh-REE-yuh)—passing loose, watery stools.

enema (EN-uh-muh)—a liquid put into a person's bottom to make him or her pass stool.

laxative (LAX-uh-tiv)—a medicine to make stools softer.

nausea (NAW-zha)—feeling like throwing up.

rectum—the last several inches of the large intestine, where stool is stored before passing out of the body.

Continued on back

What Causes Constipation?

What your child eats and *doesn't* eat.
Not getting enough fiber or liquid can make your child constipated.

Holding back, or "withholding," stool.
Your child may not want to have a BM for different reasons:

- Your child may try not to go because it hurts to pass a hard stool. (Diaper rashes can make this worse.)
- Children aged 2 to 5 years may want to show they can decide things for themselves. Holding back their stools may be their way of taking control. This is why it is best not to push children into toilet-training.
- Sometimes children don't want to stop playing to go to the bathroom.
- Older children may hold back their stools when away from home (like camp or school). They may be afraid of or not like using public toilets.

How to Prevent Constipation

- Encourage your child to drink lots of water and eat more high-fiber foods.
- Hold off on toilet-training until your child shows interest.
- Help your child set a toilet routine. Pick a regular time to remind your child to sit on the toilet daily (like after breakfast.) Put something under your child's feet to press on. This makes it easier to push BMs out.
- Encourage your child to play and be active.

What Is Encopresis?

Sometimes a child with bad constipation has BMs that look like **diarrhea***. When a child holds back stools, the stools build up and get bigger. They may get so big that the **rectum*** stretches. Then the child may not feel the urge to go to the bathroom. The stool gets too big to pass without an enema, laxative, or other treatment.

Sometimes only liquid stool can come out, and leaks onto the underwear.

This is called encopresis (en-koh-PREE-sis). Talk with your child's doctor about treatment. It can get better, but it takes months.

Getting Enough Fiber

How Much Fiber Does My Child Need?

Here is an easy way to figure how much fiber your child needs each day. Start with 5 grams. Then add your child's age. The answer is the number of grams your child needs each day.

$$ \_\_\_\_\text{years old} + 5 = \_\_\_\_ $$

Child's Age		Grams of Fiber Your Child Needs Each Day
Your Child's Age	Grams of Fiber	Grams of Fiber Each Day
2	+5	= 7
5	+5	= 10
13	+5	= 18

Read Food Labels

Check for **"Dietary Fiber"** on the *Nutrition Facts* label. Look for foods with at least 2 grams of fiber per serving.

This food has 3 grams of fiber per serving.

Nutrition Facts
Serving Size ½ cup (114g)
Servings Per Container 4

Amount Per Serving

Calories 90   Calories from Fat 30

	% Daily Value*
Total Fat 3g	5%
Saturated Fat 0g	0%
Cholesterol 0mg	0%
Sodium 300mg	13%
Total Carbohydrate 13g	4%
Dietary Fiber 3g	12%
Sugars 3g	
Protein 3g	

Source: US Food and Drug Administration

Some foods are high in fiber. Try beans, vegetables, fruits, and whole grains.

To learn more, visit the American Academy of Pediatrics (AAP) Web site at www.aap.org.

Your child's doctor will tell you to do what's best for your child.
This information should not take the place of talking with your child's doctor.

Adaptation of the AAP information in this handout into plain language was supported in part by McNeil Consumer Healthcare.

© 2008 American Academy of Pediatrics

American Academy of Pediatrics
DEDICATED TO THE HEALTH OF ALL CHILDREN™

Estreñimiento (Constipation)

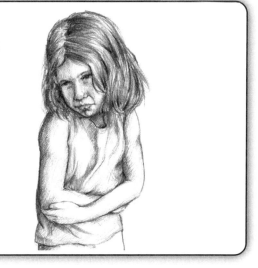

El estreñimiento es un problema común. El niño con estreñimiento puede recibir tratamiento.

Las **evacuaciones*** en los niños son variables. Cada niño es diferente. La mayoría de los niños hacen pupú una o dos veces al día. Pero algunos niños pueden llevar tres días o más sin poder hacer pupú. Esto no significa que estén estriñidos.

Señales de estreñimiento en el niño

- Las heces son duras o salen con dolor.
- Pasan muchos días entre cada evacuación.
- Le sangra el ano o el recto.
- Le da dolores de estómago, cólicos, **náusea***.
- Mancha su ropa interior con pupú. (Vea "¿Qué es la encopresis?" en la segunda página de este folleto).

Puede ser que su niño también:

- Haga evacuaciones que tapen el baño.
- Parezca sentir dolor.
- Parezca que está tratando de empujar el pupú hacia afuera, pero realmente está tratando de aguantarse, porque le duele hacer pupú.

Llame al doctor si…

- Su niño no hace al menos una evacuación cada dos o tres días.
- Le duele hacer pupú.

Cómo aliviar el estreñimiento

El tratamiento depende de la edad de su niño y que tan serio sea el problema. Normalmente no se necesitan pruebas o exámenes especiales.

El estreñimiento puede empeorar si no es tratado. Cuanto más se aguanta el niño, más duro, seco y doloroso se pone el pupú.

Esto inicia un círculo vicioso. Como al niño le da miedo que le va a doler al evacuar, se aguanta más tiempo.

El estreñimiento en los bebés

El estreñimiento no es común en los bebés hasta que empiezan a comer alimentos sólidos. Si su bebé está estreñido su doctor puede sugerir que le dé más agua o jugo. El jugo de pera y el de ciruela funcionan bien. Puede ser que el doctor también le sugiera que le dé más alimentos con fibra.

El estreñimiento en los niños y adolescentes

La causa más común del estreñimiento en los niños y adolescentes es la falta de suficiente fibra o agua en la dieta. Generalmente el estreñimiento mejora con tan solo cambiar la dieta. Agréguele más agua y fibra a la dieta de su niño.

Qué hacer para el estreñimiento severo

Puede ser que el doctor le recete a su niño medicina para suavizar o aflojar las heces. Nunca le dé **laxantes*** ni le ponga **enemas***, a menos que lo consulte con su doctor. Estos tratamientos pueden ser peligrosos en los niños si se usan mal.

Las causas comunes del estreñimiento:

Tal vez su niño no quiera evacuar por diversas razones:

- Puede ser que su niño no quiera ir al baño porque le duele hacer pupú. (La irritación causada por el pañal empeora el dolor).

✳ Palabras que debe conocer

evacuación: Cuando el pupú sale del cuerpo de su hijo.

diarrea: Hacer pupú suelto y aguado.

enema: Un líquido que se coloca dentro del ano de una persona para hacer que salgan las heces.

laxante: Una medicina que ayuda a suavizar las heces.

náusea: Sentir ganas de vomitar.

recto: Las últimas pulgadas del intestino grueso, donde se almacenan las heces antes de sacarlas del cuerpo.

Continúa atrás

- Muchos niños entre dos y cinco años quieren demostrar que ellos pueden decidir cuándo ir al baño. Una manera de tomar el control es reteniendo las heces.
  Por esta razón, es mejor no presionar a los niños para que aprendan a usar el inodoro.
- A veces los niños no quieren dejar de jugar para ir al baño.
- Los niños mayores pueden retener el pupú cuando están lejos de casa (como en el campamento o en la escuela). Puede ser que no les gusten o que tengan temor a los baños públicos.

Cómo prevenir el estreñimiento

- Motive a su niño a tomar mucha agua y a comer más alimentos con mucha fibra.
- Espere a enseñarle a usar el inodoro hasta que muestre interés.
- Ayude a su niño a que tenga una rutina para ir al baño. Elija una hora regular para recordarle que debe sentarse en el inodoro todos los días (como, después del desayuno). Coloque algo debajo de los pies de su niño para que pueda hacer fuerza más fácilmente.
- Motive a su niño a que juegue y sea activo.

¿Qué es la encopresis?

A veces cuando el estreñimiento es serio parece que el niño tiene **diarrea***. Lo que pasa es que a medida que el excremento se acumula, el recto se va estirando. El niño pierde la sensación y ya no siente la necesidad de ir al baño. El excremento se vuelve tan grande que no se puede evacuar sin un enema, laxante u otro tratamiento. En este caso sólo las heces líquidas pueden pasar y gotear manchando la ropa interior.

A esto se le llama encopresis. Consulte con su doctor acerca del tratamiento. Puede mejorar, pero en lo general tarda varios meses.

Cómo obtener suficiente fibra

¿Cuánta fibra necesita mi hijo?

Aquí le damos una manera fácil de saber cuánta fibra necesita su niño cada día. Empiece con cinco gramos. Luego, agréguele a ese número la edad de su niño. La respuesta es el número de gramos de fibra que su niño necesita cada día

Años de edad + 5 =

Edad del niño		Gramos de fibra que su niño necesita cada día
La edad de su niño	Gramos de fibra	Gramos de fibra cada día
2	+5	= 7
5	+5	= 10
13	+5	= 18

Lea las etiquetas de los alimentos

Verifique la "fibra dietética" en la etiqueta de **Información nutricional**. Busque alimentos que tengan al menos dos gramos de fibra por por porción.

Por ejemplo, este alimento tiene tres gramos de fibra por porción.

Nutrition Facts

Serving Size ½ cup (114g)
Servings Per Container 4

Amount Per Serving

Calories 90   Calories from Fat 30

	% Daily Value*
Total Fat 3g	5%
Saturated Fat 0g	0%
Cholesterol 0mg	0%
Sodium 300mg	13%
Total Carbohydrate 13g	4%
Dietary Fiber 3g	12%
Sugars 3g	
Protein 3g	

Fuente: US Food and Drug Administration

Pruebe los frijoles (habichuelas), los vegetales, las frutas y los granos. Su doctor le puede dar más sugerencias de alimentos con alto contenido en fibra.

Para aprender más, visite el sitio de la Academia Americana de Pediatría (AAP) en www.aap.org. Su pediatra le dirá qué es lo mejor para la salud de su hijo.
Esta información no debe usarse en lugar de consultar con su doctor.
La adaptación de la información de este folleto de la AAP a lenguaje sencillo se hizo con el apoyo de McNeil Consumer Healthcare. La traducción al español fue patrocinada por Leyendo Juntos (Reach Out and Read), un programa pediátrico de alfabetización.

American Academy of Pediatrics
DEDICATED TO THE HEALTH OF ALL CHILDREN™

Croup
Laryngotracheobronchitis

Croup is a common condition that afflicts tens of thousands of children every year. These are children who—because of age or a host of other factors—respond to a respiratory viral infection by developing the characteristic barking, middle-of-the-night cough that often frightens parents. Partly because of this middle-of-the-night pattern of exacerbation, croup causes many calls to physician coverage networks and answering services, and many emergency department visits. Each contact between physician and parent or patient is an opportunity for miscommunication, which can lead to prolonged or increasingly severe symptoms and ailments, or alternatively, to unnecessary return emergency department visits if parents don't understand the nature and course of the illness, or don't feel able to assess the child's condition. The challenge of assessing the child's respiratory function over the phone is just one reason that clear patient-doctor communication matters so much.

By the same token, you can enjoy practice-related benefits when communicating clearly about this condition. For example, parental anxiety will be decreased as parents' understanding of the course of the disease and the limitations of cough suppressants improves. Additionally, if parents are better able to understand and communicate the character of the child's cough and respirations, the child may be able to get a dose of steroids at the medical visit, reducing the duration of the illness and need for emergency department visits and hospitalizations.

A Patient Story. . .

Annette Morgan has brought her 14-month-old daughter, Molly, to see Dr Alexander because the child has a fever of 101°F and a runny nose, and she isn't drinking her bottle as eagerly as usual. The doctor asks about Molly's breathing, and Mrs Morgan says it's "heavy," and that she has a harsh cough.

On examination, Molly is congested but well-hydrated, and not coughing. The pediatrician suggests that Molly's mother make sure Molly keeps drinking, and recommends a dose of antipyretic medication.

When Mrs Morgan asks about "something for her cough," Dr Alexander tells her that cough medicines are not recommended for children this age; when she asks about getting an antibiotic, the pediatrician tells her that an antibiotic would not be indicated for a viral infection.

That evening, Molly's cough becomes more and more dramatic, and finally, late at night, her mother calls Dr Alexander's office.

This time, Dr Alexander can hear the classic barking cough of croup in the background and attempts to establish whether the child is in respiratory distress. He asks if Molly is pulling in with her chest muscles, and if Mrs Morgan can hear any high-pitched noises. But Mrs Morgan just keeps repeating, frantically, that she has already given the child 2 doses of cough medicine, along with some amoxicillin left over from her last ear infection, and it didn't help at all.

Finally, Dr Alexander tells Mrs Morgan to take Molly to the emergency department.

· ·

The office visit was a missed opportunity to show Mrs Morgan how to watch for retractions, or for unusually fast respirations, or how to listen for stridor.

It would also have helped her to know what the characteristic cough of croup sounds like, and to understand that it often gets worse at night. If she had been able to convey the quality of Molly's

(continued)

(continued from previous page)

cough the night before, the pediatrician might have decided to give the child a single dose of steroids.

Furthermore, Mrs Morgan didn't really understand the pediatrician's response that antibiotics are "not indicated," and that cough medicines are "not recommended" for children Molly's age, and was perhaps frustrated that the doctor would prescribe neither. She certainly didn't understand that cough medications can actually be dangerous.

The critical variables in assessing croup have to do with describing the degree of respiratory distress and the quality of the child's breathing; parents and physicians may have completely different vocabularies for all of these parameters, which can make it very difficult to assess a child by history or over the telephone. The new recommendations against using over-the-counter cough medications in young children make it particularly essential to spend time with parents discussing how to assess and treat coughs, upper respiratory infections, and their more serious manifestations.

Common areas for miscommunication may include

- Diagnosis
- Prevention and health promotion
- Management and treatment
- Worsening condition

Ask Me 3

During your patient encounter, you should communicate using plain language and health literacy principles so that by the end of the visit, the parent or child will know the answers to the *Ask Me 3* questions.

Patient: Noah, a 3-year-old with croup	
Ask Me 3 questions	**What the parent should understand at the end of the visit**
What is my child's main problem?	My son has croup, a bad cough from an infection that makes his voice box and windpipe swollen inside.

What do I need to do?	• I need to watch him carefully to make sure he keeps drinking.
	• If he gets worse tonight, I may need to make him more comfortable by taking him outside so he can breathe the cold night air, or sitting with him in the bathroom with a hot shower running so that the bathroom gets steamy. (I will not put him in the water.)
	• I should try to keep him calm by holding him and comforting him.
	• ***I will call the doctor if he is having trouble breathing.***
	  • If he seems to be fighting to breathe
	  • If he's breathing fast
	  • If his muscles pull in every time he breathes
	  • If he can't talk or cry because he's working too hard to breathe
	  • If there's a whistling sound when he breathes in
	  • If he's turning blue around the mouth

Why is it important for me to do this?	Doing these things should help him breathe easier. But sometimes, little children can have bad trouble breathing even when they just have a cold or a cough. So I need to watch for this. If he needs extra help, there are medicines and treatments they can only get in the emergency department, which can help him get better.

Medical Terms and Plain Language Alternatives

Many of the medical terms we use every day don't mean much to many parents. Below is a list of medical terms that may be confusing or difficult to explain and suggestions for plain language alternatives.

Medical Terms	Plain Language Alternatives
Antibiotics	Medicine to get rid of the germs, called "bacteria," that cause infections. Antibiotics don't work against viruses.
Croupy cough	A loud cough that sounds like a seal barking
Cyanosis	Blue color of the tongue, lips, or body
Humidifier	Steam machine
Hypoxia	Low oxygen or air in the body
Inhale/exhale	Breathe in/breathe out
Larynx	Voice box
Mucus, sputum	Snot; phlegm; the slimy liquid that coats the inside of the nose and throat
Nebulizer	A machine that turns medicine or water into a mist that the child breathes in
Oxygen	Air
Respiratory distress	Serious trouble breathing, like • Fighting to breathe • Breathing fast • Muscles around the ribs pull in every time he breathes • A whistling sound • Turning blue around the mouth
Saliva	Spit; the watery liquid in the mouth
Steroids	A medicine that can be a pill, liquid, spray or shot; it helps croup by making the swelling in the child's windpipe get better.
Stridor	A high whistling sound every time the child breathes in
Tachypnea	Breathing a lot faster than usual
Trachea	Windpipe; airway
Virus	A germ that makes you sick; antibiotics don't usually work for viruses.
Wheeze	A whistling sound the lungs make when breathing

Confusing Terms and Concepts

With any condition, there are likely to be terms or concepts for which patients and families have a different understanding than a health care professional. These may include preventive strategies, complex disease processes, medication or treatment regimens, abstract laboratory results or measurements, technical terms, or words that have a different meaning in the health care arena than in everyday use. Cultural issues and misconceptions can also contribute to lack of understanding.

Consider the following when talking with parents about croup:

Prevention and Health Promotion

Hand-washing by all members of the family can help stop the spread of infections like croup.

Parents can prevent a more serious illness that also causes a barking cough and difficulty breathing. It is called "acute epiglottitis," and its symptoms are a lot like croup, but much worse. The good news is that the Hib vaccine can protect against this illness. Your child should get the first dose of Hib at 2 months old.

Diagnosis

Parents might not know the basics about croup. While you don't need to go into the physiology (nor should you, unless they ask, because it may confuse matters), you can explain a few simple facts about the illness.

- Croup is like a cold, but worse.
- Croup is caused by the same kind of germ that causes colds, and these germs do not get better with antibiotics. (The same germ that causes a regular cold in an older child or an adult can cause croup in a baby or a toddler.)
- Croup affects the voice box and windpipe, and causes swelling inside the child's throat where you can't see. Because the child's windpipe is so small, that swelling can make it hard for the child to breathe.
- Avoid generalities such as "a few days" when you can. Tell them how many days the cough should last—even if it's a range (2 or 3 days)—and any other symptoms they should expect. Also explain that as long as the frequency of coughing is decreasing and there are no other symptoms, the child is getting better.
- Make sure parents understand that croup is very common and, while the coughing sounds awful, it isn't usually serious. What matters most of all is how the child is breathing. Also, explain clearly the signs that may indicate a more serious illness (ie, acute epiglottitis, pneumonia, tracheitis) or a worsening condition (see page 177), in which the child's airway is even more swollen.
- Even though croup isn't usually serious, you should explain that any breathing problems can be serious in young children because their breathing tubes are so small.

- We have to watch them very carefully, especially if they were born too early, or if they have had croup or any other breathing problems before.
- Clarify the difference between upper airway congestion and noisy breathing (and how to help it with a bulb syringe and saline nose drops), and trouble breathing because of swelling or congestion farther in the child's airway (throat, windpipe, or lungs) that needs more treatment.

Symptoms

Help parents characterize the "barking" cough by asking if it sounds like a dog or a seal barking. One effective technique, if your vocal skills are equal to it, is to imitate the barking cough.

- Characterizing the level of respiratory distress is probably the most important examination room discussion you can have with parents of a child with croup. Show parents where the muscles suck in when the child has trouble breathing, and explain that they should call you or 911 if the child is

  - Breathing really fast
  - Sucking in his muscles [right here] when he takes a breath
  - Making a whistling or squeaking sound when he takes a breath
  - Breathing so hard that he can't drink his bottle and breathe at the same time
  - Having so much trouble breathing that he can't talk or cry
  - Drooling a lot more than usual, or if he looks like he has trouble swallowing
  - Fighting to breathe
  - Turning blue around the mouth

Management and Treatment

Many parents may focus on the need for cough suppression; cough suppressants have never been useful for croup and, given the young age of most children with the illness, and the recent recommendations against over-the-counter (OTC) cough medications for young children, it's especially important to explain to parents why suppressing the cough is not a goal of treatment.

- Talk with parents explicitly about not using cough medicines.
  - Cough medicine can actually make things worse because it may stop the child from coughing up mucus that needs to come out.

- The cough and cold medicines that you buy in the drugstore without a prescription can be dangerous for young children and should not be used.
- If single-dose steroids are to be given, explain what they are and how they work.
  - This medicine is called "dexamethasone"; it's a kind of steroid. I'd like to give her one dose of it to swallow [or in a shot] because that may help her get better quickly—usually within 6 hours.
  - If she doesn't get better after she takes the medicine, we'll have you take her to the hospital because she may need to have an x-ray and get some other medicines, and even stay in the hospital for a little while.
- Make sure to review the normal course of croup so that parents know what to expect.
  - Croup usually gets better in the daytime, but it can get worse again at night, and this can go on for another 2 or 3 nights.
  - Children with croup may continue to have runny noses and fever, in addition to the cough.
- Emphasize what parents can do at home to make the child more comfortable and help him or her breathe.
  - Give your baby a lot of liquid to drink, even if he only wants to take a little at a time. More liquids will make him more comfortable and keep his body from drying out.
  - Comfort him and help him stay calm—crying can make things worse. So hold him and sing to him and comfort him.
  - Some children are more comfortable if their heads are up higher, so try holding him in a sitting-up position; you can also try letting him sit in his car seat to see if he likes that.
  - Some children get better if you take them outside in the cool air for a while.
  - Some children seem to breathe better if the air has more moisture in it, so you might want to try a humidifier in the room. Cool-mist humidifiers are safer because the ones that make hot steam can burn a child.
  - Another way to get the baby to breathe in moisture is to take her in the bathroom and turn on the shower with hot water so the air gets steamy. Don't sit her in the shower, but hold her on your lap, and see if the steam in the air helps her breathe.

- You do need to watch the child closely and see if his breathing gets any worse. Consider sleeping in the same room so you can check for all the breathing problems we talked about.

Cultural Beliefs

Families from different cultures may have their own ideas of what causes the symptoms of cough and noisy breathing, and what the best treatments are. Extended family members may play an important role in decision-making and management, and may urge either OTC medications or traditional remedies. This can result in confusion or lack of adherence to suggested management.

Explore potential cultural ideas by asking the parent what they think is causing the condition and what they think will make it better. This will increase your understanding of their culture while uncovering possible roadblocks or cultural issues with treatment before they arise.

Usually the parents' or families' beliefs will pose no harm to the child. Try to incorporate their beliefs into your treatment plan.

Worsening Condition

Parents may not fully understand how dangerous respiratory symptoms can be in a young child; they may not understand, for example, that when croup gets very severe, the child may cough less, rather than more, and that a child whose respiration efforts appear to be decreasing may be more severely ill.

In addition to reviewing the signs of respiratory distress, as above, reiterate to parents

- Breathing problems can be very serious in small children because their breathing tubes are so small to begin with, so if you think he is getting worse, please call and tell me right away. If you think his breathing is much worse, call 911 and go to the emergency department.

- If he looks like he's getting tired from breathing so hard, if he seems much less active than usual, or if he seems very anxious— like it's hard for him to get enough air—or if his color changes so he looks at all blue, call 911 right away.

Behavior Change

Behavior change is a key element in preventing and managing many pediatric conditions. Shifting from paternalistic advice that is either too vague or too complicated to a patient- or family-centered approach that incorporates elements of motivational interviewing and goal-setting, and that makes use of plain language, can be an effective way to empower patients and families to make changes and improve their health.

Urge families to get the Hib vaccine for their young children to protect them from more serious diseases, including meningitis and epiglottitis.

And explain how important it is for everyone in the family to keep their hands clean, especially before and after diaper changing or going to the bathroom, and before preparing food or eating. Stress the importance of hand-washing in terms of making sure the rest of the family doesn't get sick too—not just with croup, but with many common and potentially serious illnesses.

Child Involvement

Including the child, to the extent possible, is respectful and patient-centered and can contribute to developing health literacy skills as the child moves toward managing his or her own health as an adolescent and an adult. It can include direct, age-appropriate statements to the child, and also ways for the child to be involved in his or her health.

It is important to engage children in assisting with their care as they are able, but because children who get croup are usually very young and feeling very sick, there are limited ways to involve them in their care. However, croup is one of the illnesses that can be avoided with frequent hand-washing.

For example, even children younger than 2 years can be taught how to wash their hands with help. Older children can easily be given the responsibility of washing their hands too. As children become preschool age, they may be encouraged to wash their hands often and, when they're sick, to rest or drink fluids as they are able.

Involvement of children during an acute episode of croup mostly involves keeping them calm and reassured. Parents should make sure to remain calm and communicate what they are doing, such as

- Melissa, Mommy is going to take you into the bathroom and sit with you to see if turning the shower on in the room will make you feel better.
- Demetrius, Mommy will hold you and sing to you and maybe that will help you feel better.

Teach-back

The concept of teaching back entails asking parents or patients to demonstrate understanding *using their own words*, not simply asking whether they have questions or whether they understand, because that may not elicit lack of understanding. Having patients explain in their own words not only assesses their understanding, but it reinforces the information by repeating it and internalizes it for the patient. When there is a lot of information, go over each concept and elicit a teach-back before moving to the next idea.

When using teach-back, it's important to keep the burden on yourself. Avoid the perception that you are quizzing the parent or patient—emphasize that you want to be sure you've explained things clearly. The practice of using teach-back can be especially important over the phone, because it may be the only way to gauge whether the parent or patient understands fully.

Here are some approaches to using teach-back when talking about croup.

- I want to make sure I was clear when I explained this to you. When you're watching Jasmine tonight, what kind of breathing would make you call us?
- What are some things you can do to make Evan more comfortable tonight?
- What are you going to tell Julian's grandmother about cough medicine?
- What would make you call 911 for an ambulance?

Key Messages for Use by All Members of the Health Care Team

It is important to reinforce key messages for parents and children so they hear them more than once and recognize them as priorities in managing their health. In addition, families should not receive conflicting advice about their health and what to do.

Key concepts for croup are

- Croup is caused by a virus and does not need cough medicine or antibiotics, but one dose of steroids sometimes helps children get better faster.
- Croup gets better in the daytime and worse at night, so we need you to help us understand how the child was coughing and breathing last night.

- It's important for children with croup to keep drinking liquids and not get dried out.
- Sometimes cool air helps children breathe, and sometimes steam can help.
- Watch your child carefully tonight to see if he is having difficulty breathing.
- If you are ever really worried about your child's breathing, call us or call 911.
- Some children get worse, even after getting the steroid medicine. If that happens, your child may need to go to the emergency department to get some other medicines. He may even need to spend some time in the hospital, just to keep him safe, because breathing problems can be so serious in babies and small children.

Miscellaneous

Some health information is complicated but important to explain to parents. For example, when a child has croup, some parents might want to know where the child got the infection, or what physiologic process causes the stridor, or whether it will lead to asthma. You can always explain more to parents if they are asking questions or you can ask them if there are other questions that they have. But it is essential that all parents leave the office with the basic key concepts as noted above, and with a clear understanding of the importance of the child's respiratory status and how to assess it and describe it.

References

1. DeFrances CJ, Hall MJ. *2005 National Hospital Discharge Survey. Advance Data From Vital and Health Statistics.* No. 385. Hyattsville, MD: US Department of Health and Human Services, CDC, National Center for Health Statistics; 2007:15. http://www.cdc.gov/nchs/data/ad/ad385.pdf. Accessed April 7, 2008
2. Cherry JD. Croup. *N Engl J Med.* 2008;358:384–391

Croup

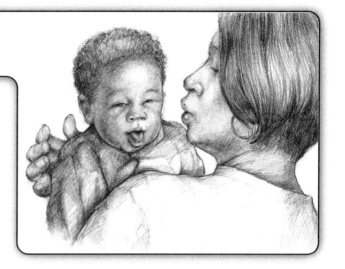

Croup is an infection that makes the inside of your child's throat swell up. This makes it hard for your child to breathe. It can be scary for both parents and children.

Croup is common in young children. Most cases of croup are mild. But croup can get worse and stop your child from breathing at all. Call the doctor if you think your child has croup and he or she is having a hard time breathing.

Croup is usually caused by a virus that infects the voice box and windpipe. The main sign of croup is a barking cough. It may start with a cold. Most children with viral croup have a low fever. But some have temperatures up to 104°F or 40°C.

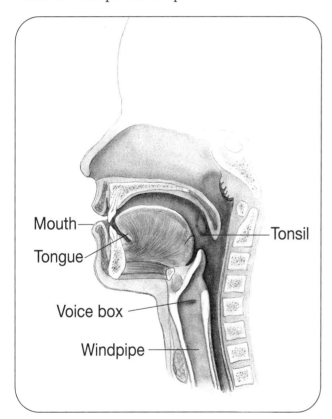

Mouth
Tongue
Tonsil
Voice box
Windpipe

Signs of Croup

Here are some signs your child may have croup:

- Barking cough
- Noisy or troubled breathing
- Hoarse voice
- Gasping for breath

What to Do for Croup

Call 911 or an Ambulance Right Away If…

…your child:

- Can't speak for lack of breath.
- Seems to be struggling to get a breath.
- Makes a whistling sound when breathing in. (This is called **stridor***.)
- Drools much more than usual or has a very hard time swallowing **saliva***.
- Has a bluish mouth or fingernails.

The above are all signs of severe croup. They may also be signs of other serious problems. Either way, if your child is having trouble breathing, you need to get him or her to the hospital.

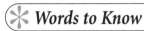 **Words to Know**

saliva (suh-LYE-vuh)—the watery liquid in your mouth.

steroids (STAIR-oydz)—a medicine that is a pill, liquid, spray you breathe in, or shot to help stop croup. It cuts down inflammation.

stridor (STRYE-dur)—a high whistling sound when your child breathes in. It is caused by something blocking the throat or voice box.

Continued on back

Call the Doctor If…

…either of these is true:

- Your child is a baby 1 year or younger.
- The cough keeps getting worse.

Try Home Treatment

Croup may wake your child up in the middle of the night. If your child is not having trouble breathing, try these home treatments.

- Steam up the bathroom by running hot water in the shower. Take your child in the bathroom to breathe the moist air for 15 or 20 minutes. Steam works for many children.
- If steam does not work, bundle your child up and go outdoors for a few minutes. The cool night air may help your child breathe more freely.
- Use a cool-mist humidifier (hyoo-MID-uh-fye-ur) in your child's room for the rest of the night. Turn it on for the next 2 to 3 nights too.

Medicines for Croup

The doctor may prescribe **steroids***. Steroids help bring down the swelling in the throat.

Antibiotics don't help because croup is almost always caused by a virus.

Cough syrups don't help either. They can even make things worse. They may keep your child from coughing up mucus (MYOO-kus) that needs to come out if there is infection.

Who Gets Croup?

Most children get croup once or twice. Some children get croup every time they get a cold or the flu. Croup can come at any time. It's most common in the winter months.

Children are most likely to get croup between 6 months and 3 years of age. After age 3, it is not as common. That's because the windpipe is larger. So swelling is less likely to get in the way of breathing.

If your child seems to get croup a lot, he or she may have another problem. Talk with your child's doctor.

Can You Prevent Croup?

You *can't* really prevent croup. But you *can* prevent a more serious illness called acute epiglottitis (uh-KYOOT epp-uh-glah-TYE-tis). Its symptoms are a lot like croup, but worse. This illness usually strikes children 1 to 5 years old.

The good news is that the Hib vaccine can protect against this illness. Your child should get the first dose of Hib at 2 months old.

To learn more, visit the American Academy of Pediatrics (AAP) Web site at www.aap.org.

Your child's doctor will tell you to do what's best for your child.
This information should not take the place of talking with your child's doctor.

Adaptation of the AAP information in this handout into plain language was supported in part by McNeil Consumer Healthcare.

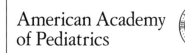

American Academy
of Pediatrics

DEDICATED TO THE HEALTH OF ALL CHILDREN™

Crup (Croup)

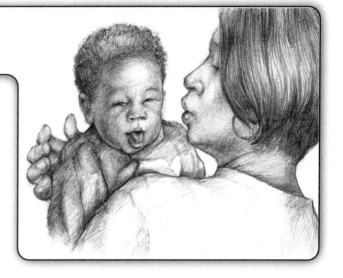

Crup es una infección que produce hinchazón dentro de la garganta de su niño. Esto dificulta la respiración de su niño. También puede asustar tanto a los padres como a los niños.

El crup es común en niños pequeños. La mayoría de casos de crup son leves. Pero el crup puede empeorar y hacer que su niño deje de respirar por completo. Llame al doctor si usted piensa que su niño tiene crup y está teniendo dificultad para respirar.

El crup es causado generalmente por un virus que infecta la caja donde se produce la voz y el tubo por donde pasa el aire. La principal señal de crup es una tos ronca que suena como un ladrido de perro. Puede comenzar con un resfriado. La mayoría de los niños con crup tienen poca fiebre. Pero algunos tienen temperaturas de hasta 104°F ó 40°C.

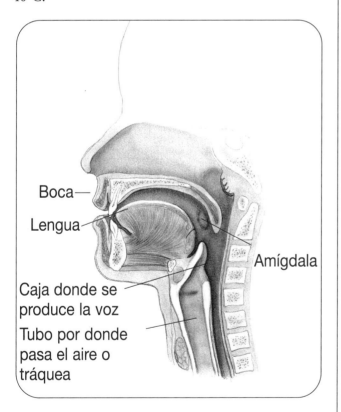

Boca—
Lengua—

Amígdala

Caja donde se produce la voz

Tubo por donde pasa el aire o tráquea

Señales de la infección crup

Estas son algunas señales que muestran que su niño puede tener crup:

- Tos ronca o áspera (como ladrido de perro)
- Respiración ruidosa o con dificultad
- Voz ronca
- Respiración con la boca abierta

Qué puede hacer cuando el niño tiene crup

Llame al 911 ó a una ambulancia si...

...su niño:

- No puede hablar por falta de respiración.
- Está batallando para poder respirar.
- Hace un sonido como silbido cuando respira. (A esto se llama **estridor***).
- Babea mucho más de lo normal o tiene dificultad para tragar la **saliva***.
- La boca o las uñas se le ponen azules.

Todos los signos mencionados antes son señales de un crup severo. También pueden ser signos de otros problemas serios. De cualquier forma, si su niño tiene problemas para respirar, usted tiene que llevarlo al hospital.

✳ *Palabras que debe conocer*

saliva: Líquido en la boca.

esteroides: Una medicina que viene en pastillas, líquido, un spray que se aspira o inyección que ayuda a eliminar los síntomas de crup. Estas medicinas bajan o reducen la inflamación.

estridor: Es un sonido de silbido alto que su niño hace al respirar. Es ocasionado por algo que bloquea la caja donde se produce la voz o la garganta.

Continúa atrás

Llame al doctor si...

...se presenta cualquiera de estas situaciones:

- Su niño es un bebé que tiene 1 año o menos.
- La tos sigue cada vez peor.

Intente un tratamiento en casa

Crup puede despertar a su niño a la media noche. Si su niño no tiene problemas para respirar, intente estos tratamientos en casa.

- Forme vapor en el baño dejando correr el agua caliente de la regadera. Lleve a su niño al baño para que respire la humedad del aire durante 15 ó 20 minutos. El vapor funciona en muchos niños.
- Si el vapor no le funciona, tape al niño y vaya afuera durante unos minutos. El aire fresco de la noche podría ayudar a que la respiración de su niño sea más fluida.
- Utilice un humidificador de vapor frío en la habitación de su niño durante el resto de la noche. Úselo durante las próximas 2 ó 3 noches.

Medicinas para la infección crup

El doctor puede prescribir **esteroides***. Los esteroides ayudan a desinflamar la garganta.

Los antibióticos no ayudan debido a que la infección crup casi siempre es causada por un virus.

Los jarabes para la tos tampoco ayudan. Éstos pueden hasta empeorar el problema. Los jarabes pueden evitar que su niño saque la flema o mucosidad, la cual es necesario expulsar si hay una infección.

¿Quién padece la infección crup?

La mayoría de los niños padecen la infección crup una o dos veces. Algunos niños padecen la infección crup cada vez que se resfrían o tienen gripe. Al niño le puede dar esta infección en cualquier momento. Pero es más común en los meses de invierno.

Los niños tienen más probabilidades de padecer la infección crup entre los 6 meses y 3 años de edad. Después de los 3 años, ya no es tan común. Esto se debe a que el tubo por donde pasa el aire o tráquea es más grande. Entonces es menos probable que la inflamación obstruya la respiración.

Si su niño padece de la infección crup muy seguido, él o ella podría tener otro problema. Consúltelo con el doctor de su niño.

¿Se puede prevenir la infección crup?

Usted no puede realmente prevenir la infección crup. Pero usted puede prevenir una enfermedad más seria llamada epiglotitis aguda. Sus síntomas son muy parecidos al crup, pero son peores. Esta enfermedad casi siempre ataca a niños de 1 a 5 años de edad.

La buena noticia es que la vacuna llamada Hib (contra la influenza tipo B) puede protegerlo contra esta enfermedad. Su niño debe recibir la primera dosis de la vacuna Hib a los 2 meses de edad.

Para aprender más, visite el sitio de la Academia Americana de Pediatría (AAP) en www.aap.org.
Su pediatra le dirá qué es lo mejor para la salud de su hijo.
Esta información no debe usarse en lugar de consultar con su doctor.
La adaptación de la información de este folleto de la AAP a lenguaje sencillo se hizo con el apoyo de McNeil Consumer Healthcare. La traducción al español fue patrocinada por Leyendo Juntos (Reach Out and Read), un programa pediátrico de alfabetización.

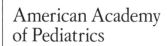

American Academy of Pediatrics

DEDICATED TO THE HEALTH OF ALL CHILDREN™

Developmental Delays and Communication Issues

Communication problems—in terms of speech, hearing, and speaking—and other developmental delays can take many forms. Here we will address some of the more common developmental delays seen in today's pediatric practice and offer some practical suggestions for helping parents and patients deal with them.

Under this topic, common areas for miscommunication may include

- Diagnosis
- Identification of symptoms
- Management and treatment

Successfully—and sensitively—caring for these families, and communicating clearly with them about the condition and available treatments and therapies, can bring potential benefits to your practice, including

- Increased likelihood of successful early screening for developmental problems and disorders
- Improved patient satisfaction resulting from addressing anxieties that may not be easy for parents to verbalize

Ask Me 3

During your patient encounter, you should communicate using plain language and health literacy principles so that by the end of the visit, the parent or child will know the answers to the *Ask Me 3* questions.

A Patient Story. . .

Donald is a 2-year-old boy brought in by his Vietnamese-speaking grandmother for his well-child visit. Dr Greene is concerned about Donald's behavior in the examination room: He doesn't seem to make eye contact, he runs in circles and screams when his grandmother tries to pick him up, and there doesn't seem to be any language.

An interpreter is called, and Dr Greene asks the interpreter to convey his concern that Donald seems to be delayed, or possibly autistic, and should be evaluated as soon as possible. Through the interpreter, Donald's grandmother says that at home the child speaks in sentences and behaves normally.

Dr Greene suggests a referral to Early Intervention, telling the grandmother that someone can come to the home to do this evaluation. The grandmother refuses, saying it isn't needed.

- -

This was a very difficult visit because it involved communicating developmental concerns across linguistic and cultural barriers. By beginning with his concerns, and invoking the words "delayed" and "autistic," which then had to be translated into Vietnamese, the pediatrician may have alarmed the grandmother into a very defensive posture.

She may also be concerned about the possibility of "evaluation," especially if it means sending an official person into the home.

It would probably make better sense if Dr Greene had begun by asking the grandmother about her perceptions of Donald's progress, and whether she was aware of any differences between his behavior and the behavior of other children his age. Dr Greene should have considered asking her to demonstrate any communication strategies that she uses with Donald.

The offer of evaluation might have been more welcome if the nature of that evaluation had been explained (that the evaluator is a speech specialist, for example) and if it had included some information about the value of starting early to help children catch up with language and communication.

Patient: Veronica, 2-year-old girl who isn't talking in sentences	
Ask Me 3 questions	**What the parent should understand at the end of the visit**
What is my child's main problem?	Veronica isn't talking as well as most children her age. She isn't yet putting words together and only seems to have a few single words.
What do I need to do?	• I need to take Veronica to get her hearing tested and then for a free evaluation of her development and her speech and language. • I need to make sure that Veronica gets help with her talking from a person with special training in speech and language of young children. • I need to learn how to talk to Veronica in a way that helps Veronica learn to speak more. I will get help from the speech and language therapist in doing this. • I need to read children's books with Veronica every day.
Why is it important for me to do this?	• If Veronica has a hearing problem, we need to find out as soon as possible to help her. • If Veronica has a speech and language problem, we will be able to help her much more if we start when she is young. • The more Veronica uses words to ask for things, the better she will get at speech and language.

Medical Terms and Plain Language Alternatives

Many of the medical terms we use every day don't mean much to many parents. The use of medical jargon or language above the comprehension level of the family confuses parents and does not allow for understanding. Below is a list of medical terms that may be confusing or difficult to explain and suggestions for plain language alternatives.

Medical Terms	Plain Language Alternatives
Autism	A problem with the brain that can hurt a child's ability to understand and be understood and to relate to people
Behavior	How a person acts
Development; maturity	Growth; growing up
Developmental delay	When a child is behind other children his age; he is unable to do the things that most other children his age can do
Developmental-behavioral specialist	An expert in the ways children grow and learn
Discipline	To correct; to teach; using ways to set limits on how a child acts, like putting a child in time-out

Early Intervention	A program for children younger than 3 years that helps them with talking and other parts of growing and learning
Referral	A note or phone call from a doctor that sends you to another doctor or specialist
Specialist	A doctor who is an expert on a subject, like allergies or hearing or feet
Speech	Talking
Speech and language therapy; speech and language therapist	Treatment for people who have trouble talking; a specially trained person who can help children learn to speak and understand words better

Confusing Terms and Concepts

With any condition, there are likely to be terms or concepts for which patients and families have a different understanding than a health care professional. These may include preventive strategies, complex disease processes, medication or treatment regimens, abstract laboratory results or measurements, technical terms, or words that have a different meaning in the health care arena than in everyday use. Cultural issues and misconceptions can also contribute to lack of understanding.

Communication Issues

Consider the following communications issues when talking with parents about developmental delays:

- Parents may overreact to the idea that their child is behind other children developmentally. Explain that children with some delays can catch up to other children, but they need parents to help them, and they may need other doctors or therapists too.

- If appropriate, explain that sometimes a child just needs to be exposed to things (like books) to understand them and become comfortable with them. There is not necessarily anything wrong with the child's ability to learn; it may just be a matter of showing more things to the child.

- Don't ever use words like "slow" or "retarded," because they can make a child feel really bad about himself. Don't allow siblings or others to use those words either.

Don't blame parents for not knowing about developmental delays or recognizing them in their child. Consider the following reasons that it can be difficult for parents to understand:

- Language about development often tends to be somewhat complex (Is the child's speech intelligible? Does he use pronouns?)

- Note: Parents who have difficulty with appropriate limit-setting or who don't have age-appropriate expectations for behavior and discipline may be at increased risk of abusing their child.
- Materials about development (like the Baby Einstein series) are often marketed to more educated parents.
- There is a lot of conflicting information in parenting books and magazines.
- Most developmental disorders include generally unfamiliar diagnostic terms, often without common plain language alternatives.
- Self-assessment forms are often used for parent-reported development screens. Some parents who aren't comfortable with their abilities may not complete the form, while embarrassment may drive other parents not to fill out the assessment forms truthfully.
- Parents may be uncertain about what skills should be expected at what age, and about what they can do to help children learn to talk or read.

Behavior Change

Behavior change is a key element in preventing and managing many pediatric conditions. Shifting from paternalistic advice that is either too vague or too complicated to a patient- or family-centered approach that incorporates elements of motivational interviewing and goal-setting, and that makes use of plain language, can be an effective way to empower patients and families to make changes and improve their health.

Parents of children with language delays can help their children with the following behaviors:

- Praise the child for any speech or communication: "Good talking!" "Good pointing." Try not to say "no" too much or to criticize the child for making mistakes. Stay away from too many commands.
- Always look directly at the child when speaking with him, so you can get his attention, and he can see you making the words.
- Expand the child's language whenever possible: "Yes, that is a ball. Look, it is a *big, blue* ball. Good talking!"
- Pronounce your words clearly, and use cheerful "motherese" when talking to young children.
- Encourage the child to use words for her wants. "I know you are excited. Can you tell me the word for what you are pointing to?"

- Read children's books to the child every day. Point to the pictures and say the words that are the names of the pictures. Encourage the child to first point to the pictures when you say their names ("Madeline, point to the picture of the apple. That's right! Great pointing!"), and then to say the names of the pictures that you are pointing to ("Madeline, what is this? Yes, that is a boy! Great talking! What is the boy doing?")
- Play naming games wherever you go, such as in the street or store.

Child Involvement

Including the child, to the extent possible, is respectful and patient-centered and can contribute to developing health literacy skills as the child moves toward managing his or her own health as an adolescent and an adult. It can include direct, age-appropriate statements to the child, and also ways for the child to be involved in his or her health.

Young children can be involved in improving development and language in a natural way.

- The parent can help the child by communicating with the child in the ways listed above.
- The child can participate in choosing which books they want to read.
- The way that children learn to speak is all about the interaction of the parent (or therapist) and the child.

Teach-back

The concept of teaching back entails asking parents or patients to demonstrate understanding *using their own words*, not simply asking whether they have questions or whether they understand, because that may not elicit lack of understanding. Having patients explain in their own words not only assesses their understanding, but it reinforces the information by repeating it and internalizes it for the patient. When there is a lot of information, go over each concept and elicit a teach-back before moving to the next idea.

When using teach-back, it's important to keep the burden on yourself. Avoid the perception that you are quizzing the parent or patient—emphasize you want to be sure you've explained things clearly.

The practice of using teach-back can be especially important over the phone, because it may be the only way to gauge whether the parent or patient understands fully.

Here are some approaches to using teach-back with respect to developmental delays.

Communication Tip

✓ Practice words and play word games, name games, rhyme games.

✓ Reading aloud to children helps them with speech and language, and helps them learn the names of things.

✓ When children don't know how to tell you what they want or what they're feeling, sometimes they get very angry and upset.

✓ Getting along with other children the same age can be harder for a child who is having trouble talking.

- We've talked about several things you can do to help Chantelle with her talking. To be sure I was clear, can you tell me 2 things you will start doing?
- How can you help Mark use his words tonight at home?
- Tell me why it's so important to check Jason's hearing?

Key Messages for Use by All Members of the Health Care Team

It is important to reinforce key messages for parents and children so they hear them more than once and recognize them as priorities in managing their health. Your staff can reemphasize the importance of care concepts. In addition, families should not receive conflicting advice about their health and what to do.

Key concepts for language delays

- When children have trouble learning to talk, the earlier we start to help them, the better.
- Children who have trouble talking can have problems getting along with other children and can feel very angry and upset.
- Most children who have trouble talking can learn to talk well and catch up, but some children have other problems learning how to behave and how to do other things and they may need more special help. Getting your child checked out now, while she's young, will mean you can find out what kind of help she needs and make sure she gets it sooner.

Miscellaneous

You may want to review the handout "What Is Your One-Year-Old Telling You?" on page 193 in more detail with the parent. Put special marks, such as stars, arrows, or underlines, on the parts of the handout you think are most important for this particular parent and child.

For parents who want more information, refer them to some reliable Web sites.

This Web site gives additional information about language delays in young children:

http://www.aap.org/publiced/BR_LanguageDelay.htm

This Web site gives additional information about autism:

http://www.aap.org/publiced/BR_Autism.htm

This Web site has links to many resources about autism:

http://www.aap.org/healthtopics/Autism.cfm

What Is Your One-Year-Old Telling You?

Language begins long before the first spoken words. Your child starts "telling" you things during the first year of life. Your child may say things with looks, smiles, movements, or sounds. These early messages are very important.

Talk with your child's doctor about how your child is growing and learning. Always tell the doctor right away if you are worried about something.

What's Normal?

Children usually can do certain things at certain ages.

By 12 months your baby should:

- Look for and find where sounds are coming from.
- Know his or her name most of the time when you call it.
- Wave goodbye.
- Look where you point when you say, "Look at the _____."
- Take turns "talking" with you. (Your child listens when you speak, then babbles when you stop.)
- Say "da-da" to Dad and "ma-ma" to Mom and at least one other word.
- Point to things he or she wants.

Between 12 and 24 months your baby should:

- Follow simple commands, like "Pick up your toy." (You may need to point to the toy at first.)
- Get things from another room when asked.
- Point to a few body parts when asked.
- Point to things or events to get you to look at them.
- Bring things to show you.
- Name a few common objects and pictures when asked.
- Enjoy pretending, like having a tea party.

By 24 months your toddler should:

- Point to many body parts and common things when asked.
- Point to some pictures in books when asked.
- Follow 2-step commands. (For example, "Get your toy and put it in the backpack.")
- Say about 50 to 100 words.
- Say many 2-word phrases like "Daddy go," "doll mine," and "all gone."

✳ Words to Know

autism (AW-tiz-um)—a long-term problem in the brain and nerves. Many people with autism have trouble understanding others and being understood. They often have trouble making friends. They may like to do one thing over and over again.

developmental-behavioral specialist (duh-vel-up-MEN-tul bee-HAY-vyer-ul SPESH-uh-list)—an expert in the ways children grow and develop.

referral (ree-FUR-ul)—a note or phone call from a doctor sending you to see someone.

speech therapy (THAIR-uh-pee)—treatment for people who have trouble talking. There are many different speech problems, and many kinds of speech therapy.

Continued on back

Signs of a Problem

Babies express themselves in many ways. Talk with the doctor if your child:

- Doesn't use any words by 18 months.
- Doesn't put 2 words in a phrase by 24 months.
- Doesn't cuddle like other babies.
- Doesn't return a happy smile back to you.
- Doesn't seem to notice if you are in the room.
- Doesn't show you things to look at together.
- Doesn't respond when you call his or her name but seems to hear other sounds.
- Prefers to play alone. Seems to "tune others out."
- Doesn't seem interested in toys, but likes to play with other things in the house.

What to Do If Your Child Isn't Talking

Many children learn to talk late. One in 5 children is slow to talk or use words.

The problem may go away on its own. Or your child may need a little extra help. Sometimes **speech therapy*** is needed.

Late talking also may be a sign of something more serious. Your child may have a hearing loss, **autism***, or other problem with growing and learning. It's important to talk with your child's doctor if you're worried.

What the Doctor May Do

After you talk about your concerns, your child's doctor may:

- Ask you some questions about your child.
- Check how your child is developing.
- Order a hearing test.
- Refer you to a speech therapist for testing. The therapist will check how well your child expresses himself or herself. The therapist will also check how well your child understands words and gestures.

- Refer you to a **developmental-behavioral specialist***. This specialist will check all areas of your child's development.

It's OK to say you are still concerned if the doctor says your child will "catch up in time." You can also ask for a **referral*** to a developmental-behavioral specialist. This specialist may refer you to others for more help.

Programs That Can Help

Your child's doctor may also refer you to a developmental or school program. These programs help children with different kinds of growing and learning problems. The program staff may want to do their own tests with your child.

If your child is younger than 3 years, the doctor may refer you to an Early Intervention Program (EIP). Or you can contact the program yourself. The government pays for these programs. EIPs help children with delays and other problems.

If your child qualifies for help, EIP staff will work with you to make a plan. This is called an Individualized Family Service Plan, or IFSP. It may include training and support for you as well as therapy, special equipment, and other services for your child. After 3 years of age, the EIP staff will refer your child to the local school district.

Remember

Follow your instincts as a parent. Ask for more testing or a referral for your child if you are still worried.

Tell your child's doctor if your child seems slow or shows any of the "Signs of a Problem" on the left. Also, tell the doctor if your baby stops talking or doing things he or she used to do.

To learn more, visit the American Academy of Pediatrics (AAP) Web site at www.aap.org.

Your child's doctor will tell you to do what's best for your child. This information should not take the place of talking with your child's doctor.

Adaptation of the AAP information in this handout into plain language was supported in part by McNeil Consumer Healthcare.

American Academy of Pediatrics

DEDICATED TO THE HEALTH OF ALL CHILDREN™

¿Qué le cuenta su niño de un año?
(What Is Your One-Year-Old Telling You?)

El lenguaje comienza mucho antes de que su niño diga las primeras palabras. Su niño comienza a "contarle" cosas durante el primer año de vida. Su niño puede decir cosas con la mirada, las sonrisas, los movimientos o los sonidos. Estos primeros mensajes son muy importantes.

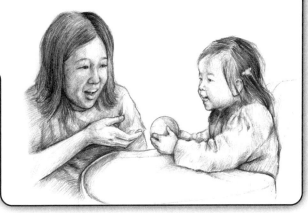

Consulte con el doctor de su niño sobre el crecimiento y aprendizaje de su niño. Siempre cuéntele al doctor de inmediato si le preocupa algo sobre su niño.

¿Qué es lo normal en su niño?

Los niños casi siempre pueden hacer ciertas cosas a ciertas edades.

A los 12 meses su bebé debería:

- Buscar y encontrar de dónde vienen los sonidos.
- Conocer su nombre la mayoría de veces cuando usted le llama.
- Decir adiós con la mano.
- Mirar hacia donde usted señala cuando usted dice "Mira ese o esa _____".
- Esperar su turno para "hablar" con usted. (Su niño escucha cuando usted habla, luego balbucea cuando usted para de hablar).
- Decir "pa-pa" a su papá y "ma-ma" a su mamá y por lo menos alguna otra palabra.
- Señalar las cosas que él o ella quiere.

Entre los 12 y 24 meses su bebé debería:

- Seguir instrucciones sencillas, como "recoge tu juguete". (Es posible que necesite señalar el juguete primero).
- Traer cosas de otra habitación cuando se le pida.
- Señalar algunas partes del cuerpo cuando se le pida.
- Señalar cosas o eventos para que usted los vea.
- Traer cosas para mostrárselas.
- Nombrar algunos objetos comunes y dibujos cuando se le pida.
- Disfrutar cuando juega dando de comer a la muñeca.

A los 24 meses su niño pequeño debería:

- Señalar muchas partes del cuerpo y cosas comunes cuando se le pregunte.
- Señalar algunos dibujos de los libros cuando se le pregunte.
- Seguir instrucciones siguiendo 2 pasos. (Por ejemplo, "recoge tu juguete y colócalo en tu mochila o bolsa").
- Decir más o menos de 50 a 100 palabras.
- Decir muchas frases de 2 palabras como "papá va," "muñeca mía" y "se acabó".

✳ Palabras que debe conocer

autismo: Un problema a largo plazo en el cerebro y el sistema nervioso. Muchas personas con autismo tienen problemas para entender a los demás y darse a entender. Con frecuencia tienen problemas para hacer amigos. Es posible que les guste hacer una misma cosa una y otra vez.

especialista en conductas de desarrollo: Es un experto en materia de desarrollo y crecimiento de los niños.

referencia o derivación: Es una nota o llamada telefónica de un doctor enviándole a ver a otro profesional.

terapia del habla: Tratamiento para las personas que tienen dificultad para hablar. Existen muchos problemas diferentes del habla y muchos tipos de terapia del habla.

Continúa atrás

Señales de que hay algún problema

Los bebés se expresan por sí solos de muchas maneras. Hable con el doctor si su niño:

- No dice ninguna palabra a los 18 meses.
- No dice 2 palabras en una frase a los 24 meses.
- No abraza como otros bebés.
- No le devuelve una sonrisa.
- No parece notar si usted está en la habitación.
- No le muestra objetos para que ustedes los vean juntos.
- No le responde cuando le llama por su nombre pero parece escuchar otros sonidos.
- Prefiere jugar a solas. Parece ser que "rechaza a los demás".
- No parece interesarse en los juguetes pero le gusta jugar con otras cosas en casa.

Qué debe hacer si su niño no habla

Muchos niños aprenden a hablar tarde. Uno de cada 5 niños es lento para hablar o emplear palabras. El problema puede desaparecer. O es posible que su niño necesite un poco de ayuda. Algunas veces la **terapia del habla*** es necesaria.

El habla tardía también puede ser señal de algo más serio. Su niño podría tener pérdida auditiva, **autismo*** u otro problema con el crecimiento y aprendizaje. Es importante que consulte con el doctor de su niño si usted está preocupada.

Lo que el doctor puede hacer por usted

Después de que usted hable acerca de sus preocupaciones el doctor de su niño puede:

- Hacerle algunas preguntas sobre su niño.
- Examinar el progreso del desarrollo de su niño.
- Ordenar una prueba de audición.
- Referirle con un terapeuta del habla para realizar una prueba. El terapeuta revisará qué tan bien se expresa su niño. El terapeuta también revisará qué tan bien comprende su niño palabras y gestos.
- Referirle a un especialista en **conductas de desarrollo***. Este especialista evaluará todas las áreas de desarrollo.

Está bien decirle que usted sigue preocupada si el doctor dice que su niño "logrará hacer las cosas a su tiempo". También usted puede pedir una **referencia*** con un especialista en conductas de desarrollo. Este especialista puede enviarla con otras personas para obtener más ayuda.

Programas que pueden ayudarle

El doctor de su niño también puede referirle un programa escolar o de desarrollo. Estos programas ayudan a los niños con diferentes tipos de problemas de crecimiento y aprendizaje. El personal del programa puede desear hacer sus propias pruebas con su niño.

Si su niño es menor de 3 años, el doctor puede referirle a un programa de Estimulación Temprana (siglas en inglés EIP). También, usted puede comunicarse con ese programa por su cuenta. El gobierno paga por estos programas. Estos programas ayudan a los niños con retrasos u otros problemas.

Si su niño es elegible para la ayuda, el personal del programa de EIP le ayudará a elaborar un plan. A esto se le llama un Plan de Servicio Familiar Individualizado (siglas en inglés IFSP). El plan puede incluir: clases de preparación, apoyo para usted, terapia, equipo especial y otros servicios para su niño. Después de que tenga más de 3 años de edad, el personal del programa referirá a su niño al distrito escolar en su área.

Recuerde

Siga sus instintos como padre o madre. Pida más pruebas o referencias para su niño si usted todavía está preocupada.

Cuéntele al doctor si su niño parece tener algún retraso o muestra alguna de las "señales de algún problema" en la lista de la izquierda. También, cuéntele al doctor si su bebé deja de hablar o de hacer cosas que él o ella acostumbraba a hacer antes.

Para aprender más, visite el sitio de la Academia Americana de Pediatría (AAP) en www.aap.org.
Su pediatra le dirá qué es lo mejor para la salud de su hijo.
Esta información no debe usarse en lugar de consultar con su doctor.
La adaptación de la información de este folleto de la AAP a lenguaje sencillo se hizo con el apoyo de McNeil Consumer Healthcare. La traducción al español fue patrocinada por Leyendo Juntos (Reach Out and Read), un programa pediátrico de alfabetización.

© 2008 Academia Americana de Pediatría

American Academy of Pediatrics

DEDICATED TO THE HEALTH OF ALL CHILDREN™

Fever

Fever is one of the most common reasons children visit the doctor. Parents are concerned that fever itself is an illness, and that the higher the fever, the sicker their child is. They may not understand that how their child acts and feels can be a better indicator of the degree of illness present.

Explaining the cause of fever, appropriate management, what to expect, and when to be concerned, along with reassuring parents, can be particularly challenging when parents are anxious and have expectations for antibiotics.

Common areas for miscommunication may include

- How to read a thermometer and take an infant's or child's temperature
- What a fever means, and what causes it
- Management and treatment
- Measures that can be taken to make the child more comfortable
- The natural course of the underlying infection and what to expect
- Signs of a worsening or more serious condition

Ask Me 3

During your patient encounter, you should communicate using plain language and health literacy principles so that by the end of the visit, the parent or child will know the answers to the *Ask Me 3* questions.

A Patient Story. . .

Miguel is a 1-year-old whose father took him to see Dr Marco because he has fever. The child's temperature has been 101.5°F rectally for the last 2 days.

There is no history of vomiting or diarrhea, but Miguel does have a cough and runny nose. His appetite is excellent and he appears to be interested in his surroundings. He smiles readily. His weight is 25 lbs (11.4 kg) and his physical examination is normal except for slight erythema of the posterior pharynx and rhinorrhea.

Dr Marco tells Miguel's father that the infant probably has a viral infection and not to worry. Dr Marco tells him to give Miguel 1 teaspoon of acetaminophen every 4 hours if his temperature is higher than 101°F, and to bring him back to the office for follow-up if he cannot be awakened easily from sleep or does not want to eat. Also, Dr Marco counsels the father to give Miguel a lot of water to drink.

Three days later, Miguel is taken to the hospital's emergency department with depressed sensorium and jaundice. The liver enzymes were markedly abnormal, and Miguel's acetaminophen levels were high.

. . . .

Miguel's father had been giving the infant 1 teaspoon of acetaminophen drops every 4 hours, as opposed to 1 teaspoon of the acetaminophen elixir. Dr Marco could have uncovered this misunderstanding through teach-back but, instead, the misunderstanding led to the father's giving the infant some infant-strength acetaminophen drops he had on hand, resulting in acute hepatic injury to his 1-year-old child.

Patient: Lucy, 3-year-old girl with a viral upper respiratory infection and fever	
Ask Me 3 questions	**What the parent should understand at the end of the visit**
What is my child's main problem?	My baby has a fever and a cold. Unless the fever is high (>101ºF) I don't have to give Lucy medicine to bring it down.
What do I need to do?	• I need to give Lucy milk or other liquids frequently so she doesn't dry out. • The acetaminophen liquid will help her fever go down and make her more comfortable. It needs to be measured carefully. [Demonstrate with a syringe and ask the mother to demonstrate how much to give.] • I need to watch her carefully over the next 3 to 4 days. If Lucy doesn't wake up easily or starts vomiting, I need to take her to a doctor right away.
Why is it important for me to do this?	• Giving her small amounts of liquids often will keep Lucy's body from drying out. • By giving acetaminophen like the doctor showed me I will help Lucy feel better.

Medical Terms and Plain Language Alternatives

Many of the medical terms we use every day don't mean much to many parents. The use of medical jargon or language above the comprehension level of the family only confuses parents and does not allow for understanding. Below is a list of medical terms that may be confusing or difficult to explain and suggestions for plain language alternatives.

Medical Terms	Plain Language Alternatives
Acetaminophen	Medicine to lower a fever and help take away pain (commonly known by the brand name Tylenol)
Anorexia or loss of appetite	Not hungry, poor feeding, or doesn't want to eat
Antibiotics	Medicine to get rid of the germs, called "bacteria," that cause infections. Antibiotics don't work against viruses.
Dehydrated	Dry; dried out. The body needs water and other liquids to stay healthy; when it doesn't have enough, it dries out, or gets "dehydrated," which can be dangerous.
Ibuprofen	Medicine for fever, aches and pains, and redness and swelling (Common brand names for ibuprofen are Motrin and Advil.)
Lethargic	Tired, sleepy, weak
Temperature; fever	The temperature is how warm or cold your body is; if the temperature is higher (hotter) than usual, you have a "fever."
Virus or bacteria	Germs that cause infections

Confusing Terms and Concepts

With any condition, there are likely to be terms or concepts for which patients and families have a different understanding than a health care professional. These may include preventive strategies, complex disease processes, medication or treatment regimens, abstract laboratory results or measurements, technical terms, or words that have a different meaning in the health care arena than in everyday use. Cultural issues and misconceptions can also contribute to lack of understanding.

Consider the following when talking with parents about fever:

Prevention and Health Promotion

Parents may not have an understanding of the factors that may increase (child care attendance and tobacco smoke) or decrease (breastfeeding, immunization against influenza) the risk of their child getting a cold or other common illness that can cause a fever. Remind them that the following steps, which they can teach their children, can help them stay healthy:

- Wash your hands with soap and water.
- Cover your mouth and nose with a tissue or your sleeve when sneezing and coughing.
- Handle food with clean hands.
- Eat a healthy diet, including fruits and vegetables.
- Get the proper amount of sleep.
- Be sure everyone in the household, including the patient, is up to date on their immunizations.

Diagnosis

Parents may lack a basic understanding of fever.

- Fever is a symptom, not an illness.
- Getting the fever to "normal," is not necessary and may not be possible.
- In most instances, fever is not serious and it's a sign the child's body is working to fight off an illness.

For many parents, a fever means an antibiotic is necessary. Because most fevers are the result of viral infections, you may need to explain to parents that viral infections are not treated with antibiotics.

- A virus is a germ that makes you sick, and antibiotics don't work to treat an infection caused by viruses.

Communication Tip

Make sure that you and the parent or caregiver are on the same page when it comes to talking about the child's temperature.

Use the American Academy of Pediatrics handout on how best to take a child's temperature, and review it with the parent in your office.

This could help you avoid mix-ups between numbers like 100.4 and 104.

Symptoms

Parents may not know how to take the child's temperature. They may be afraid to take a rectal temperature but not tell you.

Because each method is different, you should use teach-back to determine whether the parents understand how to take the child's temperature in the manner necessary.

Use the "Fever" (page 205) and "How to Take Your Child's Temperature" (page 209) handouts.

Management and Treatment

Dosing fever medicines and formulations is confusing. Be clear and precise in your instructions about medication dosage. Telling parents to give a medicine 3 times a day is too vague; it does not state how the medication is to be taken or when.

For medications that must be given multiple times in a day, work out a written schedule with the parents so the doses don't come too close together. Avoid the more vague "breakfast, lunch, dinner, and bedtime" instructions, because dinner and bedtime might be too close together, particularly for very young children. Instead, instruct them to give the medicine at 8:00 am, noon, 4:00 pm, and 8:00 pm.

To many, "day" refers to the time when it's light outside, so be sure to explain that when you say "day" you mean 24 hours, or a day and a night. If you mean only while the child is awake, say so.

Remember these kinds of simple messages, and use teach-back to make sure the parents understand your instructions.

- The medicine to make the fever go down must be given [like this] so that Ben swallows all of it.

- Do not use a regular teaspoon you eat with because it is not accurate. Use the oral syringe I give you or the measuring cup that comes with the medicine.

- Show me how you are going to measure the acetaminophen before you give it to Lynetta.

Parents may have misconceptions about medicines. Be sure they know that too much acetaminophen is dangerous, and that medicines for babies can actually be stronger than those for older children because babies can't take as much so they put more medicine in a smaller amount. Explain what strength, formulation, and dose to use for their child's age and weight.

Remind parents that many over-the-counter products (such as cold medicines and cough suppressants) contain acetaminophen, and they shouldn't give their child anything without checking the label and talking with a health professional first. Over-the-counter cold and

Did You Know...?

Mixing Meds

The popular idea of alternating doses of ibuprofen and acetaminophen is not recommended by the American Academy of Pediatrics, and may be dangerous.

cough medicines contain other drugs that can be very harmful to a young child.

Note: The popular idea of alternating doses of ibuprofen and acetaminophen is not recommended by the American Academy of Pediatrics, and may be dangerous.

Parents often treat their child's fever the way they treat their own. Explain that children don't respond the same way to medicines and treatments the same way adults do, and treatments that work for grown-ups can be extremely dangerous for children.

Ibuprofen, for example, is not recommended for infants younger than 6 months, and the use of aspirin in children is associated with the development of Reye syndrome, a potentially fatal condition. Parents should be counseled not to use any products that contain aspirin, including Alka-Seltzer, Anacin, Bufferin, Excedrin, Fiorinal, BC Powder, and Stanback Powder.

Tell parents that sponge baths—not ice baths—may also be used to reduce a high fever. Be sure to explain the proper temperature and not to use ice or the old-fashioned method of using alcohol to bathe the child.

- You may sponge an infant with water that is barely warm to your skin. Do not use alcohol to sponge because it can be absorbed through the skin and cause harm. If your child starts to shiver, take her out and dry her off.

Cultural Beliefs

Families from different cultures may have their own ideas of what causes a fever and how to treat it. Their beliefs can result in confusion and a lack of adherence to suggested management if they are not understood. Ask parents what they think is causing the fever and what they think will make it better. This will increase your understanding of their culture while uncovering possible roadblocks or cultural issues with treatment before they arise.

Usually parents' or families' beliefs will pose no harm to the child, but some remedies are potentially toxic (eg, metamizole-associated agranulocytosis). Try to incorporate their beliefs into your treatment plan when they won't be harmful to the child.

Worsening Condition

Parents may not know what to look for when determining whether their child's condition is worsening; they may not know that increasing lethargy, a significant decrease in appetite, or vomiting indicates possible systemic infection.

Parents may think that because they saw the doctor earlier in the day or yesterday there is no need to check in again, even if the child seems worse. Explain the expected course of illness. Be clear and tell them when and what should cause a call to you.

In particular, explain clearly what they should look for as signs of a more severe problem (eg, meningitis). Give them a brochure to take home if appropriate, and mark the most important parts.

Behavior Change

Behavior change is a key element in preventing and managing many pediatric conditions. Shifting from paternalistic advice that is either too vague or too complicated to a patient- or family-centered approach that incorporates elements of motivational interviewing and goal-setting, and that makes use of plain language, can be an effective way to empower patients and families to make changes and improve their health.

Preventing most of the ailments that cause fever is no different. Deliver the messages of risk factors and healthy living, just as you do with many other conditions.

Cultural Spotlight

Fever Among Some Latino Cultures

Many Latinos see fever (*calentura* or *fiebre*) as a disease, not as a symptom of broader processes, such as infection.

The presence of a fever in a young child may be a real emergency in the mind of the mother. Although other symptoms may be present, she will be most concerned with the fever. Respect this concern.

Fever may be associated in the Latino culture with *mal de ojo*, which may occur when a person glances or looks admiringly at someone without touching them. *Mal de ojo* brings with it the sudden onset of high fever, vomiting, headache, coryza, fainting, and sometimes convulsions.

Even if the parent doesn't mention *mal de ojo*, it may be helpful to address this concept.

Source: Hispanic Center of Excellence (a partnership of the Baylor College of Medicine and University of Texas-Pan American). http://www.rice.edu/projects/HispanicHealth/Courses/mod7/ojo.html. Accessed April 16, 2008.

- Child care attendance and tobacco smoke can contribute to children's illnesses, and breastfeeding and immunization can prevent them.
- Simple daily activities can help them stay healthy.
  - Wash your hands with soap and water.
  - Cover your mouth and nose with a tissue or your sleeve when sneezing and coughing.
  - Handle food with clean hands.
  - Eat a healthy diet, including fruits and vegetables.
  - Get the proper amount of sleep.

Stress the importance that everyone in the family keep their hands clean by washing them with soap and water, especially before and after diaper changing or going to the bathroom, and before preparing food or eating. Explain it in terms of making sure the rest of the family doesn't get sick too.

Explain that smoking increases the risk of getting many illnesses, and that no one should smoke around the child. There should be absolutely no smoking in the home or car, even if the child isn't there.

Child Involvement

Including the child, to the extent possible, is respectful and patient-centered and can contribute to developing health literacy skills as the child moves toward managing his or her own health as an adolescent and an adult. It can include direct, age-appropriate statements to the child, and also ways for the child to be involved in his or her health.

For example, even before age 2 years, children can be taught to cover their mouths with their sleeve or a tissue when they cough, and practice other healthful habits, such as hand-washing, that will last them into adulthood. They can be taught to wash their hands with soap and water using a simple familiar tune ("Happy Birthday" or "Twinkle, Twinkle Little Star," for example) to ensure they wash long enough.

Teach-back

The concept of teaching back entails asking parents or patients to demonstrate understanding *using their own words*, not simply asking whether they have questions or whether they understand, because that may not elicit lack of understanding. Having patients explain in their own words not only assesses their understanding, but it reinforces the information by repeating it and internalizes it for the patient. When there is a lot of information, go over each concept and elicit a teach-back before moving to the next idea.

When using teach-back, it's important to keep the burden on yourself. Avoid the perception that you are quizzing the parent or patient—emphasize that you want to be sure you've explained things clearly. The practice of using teach-back can be especially important over the phone, because it may be the only way to gauge whether the parent or patient understands.

Here are some approaches to using teach-back when managing fever.

- To make sure this plan works for you, when you get home, what medicines will you give your child and how will you give them? How much will you give at a time?
- What will you tell your husband needs to be done to help Monty through this illness?
- I want to make sure I was clear when I explained this to you. To check, can you tell me which symptoms of Jessie's will make you call me back? What things might mean that he is getting worse?

Key Messages for Use by All Members of the Health Care Team

It is important to reinforce key messages for parents and children so they hear them more than once and recognize them as priorities in managing their health. Your staff can reemphasize the importance of care concepts. In addition, families should not receive conflicting advice about their health and what to do.

Key messages for fever

- Most conditions associated with fever are caused by viruses and will not be helped by antibiotics.
- If we use antibiotics when they're not needed, it increases the chance they won't work when there's a very serious infection.
- Antibiotics are usually reserved for infants younger than 1 month and for those children with more serious illnesses caused by bacteria.
- At a well-baby visit, ideas about reducing the risk of infection, particularly those involving hand-washing and avoiding people who smoke, can be introduced and reinforced by you and the office staff.
- Fever alone won't hurt your child. You don't have to treat a fever to make your child's temperature go back to normal if she is acting normally—eating, drinking, playing, and smiling.

Mark important points on the American Academy of Pediatrics plain language handout on fever (page 205) and give it to the caregiver to take home.

Miscellaneous

Consider giving specific written and pictorial information about fever and use of acetaminophen or ibuprofen to parents as part of well-child visits and reviewing it with them during subsequent visits.

It is essential that all parents leave the office with the basic key concepts as noted above, but some parents will want to know more about their child's condition. You can always explain more to parents if they are asking questions, or you can ask them if there are other concerns that they have. Here are 2 Internet sites for parents that have in-depth discussions on fever presented at several different education levels.

- American Medical Association

  "Fever in Infants" JAMA Patient Page

  http://jama.ama-assn.org/cgi/reprint/291/10/1284.pdf
- eMedicine, as posted by Ann G. Egland, MD, consulting staff, Department of Operational and Emergency Medicine, Walter Reed Army Medical Center

  "Fever in the Young Infant"

  http://www.emedicine.com/PED/topic2698.htm

Fever

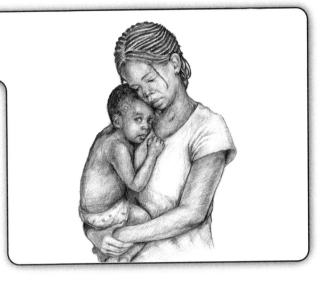

Fever is a sign that your child is fighting an infection. It is usually harmless. Your child's fever should go away in about 3 days. If it doesn't, call your child's doctor.

What Is a Fever?

A fever is a body temperature (TEM-pruh-chur) that is higher than normal. Most doctors agree that anything over **100.4°F** or **38°C** is a fever. (See "Words to Know" for **"F"** and **"C."**)

Your child may feel warm, shiver, or look flushed. You will need to take your child's temperature to know for sure. (See the AAP handout "How to Take Your Child's Temperature" if you need help.)

Fever is *not* a sickness. It is a *sign (symptom)* of sickness. It can be caused by lots of things, like a cold, the flu, or an ear infection. Look for *other* symptoms to figure out what is causing your child's fever. (Antibiotics only help if they are the right treatment for what your child has.)

Call the Doctor Right Away If…

…your child:

- Is 2 *months* or younger and has a fever, OR
- Has a high fever, over 103°F (39.4°C), OR
- Has a fever more than 3 days.

You also should call the doctor if your child has a fever and any of these signs:

- Looks very sick, is very sleepy or very fussy
- Has other symptoms, like a stiff neck, rash, bad headache, sore throat, ear pain, throwing up, or **diarrhea***

- Has had a seizure (See "What to Do for a Seizure" on the second page of this handout.)
- Has sickle cell disease, cancer, or another disease that makes it hard to fight infections
- Takes steroids
- Has been in a very hot place, like a closed car in summer

What to Do

Making children feel better helps them drink and eat. This helps them get better. They often get more active too. That's OK. They don't have to rest to get better.

To help your child feel better:

- Comfort your child.
- Give your child water, juice mixed with water, or an **electrolyte drink*** for children. Breast milk is fine for nursing babies.
- Help your child rest if he or she feels tired.
- Cool your child down if the fever is over 101°F or 38.3°C *and* your child is uncomfortable. See "Tips to Cool Down a Fever" on the second page of this handout.

✳ Words to Know

"F" stands for Fahrenheit (FER-un-hyt)—a scale of numbers to show temperature. Used mostly in the United States.

"C" stands for Centigrade (SEN-tuh-grayd)—a different scale of numbers to show temperature. Used mostly outside the United States.

acetaminophen (uh-set-tuh-MIN-uh-fin)—a medicine for pain and fever. Tylenol is one brand of acetaminophen.

diarrhea (dye-uh-REE-yuh)—passing loose, watery stools.

electrolyte (uh-LEK-troh-lyt) **drink**—a sugar and salt drink you can buy in a bottle. Pedialyte is one brand made for children.

ibuprofen (eye-byoo-PROH-fin)—a medicine for pain and fever. Advil and Motrin are brands of ibuprofen.

Continued on back

Continued from front

Tips to Cool Down a Fever

- **Give your child medicine** to bring down the fever:

    - For a baby 6 months or younger, give **acetaminophen***.

    - For a baby or child older than 6 months, give *either* acetaminophen or **ibuprofen***.

    Both of these medicines help with fever. But they are not the same. Be sure to get the right kind of medicine for your child's age. Follow what the label says. Ask your child's doctor how much to give if your child is younger than 2 years.

    Note: *Never* give your child aspirin.

- **Give your child a bath.** Try this if the fever is 104°F (40°C) or higher, *and* your child can't take fever medicine.

    The water should be cooler than your child is, but still warm (lukewarm). Sponge the water over your child's body (5 or 10 minutes is enough).

    If your child starts to shiver during the bath, then the water is too cold. And shivering can make a fever worse. Take your child out of the bath if he or she shivers.

What *Not* to Do

- Don't give your child aspirin. It's dangerous for children younger than 18 years.

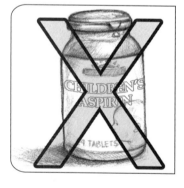

- Don't rub or bathe your child with rubbing alcohol. Rubbing alcohol can make children sick.

- Don't make your child cold enough to shiver. Shivering warms the body up more.

What to Do for a Seizure

Fever can cause a seizure (SEE-zher) in some young children. Seizures are scary, but usually harmless. Your child may look strange, shake, then stiffen and twitch. His or her eyes may roll. If this happens:

- Lay your child down on the floor or a bed.
- Turn your child's head to the side. That way, spit or vomit can drain out.
- Don't put anything in your child's mouth.
- Call the doctor.

The doctor should always check your child after a seizure.

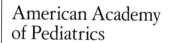

American Academy of Pediatrics

DEDICATED TO THE HEALTH OF ALL CHILDREN™

La fiebre (Fever)

La fiebre es una señal de que su niño está combatiendo una infección. Generalmente no hace daño. La fiebre de su niño deberá desaparecer en más o menos 3 días. Si no fuera así, llame al doctor de su niño.

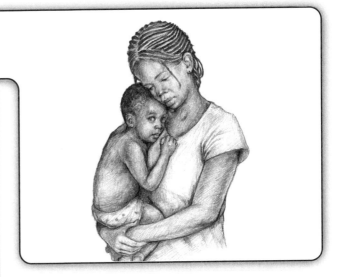

¿Qué es la fiebre?

La fiebre es la temperatura del cuerpo que es más alta de lo normal. La mayoría de médicos está de acuerdo con que cualquier temperatura arriba de **100.4°F** ó sea **38°C** es una fiebre. (Vea "Palabras que debe conocer" para aprender el significado de la "F" y "C").

Su niño puede sentirse tibio, tener escalofríos o verse colorado. Usted necesitará tomarle la temperatura para saber con seguridad si hay fiebre. (Vea el folleto de AAP "Cómo tomar la temperatura de su niño" si usted necesita ayuda).

La fiebre *no* es una enfermedad. Es una señal (*síntoma*) de enfermedad. Puede ser causada por muchas cosas, como un resfriado, la gripe o una infección de oído. Busque *otros* síntomas para averiguar qué está causando la fiebre de su niño. (Los antibióticos únicamente ayudan si son el tratamiento correcto para lo que tiene su niño).

Llame al doctor de inmediato si...

...su niño:

- Tiene 2 meses o menos y tiene fiebre, o
- Tiene fiebre alta, más de 103°F (39.4°C), o
- Ha tenido fiebre durante más de 3 días.

También deberá llamar al doctor si su niño tiene fiebre y cualquiera de estas señales:

- Se ve muy enfermo, tiene mucho sueño o está muy irritable.
- Tiene otros síntomas, como el cuello rígido, salpullido, fuerte dolor de cabeza, garganta irritada, dolor de oídos, vómitos o **diarrea***.

- Ha tenido una convulsión/ataque (Vea "Qué hacer en caso de una convulsión" en la segunda página de este folleto).
- Tiene Anemia Falciforme, cáncer u otra enfermedad que dificulte combatir las infecciones
- Toma esteroides.
- Ha estado en un lugar muy cálido como un automóvil cerrado en el verano.

Qué debe hacer

Ayudar a que los niños se sientan mejor los hace tomar líquidos y comer. Esto les ayuda a mejorarse. Con frecuencia también se ponen más activos, pero eso está bien. No tienen que reposar para sentirse mejor.

Para ayudar a su niño a sentirse mejor:

- Consuele a su niño.
- Dele a su niño agua, jugo mezclado con agua o una **bebida de electrolitos*** para niños. La leche del pecho está bien para los bebés lactantes.
- Ayude a su niño a descansar si él o ella se siente cansado.
- Refresque a su niño para bajarle la fiebre si está arriba de 101°F ó 38.3°C y su niño está molesto. Vea "Consejos para bajar la fiebre" en la segunda página de este folleto.

✳ *Palabras que debe conocer*

"F" significa Fahrenheit: Una escala de números para mostrar la temperatura. Se usa más en los Estados Unidos.

"C" significa centígrados: Una escala diferente de números para mostrar la temperatura. Se usa más fuera de los Estados Unidos.

acetaminofén: Es una medicina para el dolor y la fiebre. Tylenol es una marca de acetaminofén.

diarrea: Defecar (hacer pupú) aguado.

bebida de electrolitos: Una bebida compuesta de azúcar y sal que usted puede comprar en botellas. Pedialyte es una marca elaborada para niños.

ibuproféno: Es una medicina para el dolor y la fiebre. Advil y Motrin son marcas de ibuprofeno.

Continúa atrás

Consejos para bajar la fiebre

- **Dele a su niño medicina** para bajar la fiebre:
  - **Acetaminofén*** para un bebé de 6 meses o menos.
  - Acetaminofén **o ibuprofeno*** para un bebé o niño mayor de 6 meses.

  Ambas medicinas alivian la fiebre. Pero no son lo mismo. Asegúrese de tener la medicina apropiada para la edad de su niño. Siga lo que le indica la etiqueta. Pregúntele al doctor de su niño cuánto debe darle a su niño si es menor de 2 años.

  Nota: *Nunca le dé aspirina a su niño.*

- **Dele un baño a su niño.** Trate esto si la fiebre es de 104°F (40°C) o más, *y* su niño no puede tomar medicina para la fiebre.

  El agua debe estar más fría de lo que su niño está, pero todavía tibia (templada).
  Con una esponja moje el cuerpo de su niño (5 ó 10 minutos es suficiente).

  Si su niño comienza a tener escalofríos durante el baño, entonces el agua está muy fría. Y los escalofríos pueden empeorar la fiebre.
  Saque a su niño del baño si tiene escalofríos.

Lo que no debe hacer

- No le dé a su niño aspirina. Es peligroso para niños menores de 18 años.

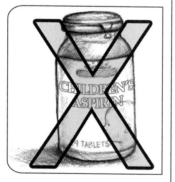

- No frote o bañe a su niño con alcohol de frotar. El alcohol de frotar puede enfermar a los niños.

- No enfríe mucho a su niño provocándole escalofríos. Los escalofríos elevan más la temperatura del cuerpo.

Lo que debe hacer en caso de una convulsión/ataque

La fiebre puede causar una convulsión en algunos niños pequeños. Las convulsiones asustan, pero en lo general no hacen daño. Su niño puede verse extraño, temblar, luego ponerse rígido y contraerse. Sus ojos pueden darse vuelta. Si esto sucede:

- Acueste a su niño en el piso o en una cama.
- Gire la cabeza de su niño hacia un lado. De esa forma, podrá escupir o vomitar.
- No coloque nada en la boca de su niño.
- Llame al doctor.

El doctor siempre debe revisar a su niño después de una convulsión.

Para aprender más, visite el sitio de la Academia Americana de Pediatría (AAP) en www.aap.org.
Su pediatra le dirá qué es lo mejor para la salud de su hijo.
Esta información no debe usarse en lugar de consultar con su doctor.
Nota: Los nombres de marca son para su información solamente.
La AAP no recomienda ninguna marca o producto de medicina específicamente.
La adaptación de la información de este folleto de la AAP a lenguaje sencillo se hizo con el apoyo de McNeil Consumer Healthcare. La traducción al español fue patrocinada por Leyendo Juntos (Reach Out and Read), un programa pediátrico de alfabetización.

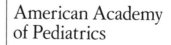

American Academy of Pediatrics

DEDICATED TO THE HEALTH OF ALL CHILDREN™

How to Take Your Child's Temperature

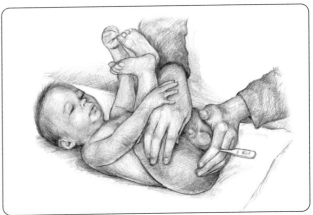

Your temperature (TEM-pruh-chur) is how warm or cold your body is. Normal temperature for a child is 98°F to 99°F or 37°C. The small circle (°) means "degrees." Anything over 100.4°F or 38°C is a fever. (See "Words to Know" for **"F"** and **"C."**)

There are many ways to check your child's temperature. *Always* use a digital (DIJ-uh-tul) thermometer (thur-MOM-uh-tur). These show the temperature in numbers in a little window.

Don't use a mercury thermometer (the kind with silver liquid inside). They are dangerous if they break.

This is how you read and say the temperature:

100.2° This means "One hundred **point** two degrees."
102° This means "One hundred **and** two degrees."

Be sure to read it carefully. There is a big difference between 100.2° and 102°.

In Child's Bottom (Rectal)

1. Turn on the thermometer.

2. Put some lubricating (LOO-bruh-kay-ting) jelly on the small end to help it slide in. KY Jelly, Surgilube, and Vaseline are brands of lubricating jelly.

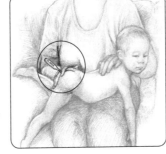

3. Lay your child across your lap or on something firm, face up or face down.

4. Put one hand on your child's back if the child is face down.

If the child is face up, bend your child's legs to his or her chest. Rest your free hand against the backs of the thighs. This will help your child hold still.

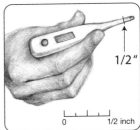

5. Gently put the small end of the thermometer in your child's bottom where poop comes out (rectum). Put it in 1/2-inch deep.

1/2"

6. Cup your hand over your child's bottom. Then hold the thermometer between the base of 2 fingers so it doesn't slip out.

7. Take it out after a minute or so, or when it signals that it is done. It may beep, stop flashing, or light up. Read the number.

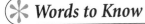
✳ *Words to Know*

"F" stands for Fahrenheit (FER-un-hyt)—a scale of numbers to show temperature. Used mostly in the United States.

"C" stands for Centigrade (SEN-tuh-grayd)—a different scale of numbers to show temperature. Used mostly outside the United States.

Continued on back

In Child's Mouth (Oral)

1. Turn on the thermometer.

2. Put the small end of the thermometer *under* your child's tongue. Put it as far back as you can without hurting your child.

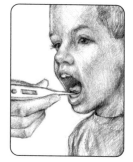

3. Have your child close his or her lips around the thermometer. Hold it there.

4. Take it out after a minute or so, or when it signals that it is done. It may beep, stop flashing, or light up. Read the number.

Under Child's Arm (Axillary)

1. Turn on the thermometer.

2. Put the small end of the thermometer in your child's armpit.

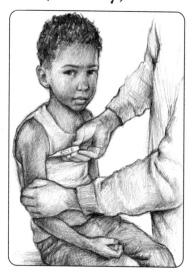

3. Hold your child's arm tightly against his or her side. With your other hand, hold the thermometer in place.

4. Take it out after a minute or so, or when it signals that it is done. It may beep, stop flashing, or light up. Read the number.

Taking Temperature by Age

Child's Age	Ways to Take Temperature
Newborn to 3 months old	In child's bottom (rectal)
3 months to 3 years old	In child's bottom (rectal) or under child's arm (axillary)*
4 to 5 years old	In child's mouth (oral) or bottom (rectal) or under child's arm (axillary)*
Older than 5 years	In child's mouth (oral) or bottom (rectal) or under child's arm (axillary)*

*Taking your child's temperature in the mouth or bottom gives a better reading than taking it under the arm.

Tips

- Wash the small end of the thermometer before and after using it. Use soap and cool water, not hot.

- Label the thermometer "oral" or "rectal." Don't use the same thermometer in both places. (You can use both kinds under the arm.)

- If your child has had a hot or cold drink, wait 15 minutes before taking your child's temperature by mouth.

- If you have questions about other kinds of thermometers, like ear or temporal (tem-PUR-ul) artery thermometers, ask your child's doctor.

- Remember: A fever is anything over 100.4°F or 38°C.

To learn more, visit the American Academy of Pediatrics (AAP) Web site at www.aap.org.

Your child's doctor will tell you to do what's best for your child. This information should not take the place of talking with your child's doctor.

Note: Brand names are for your information only. The AAP does not recommend any specific brand of drugs or products.

Adaptation of the AAP information in this handout into plain language was supported in part by McNeil Consumer Healthcare.

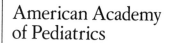

American Academy of Pediatrics

DEDICATED TO THE HEALTH OF ALL CHILDREN™

Cómo tomarle la temperatura a su niño

(How to Take Your Child's Temperature)

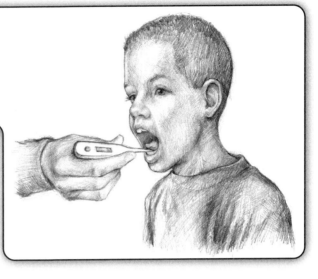

Tomar la temperatura es saber qué tan caliente o frío está su cuerpo. La temperatura normal de un niño es de 98°F a 99°F ó 37°C. El círculo pequeño (°) significa "grados". Cualquier temperatura más alta de 100.4°F ó 38°C es fiebre. (Lea en "Palabras que debe conocer" para saber que es la letra **"F"** y **"C"**).

Hay muchas formas de saber la temperatura de su niño. *Siempre* use un termómetro digital. Estos muestran los números de la temperatura en una pantalla pequeña.

No use un termómetro de mercurio (los que tienen líquido plateado adentro). Estos son peligrosos si se quiebran.

Cómo se lee y se indica la temperatura:

100.2° Esto significa "Cien **punto** dos grados."
102° Esto significa "Ciento dos grados."

Lea la temperatura con cuidado. Hay una gran diferencia entre 100.2° y 102°.

Tomar la temperatura en el recto de su niño (rectal)

1. Encienda el termómetro.

2. Ponga un poco de lubricante en la punta del termómetro para que deslice suavemente. Los productos KY Jelly, Surgilube y Vaseline son marcas de lubricantes.

3. Acueste a su niño en sus piernas o en una superficie firme, boca arriba o boca abajo.

4. Ponga una mano en la espalda de su niño si el niño está boca abajo.

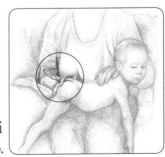

Si el niño está boca arriba, doble las piernas de su niño hacia el pecho. Descanse su mano libre contra la parte de atrás de los muslos. Esto ayudará a que su niño se quede tranquilo.

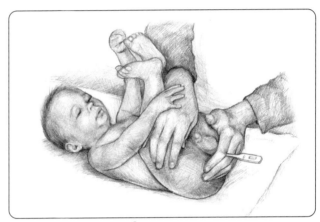

5. Suavemente meta la punta pequeña del termómetro en el recto de su niño. Métala a una profundidad de 1/2 pulgada.

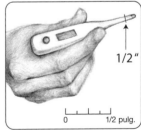

6. Ponga la mano sobre las nalgas de su bebé. Luego sostenga el termómetro entre la parte baja de dos de los dedos de modo que no se salga.

7. Sáquelo después de más o menos un minuto, o cuando muestre señal de estar listo. Puede ser que suene (bip), o deje de apagar y encender, o encienda una luz. Observe el número.

✳ *Palabras que debe conocer*

"F" significa Fahrenheit: Una escala de números para mostrar la temperatura. Se usa más en los Estados Unidos.

"C" significa centígrados: Una escala diferente de números para mostrar la temperatura. Se usa más fuera de los Estados Unidos.

Continúa atrás

En la boca de su niño (oral)

1. Encienda el termómetro.

2. Coloque el extremo pequeño del termómetro *debajo* de la lengua del niño. Colóquelo lo más adentro posible sin que lastime a su niño.

3. Haga que su niño cierre sus labios alrededor del termómetro. Sosténgalo allí.

4. Retírelo después de más o menos un minuto, o cuando muestre la señal de estar listo. Este puede hacer un sonido de bip, o dejar de iluminarse, o encenderse. Observe el número.

Debajo del brazo del niño (axilar)

1. Encienda el termómetro.

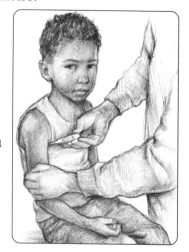

2. Coloque el pequeño extremo del termómetro en la axila de su niño.

3. Sostenga el brazo de su niño apretándolo contra su cuerpo. Con la otra mano, sostenga el termómetro en su lugar.

4. Retírelo después de más o menos un minuto, o cuando muestre la señal de estar listo. Éste puede hacer un sonido de bip, o dejar de iluminarse, o encenderse. Observe el número.

Toma de la temperatura según la edad

Edad del niño	Formas de tomar la temperatura
De recién nacido a 3 meses de edad	En el recto del niño (rectal)
De 3 meses a 3 años de edad	En el recto del niño (rectal) o debajo de la axila (axilar)*
De 4 a 5 años	En la boca del niño (oral) o en el recto (rectal) o abajo de la axila (axilar)*
Mayor de 5 años	En la boca del niño (oral) o en el recto (rectal) o abajo de la axila (axilar)*

*Tomar la temperatura al niño en la boca o en el recto le da un mejor resultado que tomarla debajo del brazo.

Consejos

- Lave el extremo pequeño del termómetro antes y después de utilizarlo. Utilice jabón y agua fría, no caliente.

- Póngale un rótulo el termómetro "oral" o "rectal." No utilice el mismo termómetro en ambas partes. (Usted puede utilizar ambos tipos debajo del brazo).

- Si su niño ha tomado una bebida caliente o fría, espere 15 minutos antes de tomar la temperatura de su niño por la boca.

- Si usted tiene preguntas sobre otros tipos de termómetros, pregúntele al doctor de su niño. Algunos de estos son los termómetros de oído y los arteriales temporales.

- Recuerde: Una fiebre es cualquier temperatura arriba de 100.4°F ó 38°C.

Para aprender más, visite el sitio de la Academia Americana de Pediatría (AAP) en www.aap.org.
Su pediatra le dirá qué es lo mejor para la salud de su hijo.
Esta información no debe usarse en lugar de consultar con su doctor.
Nota: Los nombres de marca son para su información solamente.
La AAP no recomienda ninguna marca o producto de medicina específicamente.
La adaptación de la información de este folleto de la AAP a lenguaje sencillo se hizo con el apoyo de McNeil Consumer Healthcare. La traducción al español fue patrocinada por Leyendo Juntos (Reach Out and Read), un programa pediátrico de alfabetización.

American Academy of Pediatrics

DEDICATED TO THE HEALTH OF ALL CHILDREN™

Gastroenteritis
Dehydration, Vomiting, Diarrhea

This section focuses on gastroenteritis—the symptoms of which prompt many calls to pediatricians. Because there are estimated to be more than 20 million episodes of acute diarrhea among children younger than 5 every year (accounting for nearly 4 million physician visits annually), the potential for miscommunication—and its inherent harm—is great.[1]

There are many opportunities for misunderstanding the health care provider's directions for managing gastroenteritis, which can lead to prolonged or increasingly severe symptoms.

Common areas for miscommunication may include

- Diagnosis
- Frequency and severity of symptoms
- Feeding through the illness
- Treatment
- Indicators that a child is getting worse and needs attention

Ask Me 3

During your patient encounter, you should communicate using plain language and health literacy principles so that by the end of the visit, the parent or child will know the answers to the *Ask Me 3* questions.

A Patient Story...

Mario is an 18-month-old healthy male who vomited 3 times yesterday and had a fever of 101°F and decreased solid intake. Today he vomited 4 times.

Mario's mother called the pediatrician, who said that if vomiting continued to give Mario small amounts of Pedialyte or other clear liquids. The doctor said if Mario got better, then the mother could advance him back to his regular diet after 24 hours.

Mario refused the Pedialyte, so his mother gave him sippy cups filled with apple juice for 24 hours and his vomiting decreased to 2 episodes the next day. That evening, Mario complained that he was hungry, so his mother served him his favorite dish: a beef and bean burrito.

Mario's mother called the pediatrician the next morning to say that Mario's vomiting had returned.

. . . .

Mario's mother did not understand that the clear fluids shouldn't be juice. It wasn't made clear to her that liquids should be administered in small amounts, starting with sips every 10 to 15 minutes, and increasing by only 2 ounces at a time. Further, she didn't know that food should be reintroduced gradually and gently. Inappropriate treatment of gastroenteritis is common and is often due to misunderstood directions from the health professional.

Patient: Anthony, 13-month-old boy with vomiting	
Ask Me 3 questions	**What the parent should understand at the end of the visit**
What is my child's main problem?	Anthony has a stomach infection that is making him throw up.
What do I need to do?	• I should give him sips of a clear liquid (like Pedialyte) every 10 to 15 minutes. • If he throws that up, but isn't dried out, then I'll try again after an hour or two. ***If he keeps throwing up, I should stop and call the doctor.*** • If he keeps the liquid down for 1 to 2 hours and wants to eat, then I can give him small amounts of simple foods like the ones on the list the doctor gave me. If he doesn't throw that up, I can slowly give him more food.
Why is it important for me to do this?	Giving him small amounts of liquids often and feeding him simple foods will keep Anthony's body from drying out and help him get better faster.

Patient: Mary, 4-year-old girl with moderate diarrhea	
Ask Me 3 questions	**What the parent should understand at the end of the visit**
What is my child's main problem?	Mary has a stomach infection that's causing diarrhea, and we have to make sure her body doesn't get dried out.
What do I need to do?	• I need to give Mary special electrolyte drinks that I can buy in a bottle. (One common brand name is Pedialyte.) • I can feed her simple foods like the ones on the handout the doctor gave me. • I shouldn't give her anything too sweet, salty, or fatty—no soups, juices, or soda pop for a few days.
Why is it important for me to do this?	Mary needs special liquids to keep her body from drying out and simple foods to help her fight the infection. I'll watch for the warning signs on the sheet the doctor gave me to make sure her body isn't drying out (like not drinking or peeing very much). If I see those signs, or if she keeps having diarrhea after a week, I'll call the doctor. As long as the number of times she has diarrhea in a day is going down, and as long as her body isn't dried out, then she is getting better.

Medical Terms and Plain Language Alternatives

Many of the medical terms we use every day don't mean much to many parents. Below is a list of medical terms that may be confusing or difficult to explain and suggestions for plain language alternatives.

Medical Terms	Plain Language Alternatives
Advance	Gradually increase or slowly go back to normal
Day	24 hours or daytime versus nighttime
Dehydrated	Dry; dried out. The body needs water and other liquids to stay healthy; when it doesn't have enough, it dries out, or gets dehydrated, which can be dangerous.
Diarrhea	Watery poop (stool)
Fluids	Liquids or things to drink or swallow without chewing (like soup)
Gastroenteritis	Stomach infection, or stomach flu, that causes you to throw up and have diarrhea. This is different from influenza
Hematochezia	Bright red blood in the poop (stool)
Lethargic	Tired, sleepy, weak
Melena	Dark blood in the poop (stool)
Nauseous/nauseated	Feeling sick to your stomach
Rehydration formulas	Special electrolyte fluids like Pedialyte that a child should drink when he or she is dried out
Urine	Pee, pee-pee, number 1
Vomiting	Throwing up

Confusing Terms and Concepts

With any condition, there are likely to be terms or concepts for which patients and families have a different understanding than a health care professional. These may include preventive strategies, complex disease processes, medication or treatment regimens, abstract laboratory results or measurements, technical terms, or words that have a different meaning in the health care arena than in everyday use. Cultural issues and misconceptions can also contribute to lack of understanding.

Consider the following when talking with parents about gastroenteritis:

Diagnosis

Parents may not know what a virus is or that viruses do not respond to antibiotics. You may need to explain that a virus is a germ that makes you sick and that antibiotics don't usually work for viruses.

Some refer to gastroenteritis as the "stomach flu," but it has no relation to influenza, which is caused by influenza viruses. Gastroenteritis is an infection caused by a variety of viruses (including rotaviruses and noroviruses).

Avoid generalities such as "a few days" when you can. Tell them how many days the diarrhea should last—even if it's a range (2 or 3 days)—and the number of stools per day they should expect. Also explain that as long as the frequency of diarrhea is decreasing and there are no signs of blood or dehydration, the child is getting better.

Symptoms

Sometimes, when a parent is asked the number of times a child has had loose stools or urinated in a day, the parent's answer is based only on daylight hours. Make sure the parent knows you're asking about a 24-hour period or "a day and a night."

In some families, parents do not have an understanding of what normal stool looks like, and they don't know how much is too much. They may have difficulty quantifying the diarrhea—for example, they may report the absolute number of diaper changes, even though some of the diapers had only a small amount of stool in them.

Ask parents to describe what the child's stool looks like. Remember that terms such as "a lot" or "a little" may have different meanings to the parent and the doctor, so ask about the quantity and frequency of the stools, and ask them for specific times.

Management and Treatment

Parents may not understand how long to continue a clear liquid diet. Be clear and explicit about how long you want them to use the clear liquid diet before adding other foods or before calling you back.

Some parents make their own "special fluid," which may not have the right amount of electrolytes in it. Explain to parents that special prepackaged drinks they can purchase are the safest for their child because they have the right amount of salt, water, and sugar to protect the child from getting sicker.

Tell parents not to use antidiarrhea medications unless they talk to you first because such medicines can hurt the child.

Parents and doctors may not have a shared understanding of what types of foods to give a child who has gastroenteritis. The usual food for a family might not be food that the physician would recommend. Explain what kinds of foods are best for the child, and give specific examples and a handout to take home.

Make sure you emphasize that it's OK for the child to eat the foods you're recommending, even though they're having diarrhea. You may also need to tell them that if they are breastfeeding the child, they can continue despite the diarrhea.

Also, make note of foods they probably shouldn't give the child: fatty foods, sugary drinks, juice, soda, salty soups, etc.

Did You Know...?

One recent study found that more than 75% of people were unable to follow directions correctly to prepare an oral rehydration solution for a child with diarrhea.

Source: Schwartzberg JG. *Understanding Health Literacy.* Chicago, IL: AMA Press; 2005.

Cultural Beliefs

Families from different cultures may have their own ideas of what causes the symptoms of diarrhea and vomiting. Extended family members may play an important role in decision-making and management. This can result in confusion or lack of adherence to suggested management. Explore this by asking the parent what they think is causing the condition and what they think will make it better. This will increase your understanding of their culture while uncovering possible roadblocks or cultural issues with treatment before they arise.

Usually the parents' or families' beliefs will pose no harm to the child. Try to incorporate their beliefs into your treatment plan.

Worsening Condition

Parents may not know what to look for when determining whether their child's condition is worsening; they may not know that fussiness or decreased tears can indicate that a child is dehydrated.

Sometimes they may think that because they saw the doctor earlier in the day or yesterday there is no need to check in again, even if the child seems worse, so be clear and tell them when and what triggers should cause a call to you. In particular, explain clearly what they should look for as signs of dehydration, and give them a handout they can take home and mark the important information.

Behavior Change

Behavior change is a key element in preventing and managing many pediatric conditions. Shifting from paternalistic advice that is either too vague or too complicated to a patient- or family-centered approach that incorporates elements of motivational interviewing and goal-setting, and that makes use of plain language, can be an effective way to empower patients and families to make changes and improve their health.

Discuss the importance of all family members' washing their hands before and after diaper changing or going to the bathroom, and before preparing food or eating. Stress its importance in terms of making sure the rest of the household doesn't get sick too.

Child Involvement

Including the child, to the extent possible, is respectful and patient-centered and can contribute to developing health literacy skills as the child moves toward managing his or her own health as an adolescent and an adult. It can include direct, age-appropriate statements to the child, and also ways for the child to be involved in his or her health.

For example, beginning at preschool age, children with gastroenteritis can be told they need to drink the special electrolyte fluids to feel better.

Teach-back

The concept of teaching back entails asking parents or patients to demonstrate understanding *using their own words,* not simply asking whether they have questions or whether they understand, because that may not elicit lack of understanding. Having patients explain in their own words not only assesses their understanding, but it reinforces the information by repeating it and internalizes it for the patient. When there is a lot of information, go over each concept and elicit a teach-back before moving to the next idea.

When using teach-back, it's important to keep the burden on yourself. Avoid the perception that you are quizzing the parent or patient—emphasize that you want to be sure you've explained things clearly.

The practice of teaching back can be especially important over the phone, because it may be the only way to gauge whether the parent or patient understands fully.

Here are some approaches to using teach-back when managing gastroenteritis.

- To make sure this plan works for you, when you get home, what foods will you feed Sonia? What things will you give her to drink? How much will you give at a time?
- What will you tell your husband needs to be done to help Logan through this sickness?
- I want to make sure I was clear when I explained this to you. To check, can you tell me which symptoms of John's will make you call me back? What things might mean he is getting worse?

Key Messages for Use by All Members of the Health Care Team

It is important to reinforce key messages for parents and children so they hear them more than once and recognize them as priorities in managing their health. In addition, families should not receive conflicting advice about their health and what to do.

Key concepts for gastroenteritis and dehydration are

- Gastroenteritis is usually caused by a virus and does not need medicine but will get better by itself.
- If the diarrhea is mild, parents should try to feed the child through the illness to help them get better faster.
- Provide information on specific simple foods that the parents can try.
- Sometimes the child may need special electrolyte fluids like Pedialyte.
- For children who are vomiting, frequent small sips of fluid are important.
- If the parent does not think that the child can start other foods after 24 hours, they need to call the doctor's office.
- Some children become dried out and need to be seen again. If there is decreased urine, the mouth looks dry, there are few tears with crying, or a child is very tired, the parent needs to call the doctor.

Miscellaneous

Some health information is complicated but important. For example, when a child has gastroenteritis, some parents might want to know what the likely infectious agent is, what is happening at the intestinal mucosa level, or why some children will not tolerate milk. You can always explain more to parents if they are asking questions, or you can ask them if there are other questions that they have. But it is essential that all parents leave the office with the basic key concepts as noted above.

Reference

1. Glass RI, Lew JF, Gangarosa RE, LeBaron CW, Ho MS. Estimates of morbidity and mortality rates for diarrheal diseases in American children. *J Pediatr.* 1991;118 :S27–S33

Diarrhea, Vomiting, and Water Loss (Dehydration)

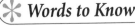

Diarrhea (loose poop) and vomiting, or "throwing up," are why many parents call the doctor. Your child's doctor may call this gastroenteritis (GAS-troh-en-tur-EYE-tis). These symptoms are often caused by a **virus***.

Your child may first have a fever and some vomiting. Diarrhea often starts later. The symptoms usually go away in a day or two. But they can last a week before getting better.

One danger with diarrhea and vomiting is that your child's body can get dried out or dehydrated (dee-hye-DRAY-dud). This happens when the body loses too much water.

Call the Doctor If…

…your child has diarrhea, vomiting, and is younger than 6 months or your child has:

- A fever over 102°F or 39°C.
- Blood in the stool (poop) or vomit.
- Green vomit.
- Vomiting for more than 12 hours or diarrhea for more than 2 days.
- Belly pain.

Also Call the Doctor If…

…your child has any of these signs of being too dry:

- Pees very little (wets fewer than 6 diapers per day)
- Has no tears when crying
- Can't or won't drink anything or feels very thirsty
- Has a dry, sticky mouth, or dry lips
- Looks like he or she has lost weight
- Has sunken eyes or sunken soft spot on head (for babies)
- Acts very tired or strange

Most of the time you can treat this by getting your child to drink something and eat simple foods. (See the list below.)

But your child may need a special fluid that you can buy in a store. It's called an **electrolyte drink***. If your child can't drink this, then he or she may need to go to the hospital.

Call your child's doctor if vomiting or diarrhea won't go away. The doctor may want to check your child.

What Can You Give Your Child When He or She Has Diarrhea?

For children 1 year old or older, these simple foods and drinks are fine:
- Rice
- Wheat bread or pasta
- Boiled or baked potatoes
- Cereal, like oatmeal
- Boiled egg
- Lean meat like chicken
- Fruits and vegetables (cooked)
- Bananas and applesauce
- Yogurt or milk
- Breast milk or infant formula
- Special electrolyte drinks

For all ages, don't give these foods or drinks:
- Fatty foods like French fries, chips, ice cream, cheese, or fried meats
- Sugary foods like candy, cookies, or cake
- Sugary drinks like juices or soda pop or very salty broths or soups when diarrhea is bad
- *Never* give boiled milk.

For children younger than 1 year check with your child's doctor.

✳ Words to Know

electrolyte (uh-LEK-troh-lyt) **drink**—a special sugar and salt drink you can buy in a bottle. These drinks are very helpful for diarrhea. Pedialyte is one brand made for children.

virus (VYE-ris)—a kind of germ that causes infection. Antibiotics do not work against viruses. The body usually needs to get over the virus on its own.

Continued on back

What to Do for Vomiting

- Give small sips of clear fluids every 10 to 15 minutes.
- If your child keeps vomiting but is NOT dry, wait 1 to 2 hours before trying again. Stop if your child starts to throw up again, and call the doctor.
- If your child is keeping down fluids and wants to eat, try giving small amounts of simple foods. See the chart on simple foods on the first page of this handout.

Remember, if you are worried or don't know what to do, call your child's doctor.

What to Do for Diarrhea

Most diarrhea lasts 3 to 6 days or even longer. Don't worry as long as your child acts well and is eating and drinking and peeing like usual.

Mild Illness

Most children should keep eating normal foods when they have mild diarrhea.

The doctor may suggest changing what your child eats for a few days. This might mean stopping cow's milk, but breastfeeding your baby is fine.

Moderate Illness

Children with moderate diarrhea can be cared for at home.

- They need special fluids, like electrolyte drinks. Talk with the doctor about how much and how long to give these and which to buy.
- Some children can't handle cow's milk when they have diarrhea. They may need to stop drinking it for a few days. Breastfeeding is fine for babies.
- As your child gets better, he or she can go back to normal foods.

Severe (Very Bad) Illness

See the "Call the Doctor If" list. Call the doctor right away if your child shows any of those warning signs. You may need to take your child to the emergency room for treatment.

Answers to Common Questions

Q. What should you do when your child is vomiting?

A. Try to give small sips of clear fluids every 10 to 15 minutes. If vomiting continues, call your child's doctor.

Q. Should you keep a child with diarrhea from drinking or eating?

A. A child with diarrhea can usually drink and eat most foods. If there is enough diarrhea to make your child very thirsty, he or she needs a special fluid called an electrolyte drink.

Soda pop, soups, and juices are OK for a child with mild diarrhea. But don't give these to a child with bad diarrhea. They have the wrong amounts of sugar and salt and can make your child sicker. Boiled skim milk is dangerous for all children. Sports drinks may be used for school-aged children.

As soon as the dryness (dehydration) clears up, let children eat simple foods. See the list of foods on the first page of this handout. They can have as much as they want.

Q. What about diarrhea medicines?

A. These do *not* help in most cases. They can sometimes be harmful. Never use them unless your child's doctor tells you to.

Remember These Dos and Dont's

- Do watch for signs of dehydration.
- Do call the doctor if your child has a high fever, has blood in his or her stool (poop), or starts acting different than normal.
- Do keep feeding your child if he or she is not throwing up.
- Do give your child special electrolyte drinks if your child is thirsty.
- Don't try to make your own electrolyte drinks.
- Don't give your child boiled milk.
- Don't use "anti-diarrhea" medicines unless told to by the doctor.

To learn more, visit the American Academy of Pediatrics (AAP) Web site at www.aap.org.

Your child's doctor will tell you to do what's best for your child.
This information should not take the place of talking with your child's doctor.

Note: Brand names are for your information only. The AAP does not recommend any specific brand of drugs or products.

Adaptation of the AAP information in this handout into plain language was supported in part by McNeil Consumer Healthcare.

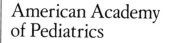

American Academy
of Pediatrics

DEDICATED TO THE HEALTH OF ALL CHILDREN™

Diarrea, vómitos y pérdida de líquidos (deshidratación)
(Diarrhea, Vomiting, and Water Loss (Dehydration))

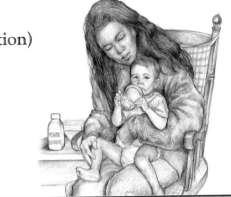

La diarrea (heces aguadas) y los vómitos causan que muchos padres llamen al doctor. El doctor puede llamarle a este problema gastroenteritis. Estos síntomas frecuentemente son causados por un **virus***.

Al principio su niño podría tener fiebre y algunos vómitos. La diarrea aparece hasta después. Los síntomas normalmente se van en un día o dos. Pero puede ser que duren una semana antes de que su niño se sienta mejor.

Un peligro con la diarrea y los vómitos es que el cuerpo del niño se puede deshidratar. Esto sucede cuando el cuerpo pierde mucha agua.

Llame al doctor si…

…su niño de 6 meses o menos tiene diarrea, vómitos o:

- Tiene fiebre más alta de 102°F ó 39°C.
- Tiene sangre en las heces o en el vómito.
- Vomita de color verde.
- Vomita durante más de 12 horas o tiene diarrea por más de 2 días.
- Tiene dolor de estómago.

Llame también al doctor si…

…su niño tiene algún signo de resequedad:

- Orina muy poco (moja menos de 6 pañales al día)
- No tiene lágrimas cuando llora
- No puede o no quiere beber o tiene mucha sed
- Tiene la boca seca y pegajosa o los labios resecos
- Parece que ha perdido peso
- Tiene los ojos hundidos. O, tiene el área blanda de la cabeza (mollera o fontanela) hundida. (Sólo los bebés)
- Se ve muy cansado o extraño

La mayoría de las veces, el tratamiento es darle a su niño alimentos simples. (Vea la lista de abajo).

Tal vez su niño necesite una bebida especial que usted puede comprar. Se llama **bebida con electrolitos***. Si su niño no puede tomar esta bebida, tal vez haya que llevarlo al hospital.

Llame al doctor de su niño si los vómitos y la diarrea no se van. Tal vez le diga que lo lleve a la clínica del doctor.

¿Qué le puede dar al niño que tiene diarrea?

Para los niños de 1 año de edad o mayores, estos alimentos y bebidas simples funcionan:	Para niños de todas las edades, no les dé estos alimentos ni estas bebidas:
- Arroz - Pan integral o pasta - Papas horneadas o cocidas - Cereal, como la avena - Huevos hervidos - Carne sin grasa (pollo) - Frutas y vegetales (cocidos) - Banana y jugo de manzana - Yogurt o leche - Leche materna o leche de fórmula (bebés) - Bebidas con electrolitos	- Alimentos con grasa como las papas fritas, helado, queso, o carnes grasosas - Alimentos con azúcar como dulces, galletas, o bizcochos - Bebidas con azúcar como la soda o líquidos con mucha sal como el caldo o las sopas (cuando tienen mucha diarrea) - Nunca les dé leche hervida

Pregúntele al doctor qué puede darle a los niños menores de 1 año de edad.

* Palabras que debe conocer

bebida con electrolitos o suero oral: Una bebida especial que contiene azúcar y sal. Usted puede comprarla en botellas. Esta bebida ayuda mucho a los niños con diarrea. Pedialyte es una marca de esta clase de bebida para niños.

virus: Es un tipo de germen que causa infección. Los antibióticos no funcionan contra los virus. El cuerpo necesita deshacerse del virus por sí sólo.

Continúa atrás

Qué hacer cuando el niño vomita

- Dele pequeños tragos de líquidos claros cada 10 ó 15 minutos.

- Si su niño continúa vomitando pero NO está deshidratado, espere de 1 a 2 horas antes de probar nuevamente. No le dé más líquido si su niño comienza a vomitar otra vez y llame al doctor.

- Si su niño ya no vomita los líquidos y desea comer, pruebe darle pequeñas cantidades de alimentos simples. Vea la lista de alimentos simples en la primera página de este folleto.

Recuerde, si usted está preocupada o no sabe qué hacer, llame al doctor de su niño.

Qué hacer si tiene diarrea

Por lo normal la diarrea dura de 3 a 6 ó hasta más días. No se preocupe si su niño actúa normal, está comiendo, tomando líquidos y orinando como de costumbre.

Enfermedad leve

La mayoría de los niños deben seguir comiendo sus alimentos normales cuando tienen diarrea leve.

Tal vez su doctor le sugiera cambiar la comida de su niño durate algunos días. Esto quiere decir, no darle leche de vaca, pero sí está bien darle leche de pecho.

Enfermedad moderada

Los niños con diarrea moderada pueden atenderse en la casa.

- Deles líquidos especiales, como las bebidas con electrolitos. Pregúntele al doctor qué cantidad y por cuánto tiempo debe darle esta bebida y cuál debe comprar.

- Algunos niños con diarrea no toleran la leche de vaca. Tal vez no deba darle leche de vaca, pero está bien darle leche de pecho.

- A medida que su niño se sienta mejor, puede volver a darle alimentos normales.

Enfermedad severa (muy mala)

Vea la lista "Llame al doctor si". Llame al doctor de inmediato si su niño muestra alguna de las señales de alarma. Puede ser que tenga que llevar a su niño a la sala de emergencia para tratamiento.

Respuestas a las preguntas comunes

P. ¿Qué debo hacer cuando mi niño está vomitando?

R. Trate de darle pequeños sorbos de líquidos claros cada 10 a 15 minutos. Si continúa vomitando, llame al doctor de su niño.

P. ¿Debo evitar que mi niño tome líquidos o alimentos cuando tiene diarrea?

R. Casi todos lo niños con diarrea pueden tomar y comer la mayoría de los alimentos. Si el niño tiene mucha diarrea y esto le da mucha sed, el niño necesita la bebida de electrolitos.

Le puede dar sodas, sopas y jugos al niño que tiene diarrea moderada. Pero **NO** se los dé al niño que tiene mucha diarrea. Éstos tienen una cantidad errónea de azúcar y sal y pueden enfermar más a su niño. La leche sin grasa hervida es dañina para todos los niños. A los niños que ya van a la escuela puede darles bebidas para deportistas (con electrolitos).

Tan pronto como la resequedad (deshidratación) se haya ido, deje a los niños comer alimentos simples. Vea la lista de alimentos en la primera página de este folleto. Pueden darle tanto como el niño desee.

P. ¿Qué debo saber sobre las medicinas para la diarrea?

R. Estas no ayudan en la mayoría de los casos. Algunas veces pueden hacer daño. Nunca las utilice a menos que el doctor de su niño así se lo indique.

Recuerde qué debe y qué no debe hacer

- Observe si hay señales de deshidratación.
- Llame al doctor si su niño tiene fiebre alta, hace heces con sangre, o comienza a actuar fuera de lo normal.
- Siga alimentando a su niño si no está vomitando.
- Dele a su niño bebidas con electrolitos si tiene sed.
- No trate de hacer usted mismo sus propias bebidas con electrolitos.
- No le dé a su niño leche hervida.
- No le dé a su niño medicinas "anti-diarrea" a menos que se lo indique el doctor.

Para aprender más, visite el sitio de la Academia Americana de Pediatría (AAP) en www.aap.org.
Su pediatra le dirá qué es lo mejor para la salud de su hijo.
Esta información no debe usarse en lugar de consultar con su doctor.
Nota: Los nombres de marca son para su información solamente.
La AAP no recomienda ninguna marca o producto de medicina específicamente.
La adaptación de la información de este folleto de la AAP a lenguaje sencillo se hizo con el apoyo de McNeil Consumer Healthcare. La traducción al español fue patrocinada por Leyendo Juntos (Reach Out and Read), un programa pediátrico de alfabetización.

American Academy of Pediatrics

DEDICATED TO THE HEALTH OF ALL CHILDREN™

Medication and Dosing
Over-the-Counter and Prescription

Medication errors concerning prescriptions are common among children in pediatric practices, occurring in as many as 1 of 6 children treated. Unlike medication errors for inpatient children, which occur primarily during ordering, outpatient errors usually occur at the point of administration by parents. About one-fifth of the errors related to prescription medications were preventable by better communication between pediatric providers and pharmacists with families.[1] Errors due to over-the-counter (OTC) medications have been less well studied but are likely to be substantial. Recent reports from the US Food and Drug Administration (FDA) about the dangers of non-prescription cough and cold medications, especially for young children, underscore the danger of these medication errors,[2] including infant deaths.[3]

Although drug information can be found easily online or in the printed materials provided by pharmacies, the information varies in quality and depth. And it's typically written at the college reading level, making it too difficult for many parents to understand.[4] That means health care providers must step in and explain clearly and thoroughly to patients or their parents about the medication the child needs, its possible side effects, and how to administer it.

Perhaps more than any other advice that health care professionals give patients, the information given to families about how and why to take medications is crucial. There is a great amount of information that parents need to know that will affect efficacy, as well as safety, and there are many areas for potential confusion.

- Different brand and generic names for the same medication
- Same medication may look different depending on the manufacturer

---

A Patient Story...

Jewel is a 4-year-old whose mother has brought her to see Dr Klein for a suspected ear infection. Jewel, indeed, has an ear infection with high fever and severe ear pain, so Dr Klein writes a prescription for amoxicillin and tells Jewel's mother to give the toddler Tylenol as needed for pain.

Two days later, Dr Klein is paged by emergency department staff: Jewel is suffering from an overdose of acetaminophen and her ear infection has worsened.

Jewel's mother gave her Tylenol hourly because the child's pain didn't go away. And she put the amoxicillin drops directly into the child's infected ear, thereby not treating the infection.

. . . .

Because the diagnosis was routine and the problem relatively minor, Dr Klein didn't spend time explaining his instructions.

If he had worked out a dosage schedule with Jewel's mother and used teach-back to see how she would give the child the antibiotic, he could have prevented what could be serious injuries to the child.

How Big Is the Problem?

- Different methods of delivery (orally, metered-dose inhaler, nebulizer, drops to eyes/ears/nose, suppositories, creams, etc)
- Large variety of OTC medications for the same things
- Same brand name for different nonprescription medications (eg, Tylenol, Tylenol Plus Cold)
- Potential drug interactions
- Side effects
- Sound-alike and look-alike names (eg, antiepileptic drug Lamictal and the antifungal drug Lamisil)
- Duration of treatment (eg, must complete course of antibiotics, but antihistamines are used as needed)
- Different medications covered under different, and often changing, formularies (eg, some not covered by public aid or insurance) and other cost- and coverage-related issues
- Timing for taking medicines (eg, the difference between "every 8 hours" and "3 times a day")
- Precautions (such as "take on empty stomach" and "avoid sunlight")
- Chronic medications and concerns about "addiction"
- Home remedies and cultural issues
- Dosing (tsp, mL, Tbsp, by weight or by age? What *is* a teaspoon?)
- Different concentrations of medications (syrup versus drops)
- Difficulties in administering medicines to children (eg, What if the patient spits it out? Can it be mixed with juice?)
- Overdose/safety/poison control
- Refills

Parental concerns about any of the above topics can lead to nonadherence with the prescribed regimen. With millions of children taking medicines every day, and each time representing the potential for an adverse event, the importance of proper medication use cannot be overstated.

Ask Me 3

During your patient encounter, you should communicate using plain language and health literacy principles so that by the end of the visit, the parent or child will know the answers to the *Ask Me 3* questions.

Patient: Carly, a 6-year-old girl with strep throat	
Ask Me 3 questions	What the parent should understand at the end of the visit
What is my child's main problem?	Carly has strep throat and needs medicine to get better.
What do I need to do?	• I need to give her amoxicillin for 10 days and not stop, even if she feels better. I will give her one measured teaspoon to drink at 8 o'clock in the morning and one more at 8 o'clock at night. 1 tsp → ← 5 mL • Show teaspoon mark on a dosing spoon/syringe/cup, or on a picture of one, like the one on the right. • *I will call the doctor if…*Carly's throat isn't feeling better within 3 days, because she might need different medicine.
Why is it important for me to do this?	• This medicine will cure Carly's infection, but if I don't give her the whole amount, Carly could get sick again.

Patient: Moby, a 9-month-old boy with a cold and fever	
Ask Me 3 questions	What the parent should understand at the end of the visit
What is my child's main problem?	Moby has a fever from a cold virus.
What do I need to do?	• I will give him Tylenol only when he has a fever or seems to be uncomfortable, but I'll wait at least 4 hours before giving him more. I can give him one dropper. 0.8 mL • *I will call the doctor if…*Moby sleeps too much, dries out, vomits or has trouble breathing.
Why is it important for me to do this?	• This medicine will not cure the infection, but will make him feel better. And I have to remember that giving him too much Tylenol can seriously hurt him.

Medical Terms and Plain Language Alternatives

Many of the medical terms we use every day don't mean much to many parents. The use of medical jargon or language above the comprehension level of the family only confuses parents and does not allow for understanding. Below is a list of medical terms that may be confusing or difficult to explain and suggestions for plain language alternatives.

Medical Terms	Plain Language Alternatives
2 puffs twice a day	2 puffs in the morning and 2 puffs in the evening, so 4 puffs total.
Acetaminophen	Medicine for fever and for aches and pains (A common brand name for acetaminophen is Tylenol.)
Antibiotics	Medicine to get rid of the germs, called "bacteria," that cause infections. Antibiotics don't work against viruses.
Complete full course	Give it for the whole [10] days, that means [30] times, even if your child is feeling better.
Dose	The amount of medicine you give your child (each time you are supposed to give it)
Ibuprofen	Medicine for fever, aches and pains, and redness and swelling (Common brand names for ibuprofen are Motrin and Advil.)
Metered-dose inhaler (MDI)	Puffer, inhaler, breathing/asthma medicine
Nebulizer	A machine that turns medicine or water into a mist that the child breathes in
Over-the-counter (OTC)	Medicine you can get without a prescription
Pharmacist	A person who has special training to fill prescriptions and teach people about their medicine
Pharmacy	Drug store
Prescription	Script, doctor's order; a note from the doctor that you take to the drugstore to get certain kinds of medicine
PRN (as needed)	Use only when your child is having the condition/symptom (fever, cough, congestion, etc).
Reaction/side effect	A symptom that comes from taking a drug but isn't part of the treatment. For example, some medicines might make you feel sick to your stomach.
Refill	More medicine. The number of refills is the number of times you can get more of the same medicine without getting another prescription from the doctor.
Take 4 times a day	Give in the morning, noon, early evening, and at night before bed.
Take every 4 hours as needed	Wait 4 hours between doses. For example, if you give it at 8:00 am, then the next dose you can give, if you need to, is at noon.
Take on an empty stomach	Give the medicine at least 1 hour before the child eats a meal (breakfast, lunch, dinner), and at least 2 hours after the child eats a meal.
Temperature; fever	The temperature is how warm or cold your body is; If the temperature is higher (hotter) than usual, you have a fever.
Vomiting	Throwing up

Confusing Terms and Concepts

With any condition, there are likely to be terms or concepts for which patients and families have a different understanding than a health care professional. These may include preventive strategies, complex disease processes, medication or treatment regimens, abstract laboratory results or measurements, technical terms, or words that have a different meaning in the health care arena than in everyday use. Cultural issues and misconceptions can also contribute to lack of understanding.

Consider the following when talking with families about medications:

Communications Issues

Parents may not fully understand the instructions you give them with regard to their child's medicine. So write down important instructions clearly. Using words and pictures, or pictograms such as the one on the right, can help. This pictogram illustrates the concept of "3 times a day" with text in English and Spanish.

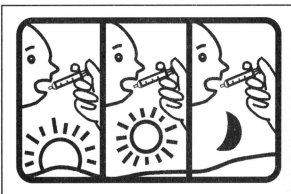

Take **3 times a day** by mouth

Tome **3 veces al día** por la boca

Consider having someone translate common instructions into other languages used in your area so you can show parents the instructions you want the patient to follow.

Confusion about dosing schedules can be caused by vague instructions on prescription labels (eg, 3 times a day).

For medications that must be given multiple times in a day, work out a written schedule with the parents. Avoid the more vague "breakfast, lunch, dinner, and bedtime" instructions, because dinner and bedtime might be too close together, particularly for very young children. Instead, instruct them to give the medicine at 8:00 am, noon, 4:00 pm, and 8:00 pm.

Parents may be confused about the meaning of the word "day."

For example, explain that "3 times a day" means 3 times before the child goes to sleep at night.

When medication needs to be given, even during the middle

Cultural Spotlight

Perceptions About Medicine

Families have varied attitudes toward medications, regardless of their ethnic or cultural background.

On the one hand, some families worry about giving too much medication, especially in cases where preventive medicines are prescribed, such as controller medicines for asthma or for attention-deficit/hyperactivity disorder. They may worry about the potential side effects or that their child will become "addicted."

On the other hand, some families want medications, instead of following other lifestyle recommendations like dietary changes for obesity, or they want antibiotics for viral infections.

There may be a misperception that if some medicine works for a condition, then more medicine will work faster and better. Some patients double the first dose to jump-start the effects. Others, if they miss one dose, will double the next one.

Patients also may not understand about potential drug interactions and may not be aware that different over-the-counter medications can contain the same active ingredient (eg, Tylenol and Tylenol Cold and Sinus).

This creates the potential for overdosing on a medication, or not getting enough of another.

Because every family has different ideas about medications, try to uncover misperceptions they may have before they leave your office.

A Few Words From the American Academy of Pediatrics

About Cough Medicine

In 2004 to 2005 an estimated 1,519 children younger than 2 years were treated for adverse events from over-the-counter cold and cough medications. Also in 2005, the Centers for Disease Control and Prevention identified 3 cases of infant deaths that were determined to have been caused by these medications.*

On January 17, 2008, the US Food and Drug Administration (FDA) issued a public health advisory saying that over-the-counter cough and cold medications should *not* be given to children younger than 2 years because of the possibility of serious and life-threatening side effects. The FDA is studying what should be done about these medications for 2- to 11-year-olds.

AAP Position**

- Over-the-counter cough and cold medicines do not work for children younger than 6 years and, in some cases, may pose a health risk.

- The efficacy and risk of such medications needs to be studied in children. As the AAP has testified, "If a medicine will be used in children, it should be studied in children. Cough and cold medications should not be exceptions to this rule."

- The labeling needs to reflect what we know: The medications are not effective for children younger than 6 years and their use and misuse could cause serious, adverse side effects.

- Dosage information for these cough and cold medicines is based on adult experience. But children are NOT little adults, and studies show their bodies handle the medications differently. That alone raises the risk of dosing errors.

- While the FDA action is a start, more needs to be done; the medications' efficacy and risks need to be studied in older children.

* Infant deaths associated with cough and cold medications—two states, 2005. *MMWR Morb Mortal Weekly Rep.* 2007;56(1):1–4.

** AAP Committee on Drugs. The use of codeine and dextromethorphan-containing cough remedies in children. *Pediatrics.* 1997;99:918–920.

of the night (ie, 24 hours a day), the prescription will read "give every 8 hours," and you should explain that you want the parent to wake the child up to give the medicine.

Some families may not be able to afford the medicines, so they don't fill the prescriptions you give them, or they don't give the child enough medicine, hoping to stretch it out.

Let families know that if they have any problems filling the prescription (due to cost or questions that emerge) they should call your office right away. There are programs that can help with free or discounted medications.

Sometimes people stop giving the medication because it looks different than what they are used to (eg, different generic versions of the same medication may look different). Ensuring that patients call or ask the pharmacist if the medicine looks different will help avoid this.

Adherence to steroids may be poor because parents confuse them with sports-enhancing hormones, which are also called steroids. Parents have concerns about addiction or using medications when they don't appear to be needed.

Explain that the kinds and amount of steroids used for diseases like asthma are not the same as the steroids parents may have heard about on the news. When applicable, tell parents that the medications in this dosage are not addictive, and they do not make the child feel "high." The child must have these medicines so he or she can stay healthy.

Stress the importance of completing a full course of antibiotics, because it's hard for some parents to understand the concept of giving medicine to a child who feels fine.

- Alfie must take all of the medicine [or take it for a certain number of days (or doses)] for the medicine to do its job and keep him healthy.
- Even though Inge will start feeling better in 2 or 3 days, you must give her the medicine for 10 days straight so we can make sure we kill all the germs that made her sick.

Behavior Change

Behavior change is a key element in preventing and managing many pediatric conditions. Shifting from paternalistic advice that is either too vague or too complicated to a patient- or family-centered approach that incorporates elements of motivational interviewing and goal-setting, and that makes use of plain language, can be an effective way to empower patients and families to make changes and improve their health.

Remind parents to store medicines according to instructions (which can include keeping them in the refrigerator, or a dark place, etc), but *always* out of their children's reach.

Make sure the parent and child know the best ways to measure and administer the medicine. Explain that an ordinary spoon isn't a good measure for medicine, and remind parents to ask the pharmacist for a measuring spoon or dropper to make sure they can give the correct dose of medicine. Demonstrate how to use other tools (like syringes, dosing spoons, or droppers), and show them the best ways to make sure the child takes all the medicine prescribed. For some parents, it may be better for you to provide the dosing tool so you can be sure they receive it and really understand how to use it.

Child Involvement

Including the child, to the extent possible, is respectful and patient-centered and can contribute to developing health literacy skills as the child moves toward managing his or her own health as an adolescent and an adult. It can include direct, age-appropriate statements to the child, and also ways for the child to be involved in his or her health.

Messages for Young Children

- This medicine will help you feel better.
- Medicines are not candy.

Involving School-aged Children

School-aged children are curious and interested in understanding how things work and why things happen. They should be given information about the medication they are taking including

- What are medicines? What kind of medicine am I taking and how do I take or use it?
- Why am I taking this medicine?
- How do I take the medicine? What is the dose, when do I take it, how do I store it, and how is it going to make me feel (including side effects)?
- Make sure they take home this key point: My parents will be giving me the medicine. I should not be taking it myself unless my parents tell me to do so.

Treating Adolescents

Studies have demonstrated that adolescents report beginning to self-administer medication between the ages of 11 and 12 years.[5] Therefore, it is critical to give educational information about medication that is age-appropriate to young teens.

- Take-home messages for adolescents
  - Ask your parents before you take medicine.

Did You Know...?

Remember...

Adolescents comprise a significant population that uses over-the-counter (OTC) medications.

One international survey found that in the United States, 48% of boys between ages 11 and 15 and 66% of girls had taken an OTC medication for headache at least once in the previous month, and 20% of boys and 35% of girls the same age had taken OTCs for stomach pain.

Girls' overall use of OTCs increased with age for headaches and stomach pain, and boys' use increased with age for headaches.

Source: Hansen EH, Holstein BE , Due P, Currie CE. International survey of self-reported medicine use among adolescents. *Ann Pharmacother.* 2003; 37(3):361–366.

- Know the possible side effects and risks of overdose.
- Read medication labels.
- Never take medicines offered to you by friends or share your medicines with others.

Teach-back

The concept of teaching back entails asking parents or patients to demonstrate understanding *using their own words*, not simply asking whether they have questions or whether they understand, because that may not elicit lack of understanding. Having patients explain in their own words not only assesses their understanding, but it reinforces the information by repeating it and internalizes it for the patient. When there is a lot of information, go over each concept and elicit a teach-back before moving to the next idea.

When using teach-back, it's important to keep the burden on yourself. Avoid the perception that you are quizzing the parent or patient—emphasize that you just want to be sure you've explained things clearly. The practice of using teach-back can be especially important over the phone, because it may be the only way to gauge whether the parent or patient understands.

Here are some approaches to using teach-back when talking about medication.

- Just to be sure I explained things clearly, how will you give this medicine when you get home?
- What will you tell Stewart's child care provider about when he needs his medicine and how to give it?
- How many times a day will Jocelyn receive her medicine? For how long?
- Can you please show me how much medicine you will give Rene for her fever?
- Using an inhaler the first time is harder than it sounds. To be sure I explained it well and make sure you get the medicine you need—and in the right place—can you please show me how you will use your inhaler?

Key Messages for Use by All Members of the Health Care Team

It is important to reinforce key messages for parents and children so they hear them more than once, and recognize them as priorities in managing their health. In addition, families should not receive conflicting advice about their health and what to do.

Key concepts for medication[2] are

- Before you leave the clinic or the pharmacy, make sure you understand what medicines your child should take, how to take them, and why.
- Read the label, or ask someone to read it to you.
  - Make sure you follow the directions.
  - Make sure the medicine is for your child.
- Give the correct amount or dose.
  - Giving more medicine will not make your child better faster.
  - If you give less, your child may not get better.
- Give it the correct way.
  - If the label says to take the medicine by mouth or with food, give it that way.
- Put the medicine away in a safe place, away from children, after you give the dose. Find out from your doctor or pharmacist whether you need to keep the medicine in a refrigerator or dark place.
- Write down the time you gave the medicine to your child.
  - You may need to check the time later on.
- Watch for side effects like feeling tired, feeling dizzy, or having a rash.
  - Side effects can happen often or not at all.
- Give the medicine for as long as the doctor tells you to.
  - For some medicines it is important to give all of it even if your child feels better before it is finished.
- Call the clinic or ask your pharmacist if you are not sure about how to give the medicine, or if you have any questions.

Miscellaneous

One way to make sure parents are administering medications appropriately is through a medication review, in which you ask them to bring all medications they give the child, and then have them explain exactly how and when they give them. This is helpful for all patients, but especially for those with chronic illnesses requiring daily medicines, or complex medical problems requiring multiple medications.

In addition to helping with medication reconciliation and identifying duplications or drug-drug interactions, medication reviews can help in 2 ways.

1. To determine if the parent is dosing medicines correctly and as prescribed. Ask, "What do you use to measure how much medicine to give?"

2. To identify parents with low literacy, who—instead of reading the label on the bottle—might instead open it and look inside the bottle at the color/shape of a pill. You might also ask, "How do you know which medicine is which?"

Medication reviews can be done by nursing staff or medical assistants and then reviewed by the provider. Nurses and health educators can also explain to parents what the parts of the prescription label mean. This can be done using a sample bottle or with a pictogram, such as the one below.

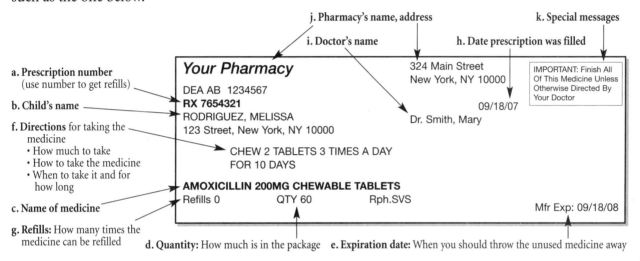

For OTC medications, refer patients to the drug facts label. This label is required by law to have a standard format and content for all OTC medications. In plain language, the label includes

- Product Name: Name of medicine

- Active Ingredients: The part that makes the medicine work, and how much medicine is in each pill or teaspoon (5 mL)

- Purpose: Type of medicine (such as antihistamine, antacid, or cough suppressant)

- Uses: What the medicine treats or prevents

- Warnings: When not to use it, when to stop taking it, when to see a doctor, and how the medicine might make you feel

- Directions: How much to take, how to take it, and how long to take it

- Other Information: Such as where to keep the medicine

- Inactive Ingredients: Other things the medicine has in it. They don't make the medicine work, but can make it last longer, taste better, etc.

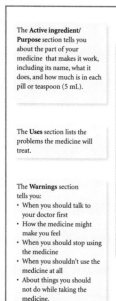

The **Active ingredient/ Purpose** section tells you about the part of your medicine that makes it work, including its name, what it does, and how much is in each pill or teaspoon (5 mL).

The **Uses** section lists the problems the medicine will treat.

The **Warnings** section tells you:
• When you should talk to your doctor first
• How the medicine might make you feel
• When you should stop using the medicine
• When you shouldn't use the medicine at all
• About things you should not do while taking the medicine.

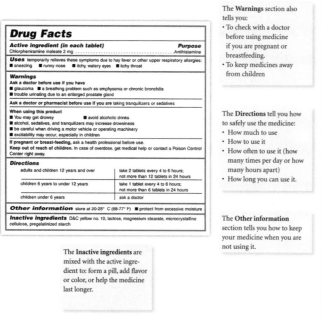

Drug Facts

Active ingredient (in each tablet) **Purpose**
Chlorpheniramine maleate 2 mg . . . . Antihistamine

Uses temporarily relieves these symptoms due to hay fever or other upper respiratory allergies:
■ sneezing ■ runny nose ■ itchy, watery eyes ■ itchy throat

Warnings
Ask a doctor before use if you have
■ glaucoma ■ a breathing problem such as emphysema or chronic bronchitis
■ trouble urinating due to an enlarged prostate gland

Ask a doctor or pharmacist before use if you are taking tranquilizers or sedatives

When using this product
■ You may get drowsy   ■ avoid alcoholic drinks
■ alcohol, sedatives, and tranquilizers may increase drowsiness
■ be careful when driving a motor vehicle or operating machinery
■ excitability may occur, especially in children

If pregnant or breast-feeding, ask a health professional before use.
Keep out of reach of children. In case of overdose, get medical help or contact a Poison Control Center right away.

Directions

adults and children 12 years and over	take 2 tablets every 4 to 6 hours; not more than 12 tablets in 24 hours
children 6 years to under 12 years	take 1 tablet every 4 to 6 hours; not more than 6 tablets in 24 hours
children under 6 years	ask a doctor

Other information store at 20-25° C (68-77° F) ■ protect from excessive moisture

Inactive ingredients D&C yellow no. 10, lactose, magnesium stearate, microcrystalline cellulose, pregelatinized starch

The **Inactive ingredients** are mixed with the active ingredient to: form a pill, add flavor or color, or help the medicine last longer.

The **Warnings** section also tells you:
• To check with a doctor before using medicine if you are pregnant or breastfeeding.
• To keep medicines away from children

The **Directions** tell you how to safely use the medicine:
• How much to use
• How to use it
• How often to use it (how many times per day or how many hours apart)
• How long you can use it.

The **Other information** section tells you how to keep your medicine when you are not using it.

Further information can be obtained through the FDA Web site (http://www.fda.gov/cder/medsinmyhome), which includes an interactive educational program about safe use of OTC medications appropriate for sixth to eighth graders and adults with literacy challenges. The site also includes pamphlets you can download and print out for your patients and their families.

The FDA has developed an interactive Web site that teaches about safe use of OTC medications and how to interpret the OTC label that can be used independently by teens, or as part of a curriculum administered through the school: http://www.fda.gov/cder/medsinmyhome.

References

1. Kaushal R, Goldmann DA, Keohane CA, et al. Adverse drug events in pediatric outpatients. *Ambul Pediatr.* 2007;7:383–389

2. US Food and Drug Administration. Use caution with cough and cold medicines for children. http://www.fda.gov/consumer/updates/cold081607.html. Accessed June 20, 2008

3. Used with permission from the NYU School of Medicine HELP Project at Bellevue Hospital's Pediatric Clinic 2008. For more information on the HELP Project go to http://HELPix.med.nyu.edu.

4. Centers for Disease Control and Prevention. Infant deaths associated with cough and cold mediciations—two states, 2005. *MMWR Morb Mortal Wkly Rep.* 2007;56:1–4

5. Medication errors injure 1.5 million people and cost billions of dollars annually; report offers comprehensive strategies for reducing drug-related mistakes [press release]. Washington, DC: Institute of Medicine; July 2006. http://www8.nationalacademies.org/onpinews/newsitem.aspx?RecordID=11623. Accessed April 28, 2008

6. Chambers CT, Reid GJ, McGrath PJ, Finley GA. Self-administration of over-the-counter medication for pain among adolescents. *Arch Pediatr Adolesc Med.* 1997;151(5): 449–455

Handouts: Tracking Your Child's Medicines

Copy the handouts on pages 237 and 238 or develop your own to give your patients and their parents.

The log on page 237 will help patients and parents keep track of medicines to be taken twice day.

The log on page 238 will help patients and parents keep track of medicines to be taken 3 times a day.

✓ **Communication Tip**

Consider copying and laminating the drug facts label to use as a teaching tool with your patients.

Keeping track of your child's medicine

Name: _____

Name of medicine: _____

| Directions: _____ by mouth |
| 2 times a day for ___ days |

Date medicine started: _____

Circle the starting dose and ending dose. Check (√) the correct box each time you give your child the medicine.

Anotando las dosis de la medicina de su niño

Nombre: _____

Nombre de la medicina: _____

| Instrucciones: _____ por la boca |
| 2 veces al día por ___ días |

Día que empezó la medicina: _____

Marcar con un círculo la primera y la última dosis. Marcar (√) la casilla correcta cada vez que le dé la medicina.

Day / Día	☀	🌙
Time / Hora:		
Monday / Lunes		
Tuesday / Martes		
Wednesday / Miércoles		
Thursday / Jueves		
Friday / Viernes		
Saturday / Sábado		
Sunday / Domingo		
Monday / Lunes		
Tuesday / Martes		
Wednesday / Miércoles		
Thursday / Jueves		
Friday / Viernes		
Saturday / Sábado		
Sunday / Domingo		
Monday / Lunes		
Tuesday / Martes		
Wednesday / Miércoles		
Thursday / Jueves		
Friday / Viernes		
Saturday / Sábado		
Sunday / Domingo		

The H.E.L.P. Project   Bellevue Hospital   Pediatric Clinic
© 2008 New York University School of Medicine

Keeping track of your child's medicine

Name: _____

Name of medicine: _____

Directions: _____ by mouth
3 times a day for ___ days

Date medicine started: _____

Circle the starting dose and ending dose. Check (✓) the correct box each time you give your child the medicine.

Anotando las dosis de la medicina de su niño

Nombre: _____

Nombre de la medicina: _____

Instrucciones: _____ por la boca
3 veces al día por ___ días

Día que empezó la medicina: _____

Marcar con un círculo la primera y la última dosis. Marcar (✓) la casilla correcta cada vez que le dé la medicina.

Day / Día			
Time / Hora:			
Monday / Lunes			
Tuesday / Martes			
Wednesday / Miércoles			
Thursday / Jueves			
Friday / Viernes			
Saturday / Sábado			
Sunday / Domingo			
Monday / Lunes			
Tuesday / Martes			
Wednesday / Miércoles			
Thursday / Jueves			
Friday / Viernes			
Saturday / Sábado			
Sunday / Domingo			
Monday / Lunes			
Tuesday / Martes			
Wednesday / Miércoles			
Thursday / Jueves			
Friday / Viernes			
Saturday / Sábado			
Sunday / Domingo			

The H.E.L.P. Project   Bellevue Hospital   Pediatric Clinic
© 2008 New York University School of Medicine

Prescription Medicines and Your Child

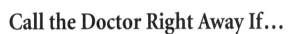

There are 2 types of medicines you can buy: 1) over-the-counter (OTC) medicines and 2) prescription medicines. OTC medicines are those you can buy without a doctor's order. Prescription medicines are those you can only buy with a doctor's order (a prescription). This handout is about prescription medicines.

Ask the Doctor or Pharmacist

Many parents have questions about their children's prescription medicines. Labels can be hard to read and understand. But it's important to give medicines the right way for your child's health and safety.

Before you give your child any medicine, be sure you know how to use them. Here are some questions you can ask the doctor or **pharmacist***:

- How will this medicine help my child?
- How much medicine do I give my child? When? For how long?
- Should my child take this medicine with food or on an empty stomach?
- Are there any **side effects*** from this medicine?
- How can I learn more about this medicine?
- When will the medicine begin to work?
- What should I do if my child misses a dose?
- What if my child spits it out?
- Can this prescription be refilled? If so, how many times?

Also, always tell your child's doctor:

- If your child is taking any other medicines (even OTC medicines) and
- If your child has any reactions to the medicines.

Call the Doctor Right Away If…

…your child throws up a lot or gets a rash after taking any medicine. Even if a medicine is safe for other children, your child may be **allergic*** to it.

Your child *may or may not* have side effects with any drug. Be sure to tell the doctor if your child has any side effects with a medicine.

Read the Label

Here is what the parts of a prescription label mean. (See example on second page of this handout.)

a. **Prescription number.** Your pharmacy will ask for this number when you call for a refill.

b. **Your child's name.**

c. **Name of the medicine.** Make sure this matches what your child's doctor told you. The strength of the medicine may also be listed (for example, 10 mg tablets).

d. **QTY.** "Quantity" or how much is in the package.

e. **Expiration date (Mfr Exp).** The medicine in this package will only work until this date. Throw away any medicine left after this date.

✳ *Words to Know*

allergic (uh-LER-jik)—to have a bad reaction to something that doesn't bother most people. For example, some people may get hives if they are stung by a bee.

pharmacist (FARM-uh-sist)—a person who has special training to fill prescriptions and teach people about their medicines.

side effects—symptoms that come from taking a drug and are not part of the treatment. For example, some medicines can make you feel sick to your stomach.

Continued on back

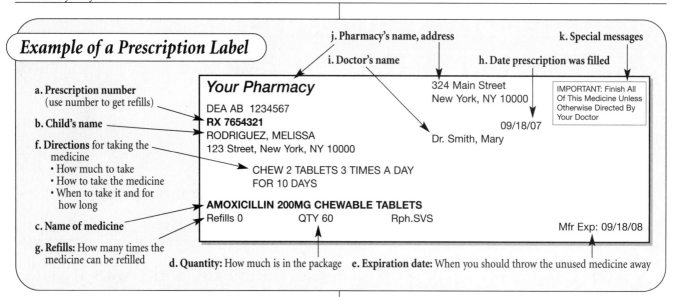

Example of a Prescription Label

a. **Prescription number** (use number to get refills)

b. **Child's name**

f. **Directions** for taking the medicine
• How much to take
• How to take the medicine
• When to take it and for how long

c. **Name of medicine**

g. **Refills:** How many times the medicine can be refilled

j. **Pharmacy's name, address**

i. **Doctor's name**

k. **Special messages**

h. **Date prescription was filled**

Your Pharmacy

DEA AB 1234567
RX 7654321
RODRIGUEZ, MELISSA
123 Street, New York, NY 10000

CHEW 2 TABLETS 3 TIMES A DAY
FOR 10 DAYS

AMOXICILLIN 200MG CHEWABLE TABLETS
Refills 0   QTY 60   Rph.SVS

324 Main Street
New York, NY 10000

09/18/07

Dr. Smith, Mary

IMPORTANT: Finish All Of This Medicine Unless Otherwise Directed By Your Doctor

Mfr Exp: 09/18/08

d. **Quantity:** How much is in the package   e. **Expiration date:** When you should throw the unused medicine away

---

f. **Directions.** This tells you how your child needs to take the medicine and what it is for. The label should match what your child's doctor told you.

Here are some examples:

• **"Take 4 times a day."** Give the medicine to your child 4 times during the day. For example, at breakfast, lunch, dinner, and before bed.

• **"Take every 4 hours."** Give the medicine to your child every 4 hours. This adds up to 6 times in a 24-hour period. For example, 6:00 am, 10:00 am, 2:00 pm, 6:00 pm, 10:00 pm, and 2:00 am. Most medicines don't have to be given at the exact time to work, but some do.

• **"Take as needed as symptoms persist."** Give the medicine to your child only when needed.

• **"Take with food."** Give the medicine to your child after a meal. This is for medicines that work better when the stomach is full.

g. **Refills.** The label will show the number of refills you can get. "No refills—Dr. authorization required" or "0" means you need to call your child's doctor if you need more. The doctor may want to check your child before ordering more medicine.

h. **Date prescription was filled.**

i. **Doctor's name.**

j. **Pharmacy's name, address.**

k. **Special messages.** The medicine may have extra bright-colored labels with special messages. For example, you may see, "Keep refrigerated," "Shake well before using," or "May cause drowsiness." Be sure to ask if you don't understand what they mean.

Tips

• **Use safety caps.** Always use child-resistant caps.

• **Store medicines in a locked, childproof cupboard** if you have children at home.

• **Store medicines in a cool, dry place.** Wetness can hurt medicines. So don't store them in a bathroom. Some medicines need to be kept in a refrigerator.

• **Never let your child take medicine alone.** Don't call medicine "candy." (If you do, your child may try to eat some when you're not around.)

• **Watch your child carefully.** Children can find medicine where you least expect it. Your child might find it in a visitor's purse or at other people's homes. On moving day, medicines and poisons may be out where children can find them.

To learn more, visit the American Academy of Pediatrics (AAP) Web site at www.aap.org.

Your child's doctor will tell you to do what's best for your child.
This information should not take the place of talking with your child's doctor.

Adaptation of the AAP information in this handout into plain language was supported in part by McNeil Consumer Healthcare.

American Academy of Pediatrics

DEDICATED TO THE HEALTH OF ALL CHILDREN™

Medicinas recetadas para su niño
(Prescription Medicines and Your Child)

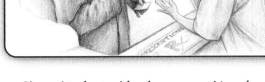

Existen dos tipos de medicinas que usted puede comprar:

1) Medicinas de venta sin receta médica: Estas son las que usted puede comprar sin que se las ordene el doctor.

2) Medicinas recetadas. Estas son las que solamente puede comprar con la receta que le da el doctor (una prescripción).

Este folleto se refiere a las medicinas con receta médica.

Pregúntele al doctor o al farmacéutico

Muchos padres tienen preguntas acerca de las medicinas recetadas para sus niños. Las etiquetas pueden ser difíciles de leer y de entender. Pero es importante darle a su niño las medicinas en la forma correcta.

Antes de darle a su niño cualquier medicina, asegúrese de saber cómo usarlas. Estas son algunas de las preguntas que puede hacerle al doctor o al **farmacéutico***:

- ¿Cómo ayudará a mi niño esta medicina?
- ¿Qué cantidad de medicina debo darle a mi niño? ¿Cuándo? ¿Por cuánto tiempo?
- ¿Debe mi niño tomar esta medicina acompañada con alimentos o con el estómago vacío?
- ¿Cuáles son los **efectos secundarios*** de esta medicina?
- ¿Dónde puedo obtener más información?
- ¿Cuándo comenzará a tener efecto?
- ¿Qué debo hacer si mi niño no toma una dosis?
- ¿Qué pasa si mi niño la escupe?
- ¿Se puede renovar esta receta? De ser así, ¿cuántas veces?

Siempre dígale al doctor de su niño:

- Si su niño está tomando otras medicinas incluyendo las que se compran sin receta.
- Si su niño ha tenido alguna reacción a las medicinas.

Llame al doctor de inmediato si...

...su niño vomita mucho o tiene alguna erupción después de tomar cualquier medicina. Puede ser que su niño sea **alérgico*** a esa medicina.

Lea la etiqueta

La etiqueta de la medicina le indica lo siguiente:

(Vea el ejemplo en la segunda página de este folleto).

a. **Número de la receta médica.** Su farmacia le pedirá este número cuando usted llame para que le renueven la medicina.

b. **Nombre de su niño.**

c. **Nombre de la medicina.** Asegúrese que sea la medicina que el doctor de su niño le recetó. Además del nombre de la medicina, la potencia puede estar especificada (por ejemplo, tabletas de 10 mg).

d. **"Cantidad"** cuánta medicina hay en el envase.

e. **Fecha de vencimiento (Mfr Exp).** La medicina solamente deberá usarse antes de la fecha de vencimiento. Descarte el resto.

f. **Instrucciones.** Esto le indica como darle la medicina a su niño. La etiqueta debe coincidir con lo que el doctor de su niño le dijo.

✳ Palabras que debe conocer

alérgico: Significa tener una mala reacción a algo que no causa problemas en la mayoría de personas. Por ejemplo, algunas personas pueden tener sarpullido si les pica una abeja.

farmacéutico: Es la persona que tiene un entrenamiento especial para preparar recetas médicas y enseñar al público acerca de sus medicinas.

efectos secundarios: Son reacciones causadas por el uso de una medicina. Por ejemplo, algunas medicinas causan dolor de estómago.

Continua atrás

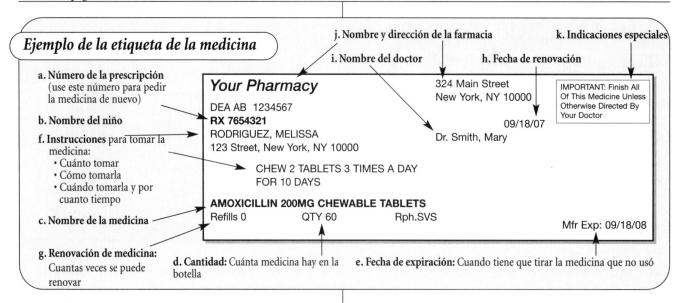

Ejemplo de la etiqueta de la medicina

a. Número de la prescripción
(use este número para pedir la medicina de nuevo)

b. Nombre del niño

f. Instrucciones para tomar la medicina:
- Cuánto tomar
- Cómo tomarla
- Cuándo tomarla y por cuanto tiempo

c. Nombre de la medicina

g. Renovación de medicina:
Cuantas veces se puede renovar

j. Nombre y dirección de la farmacia

i. Nombre del doctor

k. Indicaciones especiales

h. Fecha de renovación

Your Pharmacy
DEA AB 1234567
RX 7654321
RODRIGUEZ, MELISSA
123 Street, New York, NY 10000

CHEW 2 TABLETS 3 TIMES A DAY
FOR 10 DAYS

AMOXICILLIN 200MG CHEWABLE TABLETS
Refills 0   QTY 60   Rph.SVS

324 Main Street
New York, NY 10000

09/18/07
Dr. Smith, Mary

IMPORTANT: Finish All Of This Medicine Unless Otherwise Directed By Your Doctor

Mfr Exp: 09/18/08

d. Cantidad: Cuánta medicina hay en la botella

e. Fecha de expiración: Cuando tiene que tirar la medicina que no usó

Por ejemplo:

- **"Tómela 4 veces al día"**. Por ejemplo, con en el desayuno, almuerzo, cena y antes de ir a dormir.

- **"Tómela cada 4 horas"**. En este caso dele la medicina a su niño 6 veces en un período de 24 horas. Por ejemplo, 6:00 am, 10:00 am, 2:00 pm, 6:00 pm, 10:00 pm y 2:00 am. La mayoría de medicinas no tienen que darse a la hora exacta para hacer efecto, pero algunas sí.

- **"Tómela mientras los síntomas persisten"**. Dele la medicina sólo cuando su niño la necesita.

- **"Tómela con alimentos"**. Dele la medicina después de una comida. Algunas medicinas hacen mejor efecto cuando el estómago está lleno.

- **g. Renovación.** La etiqueta mostrará el número de veces que puede renovar la medicina antes de ordenar más medicina. "Autorización del doctor requerida" ó "0" significa que usted necesita llamar al doctor de su niño si necesita más medicina. Puede ser que el doctor quiera revisar al niño para asegurarse que todavía necesita la medicina.

- **h. Fecha en que le dieron la medicina de la receta.**

- **i. Nombre del doctor.**

- **j. Nombre y dirección de la farmacia.**

- **k. Indicaciones especiales.**
La medicina puede tener etiquetas de colores brillantes con mensajes especiales. Por ejemplo, "Manténgase refrigerado",

"Agítese bien antes de usar", o "Puede ocasionar sueño". Si no entiende las indicaciones en la receta consulte con el farmacéutico.

Consejos

- **Siempre use tapas a pruebas de niños.**

- **Guarde las medicinas bajo llave,** o en un mueble que los niños no puedan abrir.

- **Guarde las medicinas en un lugar fresco y seco.** La humedad puede dañar las medicinas. Algunas medicinas tienen que guardarse en el refrigerador (nevera).

- **Nunca deje que su niño tome la medicina solo.** Nunca le diga a sus niños que las medicinas son "dulces o caramelos". (Si lo hace, su niño querrá comerlos cuando usted no está).

- **Observe a su niño con cuidado.** Los niños son capaces de encontrar medicinas donde usted menos lo espera. Por ejemplo en el bolso de un visitante o en la casa de otros.

Para aprender más, visite el sitio de la Academia Americana de Pediatría (AAP) en www.aap.org.
Su pediatra le dirá qué es lo mejor para la salud de su hijo.
Esta información no debe usarse en lugar de consultar con su doctor.
La adaptación de la información de este folleto de la AAP a lenguaje sencillo se hizo con el apoyo de McNeil Consumer Healthcare. La traducción al español fue patrocinada por Leyendo Juntos (Reach Out and Read), un programa pediátrico de alfabetización.

© 2008 Academia Americana de Pediatría

American Academy of Pediatrics
DEDICATED TO THE HEALTH OF ALL CHILDREN™

Using Liquid Medicines

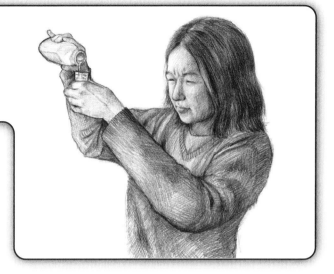

Many children's medicines come in liquid form. Liquid medicines are easier to swallow than pills. But they must be used the right way.

Types of Liquid Medicines

There are 2 types of liquid medicines:

- Medicines you can buy without a doctor's prescription (called over-the-counter or OTC)
- Medicines a doctor prescribes

OTC Medicines

All OTC medicines have the same kind of label. The label gives important information about the medicine. It says what it is for, how to use it, what is in it, and what to watch out for. Look on the box or bottle, where it says **"Drug Facts."**

Check the chart on the label to see how much medicine to give. If you know your child's weight, use that first. If not, go by age. **Check the label to make sure it is safe for infants and toddlers younger than 2 years.** If you are not sure, ask your child's doctor.

Prescription Liquid Medicines

Your child's doctor may prescribe a liquid medicine. These medicines will have a different label than OTC medicines. Always read the label before you give the medicine to your child.

With OTC or prescription medicines, be sure to call your child's doctor or **pharmacist*** if you have any questions about:

- How much medicine to give.
- How often to give it.
- How long to give it.

✳ Word to Know

pharmacist (FARM-uh-sist)—a person who has special training to fill prescriptions and teach people about their medicines.

A Word About Infant Drops

Infant drops are stronger than syrup for toddlers. Parents may make the mistake of giving higher doses of infant drops to a toddler, thinking the drops are not as strong. Be sure the medicine you give your child is right for his or her weight and age.

How to Give Liquid Medicines

Follow the directions exactly. Some parents give their children too much medicine. This will not help them get better faster. And it can be very dangerous, especially if you give too much for several days. Always read the label carefully.

How to Measure Liquid Medicines

Use the dropper, syringe (sir-INJ), medicine cup, or dosing spoon that comes with the medicine. If nothing comes with your medicine, ask your pharmacist for help. Kitchen tablespoons or teaspoons are usually not the right size.

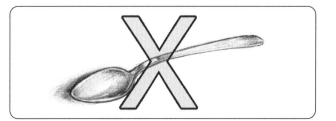

Continued on back

Medicine can be measured in different ways. You may see teaspoon (tsp), Tablespoon (Tbsp or TBSP), or milliliters (mL, ml, or mLs).

Tips

1 teaspoon (tsp) = 5 milliliters (mL)

3 teaspoons (tsp) = 1 Tablespoon (TBSP)

1 Tablespoon (TBSP) = 15 milliliters (mL)

Medicine Cups

Be sure to use the cup that comes with the medicine. These often come over the lids of liquid

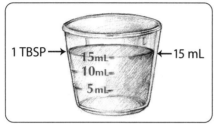

1 Tablespoon (TBSP) is the same as 15 mL.

cold and flu medicines. Don't mix and match cups to different products. You might end up giving the wrong amount.

Don't just fill it up. Look carefully at the lines and letters on the cup. Use the numbers to fill the cup to the right line. Ask your pharmacist to mark the right line for *your* child if you are not sure. Be sure the cup is level. You can check by putting it on a flat surface.

Dosing Spoons

These work well for older children who can "drink" from the spoon. Use only the spoon that comes with the medicine. Be sure to use the lines and numbers to get the right amount for *your* child. Or ask your pharmacist to mark the right line if you are not sure.

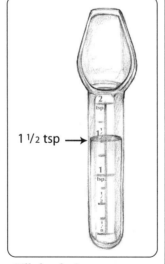

Fill the dosing spoon while holding it upright.

Droppers or Syringes

Don't just fill the dropper or syringe to the top. Read the directions carefully to see how much to give *your* child. Look at the numbers on the side of the dropper or syringe. Use the numbers to fill it to the right line. Or ask your pharmacist to mark the right line if you are not sure. (If the syringe has a cap, throw it away before you use it. The cap could choke your child.)

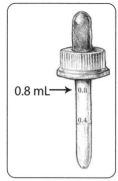

In this example, a dropper-full is the same as 0.8 mL.

Don't put the medicine in the back of the throat. This could choke your child. Instead, squirt it gently between your child's tongue and the side of the mouth. This makes it easier to swallow.

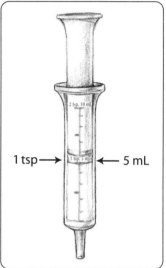

1 teaspoon (tsp) is the same as 5 mL.

To learn more, visit the American Academy of Pediatrics (AAP) Web site at www.aap.org.

Your child's doctor will tell you to do what's best for your child.
This information should not take the place of talking with your child's doctor.

Adaptation of the AAP information in this handout into plain language was supported in part by McNeil Consumer Healthcare.

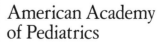

American Academy of Pediatrics

DEDICATED TO THE HEALTH OF ALL CHILDREN™

El uso de medicinas líquidas (Using Liquid Medicines)

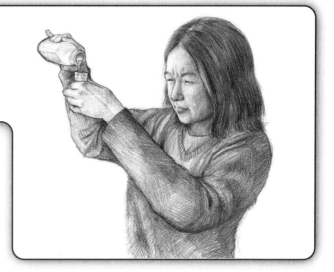

Muchas de las medicinas para niños vienen en forma líquida. Las medicinas líquidas son más fáciles de tragar que las pastillas. Estas medicinas deben usarse en forma correcta.

Tipos de medicinas líquidas

Hay 2 tipos de medicinas líquidas:

- Las medicinas que se compran sin receta (llamadas medicinas de venta sin receta médica).
- Las medicinas recetadas.

Las medicinas de venta sin receta médica

Las medicinas de venta sin receta tienen el mismo tipo de etiqueta. Allí se encuentra la información importante sobre la medicina. Esta le indica para qué sirve, cómo se usa y las precauciones que deben tomarse al usar la medicina. Lea la etiqueta donde dice **"Drug Facts"** (Propiedades de la medicina).

Lea la etiqueta para ver cuánta medicina debe darle al niño. Si sabe el peso de su niño, primero guíese por ese dato. Si no lo sabe, guíese por la edad. **Lea la etiqueta para confirmar que la medicina sea segura para bebés y para niños menores de 2 años.** Si no está seguro, consulte con el doctor de su niño.

Las medicinas líquidas con receta médica

Puede ser que el doctor de su niño le recete una medicina líquida. Siempre lea la etiqueta antes de darle la medicina.

Llame al doctor de su niño o al **farmacéutico*** si tiene alguna pregunta sobre:

- Cuánta medicina debe darle al niño.
- Con qué frecuencia debe dárlsela.
- Por cuánto tiempo debe dárlsela.

La medicina en gotas para bebés

Las gotas para los bebés contienen más medicación que la misma cantidad de jarabe. Si usted usa las gotas en lugar del jarabe le dará a su niño demasiada medicina. Asegúrese de que la medicina que usted le da a su niño sea la apropiada para su peso y su edad.

Cómo dar las medicinas líquidas

Siga bien las indicaciones. Algunos padres les dan a sus niños demasiada medicina. Esto no ayuda a que se sientan mejor más rápido. Y puede ser muy peligroso, especialmente si le da mucha medicina durante varios días. Siempre lea la etiqueta con cuidado.

Cómo debe medir las medicinas líquidas

Utilice el gotero, la jeringa, la copita o la cuchara medidora que viene con la medicina. Si no viene ningún medidor con su medicina, pídale a su farmacéutico que le ayude. Las cucharas o cucharitas de la cocina generalmente no son exactas para medir medicinas.

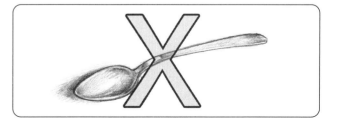

---

* Palabra que debe conocer

farmacéutico: La persona que tiene un entrenamiento especial para preparar recetas médicas e informar a la gente acerca de sus medicinas.

Continúa atrás

Viene de la página anterior

La medicina puede medirse de diferentes formas. Se puede medir en cucharaditas (tsp), cucharadas (Tbsp ó TBSP), o mililitros (mL, ml, ó mLs).

Consejos

1 cucharadita (tsp) = 5 mililitros (mL)

3 cucharaditas (tsp) = 1 cucharada (TBSP)

1 cucharada (TBSP) = 15 mililitros (mL)

Copitas para medir la medicina

Asegúrese de utilizar la copita que viene con la medicina. Éstas a menudo vienen sobre la tapa de las medicinas líquidas.

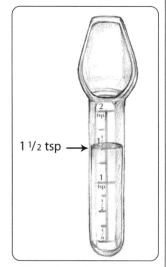

1 cucharada (TBSP) es igual a 15 mL.

No mezcle o use la misma copita para diferentes productos para evitar dar una cantidad equivocada.

Fíjese en las líneas de la copita para llenarla hasta el nivel correcto. Pídale a su farmacéutico que le marque la línea correcta para *su* niño si usted no está segura.

Cucharas medidoras

Éstas funcionan bien para los niños más grandes que pueden "tomar" de una cuchara. Solamente use la cuchara que viene con la medicina. Asegúrese de usar las líneas y los números para medir la cantidad correcta para su niño. O pídale a su farmacéutico que le marque la línea correcta si usted no está segura.

1 ½ tsp →

Llene la cuchara medidora mientras la sostiene hacia arriba.

Goteros o jeringas

No llene el gotero o la jeringa por completo. Fíjese primero cuanta medicina debe darle a su niño. Use los números en el gotero o jeringa para llenarlo hasta la línea correcta. O pídale al farmacéutico que marque la línea correcta si usted no está seguro. (Si la jeringa tiene tapa, descarte la tapa para que no se atragante su niño).

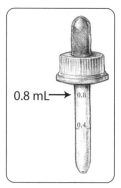

0.8 mL →

En este ejemplo, un gotero lleno es lo mismo que 0.8 mL.

No coloque la medicina hasta adentro de la garganta. Gotee la medicina suavemente entre la lengua y el lado de la boca de su niño. Evite poner la jeringa muy adentro de la garganta para que el niño no se atragante.

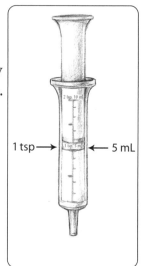

1 tsp → ← 5 mL

1 cucharadita (tsp) es lo mismo que 5 mL

Para aprender más, visite el sitio de la Academia Americana de Pediatría (AAP) en www.aap.org.
Su pediatra le dirá qué es lo mejor para la salud de su hijo.
Esta información no debe usarse en lugar de consultar con su doctor.
La adaptación de la información de este folleto de la AAP a lenguaje sencillo se hizo con el apoyo de McNeil Consumer Healthcare. La traducción al español fue patrocinada por Leyendo Juntos (Reach Out and Read), un programa pediátrico de alfabetización.

American Academy of Pediatrics

DEDICATED TO THE HEALTH OF ALL CHILDREN™

Choosing Over-the-Counter Medicines for Your Child

"Over-the-counter" (OTC) means you can buy the medicine without a doctor's prescription. Talk with your child's doctor or **pharmacist*** before giving your child any medicine, especially the first time.

All OTC medicines have the same kind of label. The label gives important information about the medicine. It says what it is for, how to use it, what is in it, and what to watch out for. Look on the box or bottle, where it says **"Drug Facts."**

Check the chart on the label to see how much medicine to give. If you know your child's weight, use that first. If not, go by age. **Check the label to make sure it is safe for infants and toddlers younger than 2 years.** If you are not sure, ask your child's doctor.

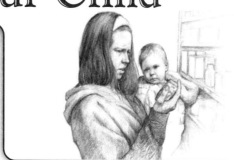

Call the Doctor Right Away If…

…your child throws up a lot or gets a rash after taking any medicine. Even if a medicine is safe, your child may be **allergic*** to it.

Your child *may or may not* have **side effects*** with any drug. Be sure to tell the doctor if your child has any side effects with a medicine.

Over-the-Counter Medicines

Type of Medicine	What It's Used For	What Else You Need to Know
Antihistamine (an-tee-HIS-tuh-meen)	Helps runny nose, itchy eyes, and sneezing from allergies. Also helps with itching from bug bites, hives, or other allergic reactions.	Can make some children sleepy. Other children may become fussy, nervous, or restless.
Aspirin		**Never** give aspirin to your child unless your child's doctor tells you it's safe. Aspirin can cause a very serious liver disease called Reye syndrome. This is especially true when given to children with the flu or chickenpox.
Cough medicine	Helps loosen mucus and phlegm (flem) so your child can cough it up OR calms a cough.	Some cough medicines help loosen mucus. Others calm a cough. Ask your child's doctor if your child needs a cough medicine and which kind to use. Doctors *don't* recommend cough medicine for coughs caused by asthma.

✳ Words to Know

allergic (uh-LER-jik)—to have a bad reaction to something that doesn't bother most people. For example, some people may get hives if they are stung by a bee.

pharmacist (FARM-uh-sist)—a person who has special training to fill prescriptions and teach people about their medicines.

side effects—symptoms that come from taking a drug and are not part of the treatment. For example, some medicines can make you feel sick to your stomach.

Continued on back

Over-the-Counter Medicines *continued*

Type of Medicine	What It's Used For	What Else You Need to Know
Cold medicine	Helps runny nose, fever, and/or cough.	Cold medicines have lots of different medicines in them. They may have antihistamine (an-tee-HIS-tuh-meen), decongestant (dee-kun-JEST-int), cough medicine, and/or fever medicine all mixed together. **Always check to see what's in a cold medicine before you give it.** Make sure you don't give fever medicine to your child *twice*—once in the cold medicine and once by itself. **This could lead to an overdose.**
Decongestant (dee-kun-JEST-int) **(liquid or pills)**	May help some cold symptoms.	Children may become fussy, nervous, or restless. Check with your child's doctor before giving this medicine. Scientists are starting to think it may not help.
Decongestant (nose drops)	Can help make breathing easier.	Never give decongestant nose drops to a baby. See "Saline (saltwater) nose drops" below instead. If your child is sleeping and eating well, there's no need to treat a stuffy nose. If your older child is using them, don't give these drops for more than 2 to 3 days. The more you use them, the less they work. And symptoms can come back worse than before.
Hydrocortisone (high-druh-KOR-tuh-zohn) **or cortisone cream**	Treats insect bites, mild skin rashes, poison ivy, and eczema (EGG-zu-muh).	Ask the doctor how often you can put it on your child's skin. Don't put any on your child's face unless the doctor says it is OK. Never use this cream on burns, infections, cuts, or broken skin.
Pain and fever medicine	Helps fever and headaches or body aches. Also can help with pain from bumps or soreness from a shot.	Examples are acetaminophen (uh-SET-tuh-MIN-uh-fin) and ibuprofen (eye-byoo-PROH-fin). Tylenol is one brand name for acetaminophen. Advil and Motrin are brand names for ibuprofen.
Saline (saltwater) nose drops	May help if your baby is having trouble eating or sleeping because of a stuffy nose.	Put 1 to 2 drops into each side of the nose. Then use a bulb syringe to suck out the drops and mucus. Using a bulb syringe can make the nose sore, so try not to use it too often.
Stomach medicines	Treats problems like heartburn, gas, not being able to pass stool (constipation), or loose, runny stools (diarrhea).	There are different kinds of medicines, depending on what the problem is. Talk with your child's doctor before using any of them. Most of these problems go away on their own. Sometimes just changing your child's diet helps. Some stomach medicines also contain aspirin, which can harm your child. See "Aspirin" on the first page of this handout.

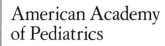

American Academy of Pediatrics

DEDICATED TO THE HEALTH OF ALL CHILDREN™

Elección de medicinas de venta sin receta para su niño (Choosing Over-the-Counter Medicines for Your Child)

La medicinas de "venta sin receta" se pueden comprar sin la orden del doctor. Hable con el doctor de su niño o **farmacéutico*** antes de darle cualquier medicina, especialmente si es por primera vez.

Las medicinas de venta sin receta tienen el mismo tipo de instrucciones en el envase. Esta información indica para qué sirven, cómo se usan, qué contienen y contraindicaciones. Lea la caja o el envase donde dice **"Drug Facts" ("Propiedades de la medicina").**

Lea la etiqueta para saber la cantidad de medicina que debe darle a su niño. Si sabe el peso de su hijo, primero guíese por ese dato. Si no lo sabe, calcule la cantidad de acuerdo a la edad.

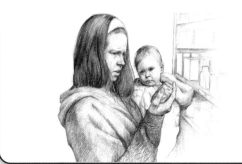

Lea la etiqueta para confirmar que la medicina sea apropiada para bebés y niños menores de 2 años. Si no está seguro, consulte con el doctor de su hijo.

Llame al doctor de inmediato si ...

...su hijo vomita mucho o le sale sarpullido después de tomar la medicina. Dígale a su doctor si el niño tiene efectos secundarios con la medicina.

Medicinas de venta sin receta

Tipo de medicina	Para qué se usa	Qué más debe saber
Antihistamínico	Controla la secreción nasal, la comezón de los ojos y los estornudos provocados por alergias. También controla la comezón por picaduras de insectos, ronchas y otras reacciones alérgicas.	A algunos niños les da sueño. A otros los inquieta o los pone nerviosos o molestos.
Aspirina		**Nunca** le dé aspirina a su hijo, a menos que el doctor le diga que es seguro hacerlo. La aspirina puede provocar una enfermedad muy seria del hígado llamada Síndrome de Reye, especialmente en niños con gripe o varicela.
Medicina para la tos	Ayuda a aflojar la mucosidad y la flema para que su hijo las pueda expulsar. También calma la tos.	Algunas medicinas ayudan a aflojar la mucosidad. Otras calman la tos. Pregúntele al doctor si su hijo necesita una medicina para la tos y qué tipo se debe usar. Los doctores *no* recomiendan usar medicina para la tos cuando ésta es causada por el asma.

✳ Palabras que debe conocer

alérgico: Tiene una mala reacción a algo que no causa problemas en la mayoría de las personas. Por ejemplo, a algunas personas les sale sarpullido cuando les pica una abeja.

farmacéutico: La persona que tiene un entrenamiento especial para preparar recetas y enseñar al público acerca de sus medicinas.

efectos secundarios: Reacciones causadas por el uso de las medicinas. Por ejemplo, algunas medicinas pueden causar dolor de estómago.

Continúa atrás

Medicinas de venta sin receta *(continuación)*

Tipo de medicina	Para qué se usa	Qué más debe saber
Medicina para el resfriado	Controla la secreción nasal, la fiebre y la tos.	Las medicinas para el resfriado contienen mezclas de diferentes medicinas. Pueden incluir: antihistamínicos, descongestionantes, medicinas para la tos o la fiebre. **Antes de administrar una medicina para el resfriado, revise siempre lo que contiene.** Asegúrese de no darle a su hijo medicina para la fiebre dos veces, una vez con la medicina para el resfriado y la otra por separado. **Podría provocar una sobredosis.**
Descongestionante (en líquido o pastillas)	Puede aliviar algunos síntomas del resfriado.	Puede ser que los niños se inquieten o se pongan nerviosos o molestos. Consulte con el doctor sobre su hijo antes de darle esta medicina. No hay evidencia de que estas medicinas le ayuden.
Descongestionante (gotas nasales)	Puede ayudar a mejorar la respiración.	Nunca le aplique gotas nasales descongestionantes a un bebé. Lea más adelante la sección "Gotas salinas (agua con sal) para la nariz". Si su hijo está durmiendo y comiendo bien, no es necesario tratar una nariz tapada. En niños mayores de 2 años, no se las aplique por más de 2 ó 3 días. Mientras más las use, menos funcionarán. Además la congestión nasal podría empeorar.
Hidrocortisona o cortisona en crema	Para el tratamiento de picaduras de insectos, sarpullidos leves, erupción causada por hiedra venenosa y eczema.	Pregúntele al doctor qué tan seguido la puede frotar en la piel de su hijo. No la use en la cara del niño, a menos que el doctor se lo recomiende. Nunca use esta crema sobre quemaduras, infecciones, cortaduras o rasguños en la piel.
Medicina para el dolor y la fiebre	Controla la fiebre, los dolores de cabeza o de cuerpo. También puede aliviar el dolor causado por golpes o inyecciones.	Algunos ejemplos son el acetaminofén y el ibuprofeno. Tylenol es una marca comercial de acetaminofén. Advil y Motrin son marcas comerciales de ibuprofeno.
Gotas salinas (agua con sal) para la nariz	Puede ser útil si su bebé tiene problemas para comer o dormir debido a que tiene la nariz tapada.	Aplique 1 ó 2 gotas en cada fosa nasal. Luego, use una pera succionadora de goma para extraer las gotas y el moco. El uso de una bomba de succión puede irritarle la nariz, así que trate de no usarla con mucha frecuencia.
Medicinas para el estómago	Pueden ser útiles para problemas coma la acidez, exceso de gas, estreñimiento o diarrea.	Existen diferentes tipos de medicinas dependiendo de cuál sea el problema. Consulte con el doctor de su hijo antes de usarlas. La mayoría de estos problemas desaparecen por sí solos. Algunas veces, se resuelven sólo con cambiar la dieta de su hijo. Algunas medicinas para el estómago también contienen aspirina, que puede hacerle daño a su hijo. Lea la sección "Aspirina" en la primera página de este folleto.

Para aprender más, visite el sitio de la Academia Americana de Pediatría (AAP) en www.aap.org. Su pediatra le dirá qué es lo mejor para la salud de su hijo.

Esta información no debe usarse en lugar de consultar con su doctor.

Nota: Los nombres de marca son para su información solamente. La AAP no recomienda ninguna marca o producto de medicina específicamente.

La adaptación de la información de este folleto de la AAP a lenguaje sencillo se hizo con el apoyo de McNeil Consumer Healthcare. La traducción al español fue patrocinada por Leyendo Juntos (Reach Out and Read), un programa pediátrico de alfabetización.

American Academy of Pediatrics

DEDICATED TO THE HEALTH OF ALL CHILDREN™

Using Over-the-Counter Medicines With Your Child

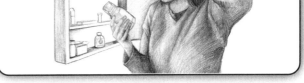

"Over-the-counter" (OTC) means you can buy the medicine without a doctor's prescription. This *doesn't* mean that OTCs are harmless. Like prescription medicines, OTCs can be dangerous if not taken the right way. Talk with your child's doctor before giving your child any medicine, especially the first time.

All OTC medicines have the same kind of label. The label gives important information about the medicine. It says what it is for, how to use it, what is in it, and what to watch out for. Look on the box or bottle, where it says **"Drug Facts."**

Ask the Doctor or Pharmacist

Check the chart on the label to see how much medicine to give. If you know your child's weight, use that first. If not, go by age. **Check the label to make sure it is safe for infants and toddlers younger than 2 years.** If you are not sure, ask your child's doctor.

Before you give your child any medicines, be sure you know how to use them. Here are some questions you can ask the doctor or **pharmacist***:

- How will this medicine help my child?
- Can you show me how to use this medicine?
- How much medicine do I give my child? When? For how long?
- Are there any **side effects*** from this medicine?
- How can I learn more about this medicine?
- What if my child spits it out?
- Does it come in **chewable tablets*** or liquid?

Also, always tell your child's doctor or pharmacist:

- If your child is taking *any* other medicines.
- If your child has any reactions to a medicine.

Call the Doctor Right Away If…

…your child throws up a lot or gets a rash after taking any medicine. Even if a medicine is safe, your child may be **allergic*** to it.

Your child *may or may not* have side effects with any drug. Be sure to tell the doctor if your child has any side effects with a medicine.

About Pain and Fever Medicines

Acetaminophen (uh-SET-tuh-MIN-uh-fin) and **ibuprofen** (eye-byoo-PROH-fin) help with fever and headaches or body aches. Tylenol is one brand name for acetaminophen. Advil and Motrin are brand names for ibuprofen.

These medicines also can help with pain from bumps, or soreness from a shot. Ask the doctor which one is best for your child.

✳ *Words to Know*

allergic (uh-LER-jik), **allergy** (AL-ur-gee)—to have a bad reaction to something that doesn't bother most people. For example, some people may get hives if they are stung by a bee.

chewable tablet—a flavored pill that a child can chew instead of drinking liquid or swallowing an adult pill.

pharmacist (FARM-uh-sist)—a person who has special training to fill prescriptions and teach people about their medicines.

side effects—symptoms that come from taking a drug and are not part of the treatment. For example, some medicines may make you feel sick to your stomach.

Continued on back

What Else You Need to Know

- *Never* give ibuprofen to a baby younger than 6 months.
- If your child has a kidney disease, asthma, an ulcer, or another chronic (long-term) illness, *ask the doctor before giving ibuprofen.*
- Don't give acetaminophen or ibuprofen at the same time as other OTC medicines, unless your child's doctor says it's OK.

A Warning About Aspirin

Never give aspirin to your child unless your child's doctor tells you it's safe. Aspirin can cause a very serious liver disease called Reye syndrome. This is especially true when given to children with the flu or chickenpox.

Ask your pharmacist about other medicines that may contain aspirin. Or, contact the National Reye's Syndrome Foundation at 1-800-233-7393 or www.reyessyndrome.org.

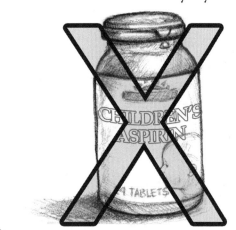

What to Do for Poisoning

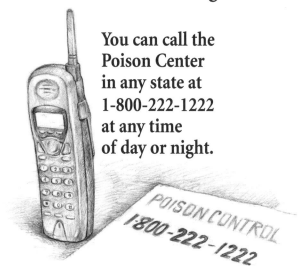

You can call the Poison Center in any state at 1-800-222-1222 at any time of day or night.

Call the Poison Center if you're not sure.

Sometimes parents find their child with something in his or her mouth or with an open bottle of medicine. The Poison Center can help you find out if this could hurt your child. Don't wait until your child is sick to call the Poison Center.

Call 911 or your local emergency number *right away* if your child:

- Is passed out and can't wake up, OR
- Is having a lot of trouble breathing, OR
- Is twitching or shaking out of control, OR
- Is acting very strange.

Don't use syrup of ipecac.

If you have syrup of ipecac in your home, flush it down the toilet and throw away the bottle. Years ago people used syrup of ipecac to make children throw up if they swallowed poison. Now we know that you should not make a child throw up.

To learn more, visit the American Academy of Pediatrics (AAP) Web site at www.aap.org.

Your child's doctor will tell you to do what's best for your child. This information should not take the place of talking with your child's doctor.

We hope the resources in this handout are helpful. The AAP is not responsible for the information in these resources. We try to keep the information up to date but it may change at any time.

Note: Brand names are for your information only. The AAP does not recommend any specific brand of drugs or products.

Adaptation of the AAP information in this handout into plain language was supported in part by McNeil Consumer Healthcare.

© 2008 American Academy of Pediatrics

American Academy of Pediatrics
DEDICATED TO THE HEALTH OF ALL CHILDREN™

Uso de medicinas de venta sin receta con su niño (Using Over-the-Counter Medicines With Your Child)

Las medicinas de "venta sin receta" se pueden comprar sin la orden de un doctor. Al igual que las medicinas de venta con receta, las medicinas de venta sin receta pueden ser peligrosas si no se toman en forma correcta. Hable con el doctor de su niño antes de darle cualquier medicina, especialmente si es por primera vez.

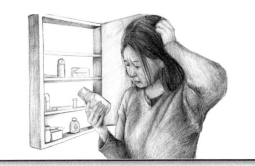

Las medicinas de venta sin receta tienen el mismo tipo de instrucciones en el envase. Esta información indica para qué sirve, cómo se usa, qué contiene y las posibles contraindicaciones. Lea la caja o el envase donde dice **"Drug Facts" ("Propiedades de la medicina")**.

Consulte con el doctor o el farmacéutico

Busque en la etiqueta la cantidad de medicina que debe darle a su niño. Si sabe el peso de su niño, primero guíese por ese dato. Si no lo sabe, calcule la cantidad de acuerdo a la edad. **Lea la etiqueta para confirmar que la medicina sea apropiada para bebés y niños menores de 2 años.** Si no está seguro, consulte con el doctor de su niño.

Antes de darle alguna medicina a su niño, confirme cómo se usa. Estas son algunas preguntas que puede hacerle al doctor o al **farmacéutico***.

- ¿Cómo le ayudará esta medicina a mi niño?
- ¿Puede enseñarme cómo se usa esta medicina?
- ¿Cuánta medicina puedo darle a mi niño?
- ¿Cuándo? ¿Por cuánto tiempo?
- ¿Cuáles son los efectos **secundarios*** de esta medicina?
- ¿Cómo puedo obtener más información?
- ¿Que hago si mi niño la escupe?
- ¿Viene en **tabletas para masticar*** o en líquido?

Siempre dígale al doctor de su niño o al farmacéutico:
- Si su niño está tomando *cualquier* otra medicina.
- Si hay alguna medicina a la que el niño sea **alérgico***.

Llame al doctor de inmediato si...

...su niño vomita mucho o le sale sarpullido después de tomar la medicina. Dígale a su doctor si el niño tiene efectos secundarios a la medicina.

Información sobre las medicinas para el dolor y la fiebre

El **acetaminofén** y el **ibuprofeno** se usan para controlar la fiebre y el dolor. Tylenol es una marca comercial de acetaminofén. Advil y Motrin son marcas comerciales de ibuprofeno.

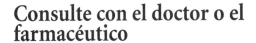

✳ Palabras que debe conocer

alérgico, alergia: Una mala reacción a algo que no causa problemas en la mayoría de las personas. Por ejemplo, a algunas personas les salen ronchas cuando les pica una abeja.

farmacéutico: La persona que tiene un entrenamiento especial para preparar recetas y para enseñar al público sobre el uso de sus medicinas.

efectos secundarios: Reacciones causadas por el uso de medicamentos. Por ejemplo, algunas medicinas causan náuseas o vómitos.

Continúa atrás

Qué más debe saber

- *Nunca* le dé ibuprofeno a un bebé menor de 6 meses.
- Si su niño tiene una enfermedad en el riñón, asma, úlcera u otra enfermedad crónica (de largo plazo), Consulte con su doctor antes de darle ibuprofeno.
- No le dé acetaminofén o ibuprofeno al mismo tiempo que otras medicinas de venta sin receta, a menos que el doctor de su niño se lo recomiende.

Una advertencia sobre la aspirina

Nunca le dé aspirina a los niños, a menos que su doctor le diga que no hay ningún peligro. La aspirina puede causar una enfermedad del hígado muy seria llamada síndrome de Reye. Puede pasarle especialmente a niños con gripe o varicela.

Pídale a su farmacéutico que le recomiende otras medicinas que no contengan aspirina. Si quiere saber más sobre el síndrome de Reye llame al 1-800-233-7393 o visite www.reyessyndrome.org.

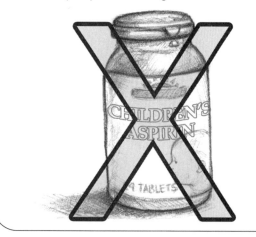

Qué hacer en caso de envenenamiento o intoxicación

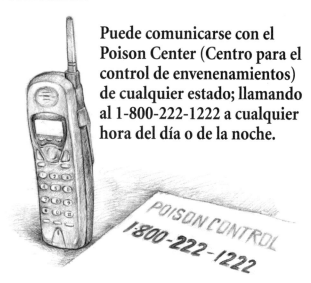

Puede comunicarse con el Poison Center (Centro para el control de envenenamientos) de cualquier estado; llamando al 1-800-222-1222 a cualquier hora del día o de la noche.

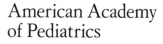

Asegúrese de guardar todas sus medicinas fuera del alcance de los niños. Si su niño toma un medicina por accidente llame de inmediato al "Poison Center" para saber qué debe hacer. Tenga a mano el nombre de la medicina. El "Poison Center" puede informarle si lo que el niño tomó puede o no ser dañino. No espere hasta que su niño se sienta mal para llamar al "Poison Center".

Llame de inmediato al 911 ó a su número local de emergencia, si su niño:

- Se desmaya o no puede despertarse
- Tiene problemas para respirar
- Tiembla y se sacude sin control
- Actúa de forma extraña.

No use jarabe de ipecacuana (ipecac).

Si tiene jarabe de ipecacuana en su casa, échelo en el inodoro y tire el envase. Por años se recomendó el uso del jarabe de ipecacuana para hacer que los niños vomitaran si tragaban veneno. Ahora se sabe que no se debe hacer que el niño vomite.

Para aprender más, visite el sitio de la Academia Americana de Pediatría (AAP) en www.aap.org.
Su pediatra le dirá qué es lo mejor para la salud de su hijo.
Esta información no debe usarse en lugar de consultar con su doctor.
Esperamos que la información en este folleto le sea útil. La AAP no es responsable por la información contenida en este folleto. Tratamos de presentar la información más actual pero a veces las recomendaciones cambian.
Nota: Los nombres de marca son para su información solamente.
La AAP no recomienda ninguna marca o producto de medicina específicamente.
La adaptación de la información de este folleto de la AAP a lenguaje sencillo se hizo con el apoyo de McNeil Consumer Healthcare. La traducción al español fue patrocinada por Leyendo Juntos (Reach Out and Read), un programa pediátrico de alfabetización.

American Academy of Pediatrics

DEDICATED TO THE HEALTH OF ALL CHILDREN™

Oral Health
Dental Hygiene

Both the American Academy of Pediatrics and the American Academy of Pediatric Dentistry recommend that children have their first dental visits around 1 year of age. However, there are currently too few pediatric dentists to see all of these patients, and many general dentists are uncomfortable seeing children younger than 3 years—or even older.

Because pediatricians and other child health professionals see children frequently during the first 3 years of life, it makes sense that they incorporate oral health risk assessment and screening for caries into their well-child visits. Early childhood caries is preventable, but too few parents get that message because they're not taking their children to see dentists, and their pediatricians don't focus on oral health.

Major areas that need to be addressed with families include

- Risk of drinking liquids frequently from a bottle or sippy cup
- Healthy dietary recommendations for children
- Importance of appropriate oral hygiene, including brushing and flossing
- Role of fluoride—systemically and topically, and in tap water

Ask Me 3

During your patient encounter, you should communicate using plain language and health literacy principles, so that by the end of the visit, the parent or child will know the answers to the *Ask Me 3* questions.

A Patient Story. . .

Dr Scrivner is seeing Martin Alvarez for his 15-month well-child visit. His weight is above the 90th percentile, suggesting high caloric intake, and he is drinking from a bottle filled with red punch.

During the physical examination, Dr Scrivner finds signs of caries. He asks Mrs Alvarez about Martin's diet, and learns that Martin's grandmother babysits him on weekdays and lets him eat a lot of candy and drink "juice" from his bottle.

Dr Scrivner noted that Martin is at very high risk for caries for the following other reasons: He is on Medicaid; his mother has visible, untreated tooth decay; his father smokes; there is no family dental home; and Martin has no fluoride in his tap water.

Dr Scrivner gives Martin's mother the following advice:

- Stop giving him drinks with sugar.
- Stop giving him a bottle.
- Fill the prescription for daily fluoride supplements and give them to Martin every day.
- Start brushing Martin's teeth twice a day.
- Call the dentist for an appointment for Martin.

At Martin's 18-month visit, Dr Scrivner sees no improvement in the toddler's oral health.

. . . .

Mrs Alvarez was not told that juice has a lot of sugar in it, and because WIC supplies juice, she started putting juice in the bottle.

Martin's grandmother ignored the advice about stopping the bottle because in her native Mexico, many children have bottles until at least age 5. Dr Scrivner could have explained to Mrs Alvarez how and why to get Martin off the baby bottle in terms that she could effectively convey to Martin's grandmother.

Mrs Alvarez said she was unable to get a dental appointment for Martin because none of the dentists would see new Medicaid patients, but Dr Scrivner could have supplied Mrs Alvarez with a list of local dentists known to take patients with Medicaid.

And, working together, the doctor and the mother could have set small, achievable goals that could have built her confidence and Martin's success.

Patient: Ramon, 4-year-old boy with cavities	
Ask Me 3 questions	**What the parent should understand at the end of the visit**
What is my child's main problem?	Ramon has cavities, or holes in his teeth.
What do I need to do?	• I should stop his bottle. • I should brush his teeth 2 times every day. • I should stop giving him sugary drinks, including juice. • I should get him a dentist appointment as soon as possible.
Why is it important for me to do this?	If Ramon's cavities get worse, he will have pain and might even need a big operation to fix them. They might even hurt his health later in his life.

Medical Terms and Plain Language Alternatives

Many of the medical terms we use every day don't mean much to many parents. Below is a list of medical terms that may be confusing or difficult to explain and suggestions for plain language alternatives.

Medical Terms	Plain Language Alternatives
Cavity; tooth decay	Tooth decay (rotting teeth) happens when germs in the mouth mix with the sugar in foods and drinks. The germs then make acids that break down the outside part of the tooth. Cavities are the holes in the enamel caused by tooth decay.
Dental	Of the teeth
Dental caries	Tooth decay; rotting teeth; cavities
Enamel	The hard outer coating that protects the tooth
Eruption	Teething; teeth coming in
Fluoride	A natural substance in water and toothpaste that helps keep teeth healthy and strong (If local tap water does not have enough fluoride, pills or drops can be given to the child every day.)
Night feedings	Any liquid other than water given to an infant or toddler at night without brushing or wiping the teeth afterward
Oral	Of the mouth
Oral abscess	An infected spot or sore in the mouth, caused by bacteria and filled with liquid/fluid/pus; similar, in some ways, to a blister on the foot or hand
Oral hygiene	Keeping the mouth and teeth clean
Primary teeth	Baby teeth
Secondary teeth	Permanent teeth; adult teeth
Sippy cup	A non-spilling cup (usually with a lid or top) that can be used for liquids with meals, but should not be carried around all day with any liquid other than water in it

Confusing Terms and Concepts

With any condition, there are likely to be terms or concepts for which patients and families have a different understanding than a health care professional. These may include preventive strategies, complex disease processes, medication or treatment regimens, abstract laboratory results or measurements, technical terms, or words that have a different meaning in the health care arena than in everyday use. Cultural issues and misconceptions can also contribute to lack of understanding.

Consider the following when talking with parents about oral health:

Prevention and Health Promotion

Explain to parents and children that keeping teeth healthy is very important, and that it's much easier to prevent a problem than to fix one. Offer some basic tips for prevention.

- Make sure there is a source of fluoride available to the child (through water, toothpaste, and/or supplements).
- Keep the child from using a baby bottle and/or sippy cup frequently during the day; allow it only at mealtime, if necessary.
- Discourage "grazing": child walking around with a container of snacks, continuously eating.
- If the child drinks a lot during the day, give her water, saving juices and milk for mealtime.
- Never put the child to bed with a bottle with milk or juice in it.
- Brush the child's teeth with plain water when younger than 2 years or fluoride toothpaste when older than 2 years twice a day, including once before bed. Don't let them eat or drink after their bedtime toothbrushing. And make sure parents know they need to brush their child's teeth after snacks such as crackers and raisins.

Parents may not understand that some of the foods they give children can harm their teeth. The usual food for a family might not be food that the physician would recommend. Explain what kinds of foods are best for the child's teeth, and give specific examples and a handout to take home.

Make note of foods they probably shouldn't give the child.

- Sugary or flavored drinks, juice, soda, and candy are obvious, but also discuss foods with "hidden carbohydrates," such as soft bakery products.
- Foods that stick to the teeth—like raisins, fruit leather, or gummy bears—are especially bad for promoting caries.

Encourage them to give the child foods that are low in sugar content, such as whole grains, fruits, and vegetables.

Did You Know...?
Bad Combination

Dental caries is an infection caused by the interaction between pathogenic oral flora (primarily *Streptococcus mutans*), poor oral hygiene, and dietary sugars.

Diagnosis

Parents may not know what dental caries are or why the child is having tooth problems. Make sure parents appreciate the importance of preventing dental caries, and the ease with which caries can be prevented.

Remain sensitive to the parents' feelings and cultural or ethnic background when you explain that caries can occur with poor diet or oral hygiene, in addition to prolonged bottle feeding.

- You may have heard of "baby bottle tooth decay," which is the same thing as caries, but that the newer term for tooth decay in children is "early childhood caries."

In some families, oral hygiene is not a priority. Take into consideration the teeth of the parent or caregiver who is with the child. Remember that children are at increased risk for early childhood caries if there is a history of untreated tooth decay in the parent or guardian, or if the family does not have a dental home or dental insurance.

Advise parents that establishing a dental home is a health priority, and that daily brushing and flossing, access to fluoride in the water or as a supplement, and a diet low in sugars are the best ways to prevent tooth decay. (See the Miscellaneous section at the end of this chapter for more information on the dental home.)

Stress the link between good oral health and good overall health, and give examples to make the point.

- Links have been established between poor oral hygiene and many common adult diseases, including diabetes, heart disease, stroke, and dementia.
- There may be a higher risk of low birth weight and preterm labor among pregnant women with poor oral hygiene.
- An untreated cavity can become an abscessed tooth. The infection associated with an abscess can spread through the whole body and cause death.

Symptoms

Parents often miss the signs of dental problems, or mistake them for other behavioral or health issues. Children may refuse to eat because it is painful, or they may act out or misbehave, not always understanding what hurts. Make sure parents understand that stubbornness isn't the only reason children refuse to eat.

- Cavities, caries, abcesses, and tooth eruption (new teeth coming in) can all cause mouth pain that can get worse with salty, acidic (sour), hot, cold, or sugary foods.
- A cavity that has grown into an abscess can be really painful— and even deadly, if its infection spreads—and should be taken very seriously.

Management and Treatment

Some families live in areas with low or no fluoride in the tap water. If you need to have a patient or parent collect a water sample to test for fluoride, be sure to explain your instructions in clear, complete, and concise terms.

If this is a common problem in your area, consider writing up simple instructions for collecting the water sample in a handout that patients can take home. And give them contact information for places to have their water tested. It's often conducted through the local health department.

- If you prescribe supplemental fluoride, use plain language dosing instructions. (See the "Medication and Dosing" topic on page 225 for tips.)

You may prefer to refer the patient to a dentist for management and treatment. In that case, give them a list of local dentists who take their insurance or Medicaid, and make the appointment for them, if necessary. Follow up with them later by phone to see if they saw a dentist or made an appointment.

Cultural Beliefs

Families from different cultures may have their own ideas of what causes oral health problems. Explore this by asking the parent what they think is causing the condition and what they think will make it better. This will increase your understanding of their culture while uncovering possible roadblocks or cultural issues with treatment before they arise.

Usually the parents' or families' beliefs will pose no harm to the child. Try to incorporate their beliefs into your treatment plan, if they're safe.

Remember: Extended family members may play an important role in decision-making and management. Their input can sometimes result in confusion or lack of adherence to suggested management.

Worsening Condition

Help parents find a dentist, and encourage them to take the child for an appointment. Follow up with them by phone later to see if they saw a dentist or at least scheduled an appointment.

How Big Is the Problem?

More than 108 million children and adults in the United States lack dental insurance, which is more than 2.5 times the number who lack medical insurance.

Source: US Department of Health and Human Services. *Oral Health in America: A Report of the Surgeon General—Executive Summary.* Rockville, MD: US Department of Health and Human Services, National Institute of Dental and Craniofacial Research, National Institutes of Health; 2000.

Cultural Spotlight

Tooth Decay in Latinos

Latino children have the highest rate of dental caries among all children living in the United States. One important factor that contributes to this problem is continuation of the bottle until age 4, or even 6.

Health care providers need to be sensitive to this cultural difference in child-rearing, but also must continue to give messages about the risks of any liquids other than water being sucked from a bottle or sippy cup throughout the day or at bedtime.

Beverages should be consumed at mealtime and not all day long because the sugar breakdown products (acids) are a major factor in the development of tooth decay.

Remind them that tooth decay in baby teeth often means tooth decay in adult teeth.

Behavior Change

Behavior change is a key element in preventing and managing many pediatric conditions. Shifting from paternalistic advice that is either too vague or too complicated to a patient- or family-centered approach that incorporates elements of motivational interviewing and goal-setting, and that makes use of plain language, can be an effective way to empower patients and families to make changes and improve their health.

Talk with the patient's parents or guardians about how everyone in the family needs to eat healthy foods and make regular trips to the dentist. The type of foods and drinks available in the home can increase or decrease the risk for both dental caries and obesity. Link the importance of the family's role in modeling healthy eating and good oral hygiene. Help them identify reasons to make changes, and build conviction and confidence using motivational interview techniques.

- How convinced are you that finding a dentist for Torey is important?
- How confident are you that you can change Pauley's bedtime bottle from milk to water over the course of the next couple of weeks?
- On a scale of 1 to 10, how confident are you that you can get Louisa to brush her teeth at least twice every day?

Child Involvement

Including the child, to the extent possible, is respectful and patient-centered and can contribute to developing health literacy skills as the child moves toward managing his or her own health as an adolescent and an adult. It can include direct, age-appropriate statements to the child, and also ways for the child to be involved in his or her health.

For example, children can be taught to brush and floss their teeth starting when they are toddlers. But, until about age 6 or 8, a parent or guardian must supervise or actually do the brushing and flossing. After that age, children will generally have the manual dexterity needed to do an adequate job of brushing.

Be sure to note that fluoride-containing toothpaste is not recommended for children younger than 2 years because the child is not generally able to spit out the toothpaste, so there is a risk of swallowing too much fluoride. There are suitable alternatives (often called "training" toothpastes) that are widely available at grocery stores and drugstores.

Children can be taught to choose sugar-free foods and treats to keep their teeth healthy, and they can be encouraged with a reward chart to make smart choices, and to brush and floss daily.

- Parents also need to make sure they do not transmit fear of the dentist to the child.

Teach-back

The concept of teaching back entails asking parents or patients to demonstrate understanding *using their own words*, not simply asking whether they have questions or whether they understand, because that may not elicit lack of understanding. Having patients explain in their own words not only assesses their understanding, but it reinforces the information by repeating it and internalizes it for the patient. When there is a lot of information, go over each concept and elicit a teach-back before moving to the next idea.

When using teach-back, it's important to keep the burden on yourself. Avoid the perception that you are quizzing the parent or patient—emphasize that you want to be sure you've explained things clearly.

The practice of using teach-back can be especially important over the phone, because it may be the only way to gauge whether the parent or patient understands fully.

Here are some approaches to using teach-back when managing oral health.

- To make sure this information works for you, when you get home, how will you decrease bottle feedings and eventually stop the bottle completely?
- What will you tell your husband about when you can start using toothpaste with fluoride in it and when Ella will be old enough to brush her teeth without help?
- I want to make sure I was clear when I explained this: Can you tell me some foods that have "hidden sugars" that should not be given to your child?

Key Messages for Use by All Members of the Health Care Team

It is important to reinforce key messages for parents and children so they hear them more than once and recognize them as priorities in managing their health. In addition, families should not receive conflicting advice about their health and what to do.

Key concepts for good oral health

- Fluoride in tap water, toothpaste, and/or supplements prevents cavities.
- Wiping or brushing teeth should begin as soon as the teeth come in.
- Bottles and sippy cups should not be used at bedtime or frequently during the daytime, unless they contain water.
- Sugar in the diet and in liquids decays teeth.
- Cavities in baby teeth are strongly linked to cavities in adult teeth.
- Patients should be in a dental home by 1 year of age.

Miscellaneous

All families are encouraged to establish a dental home. Explain to parents that you may look into the child's mouth to assess early signs of tooth decay if the child does not already have a dentist; you may also apply a concentrated fluoride varnish on the child's teeth if she is at risk for dental caries to help protect the teeth until the child gets into a dental home. But nothing you are likely to do can duplicate or replace the dental home.

The concept of the dental home is derived from the concept of the medical home, about which the American Academy of Pediatrics states

- The medical care of infants, children, and adolescents ideally should be accessible, continuous, comprehensive, family-centered, coordinated, compassionate, and culturally effective. It should be delivered or directed by well-trained physicians who provide primary care and help to manage and facilitate essentially all aspects of pediatric care.

Pediatric primary dental care needs to be delivered in a similar manner.

- The dental home is a specialized primary dental care provider within the philosophical complex of the medical home. Referring a child for an oral health examination by a dentist who provides care for infants and young children 6 months after the first tooth erupts, or by 12 months of age, establishes the child's dental home and provides an opportunity to implement preventive dental health habits that meet each child's unique needs and keep the child free from dental or oral disease.

The dental home should be expected to provide

- An accurate risk assessment for dental diseases and conditions
- An individualized preventive dental health program based on the risk assessment
- Anticipatory guidance about growth and development issues (ie, teething, digit or pacifier habits, and feeding practices)
- A plan for emergency dental trauma
- Information about proper care of the child's teeth and gingival tissues
- Information regarding proper nutrition and dietary practices
- Comprehensive dental care in accordance with accepted guidelines and periodicity schedules for pediatric dental health
- Referrals to other dental specialists, such as endodontists, oral surgeons, orthodontists, and periodontists, when care cannot be provided directly within the dental home

For more information on the dental home, visit http://aappolicy. aappublications.org/cgi/content/full/pediatrics;111/5/1113.

Caring for Your Child's Teeth

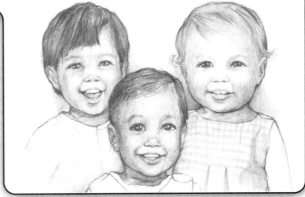

Almost 1 in 4 children in America will have a **cavity** (KA-vuh-dee) before turning 4 years of age! That's why it's very important for parents to know how to care for their children's teeth.

Things You Can Do to Care for Your Child's Teeth

Birth to 1 Year

- After feedings, gently brush your baby's gums and any baby teeth with water and a soft baby toothbrush. Or wipe them with a clean washcloth or gauze.
- After the first tooth comes in, ask your child's doctor if your child is getting enough **fluoride***.
- Your child's doctor will check your baby's mouth at well-child visits. Babies at high risk for decay will be sent to a dentist.

1 Year to 2 Years

- Brush your child's teeth twice a day with water and a soft baby toothbrush. The best times are after breakfast and before bed. Start when your child has any teeth.
- Make sure your child doesn't drink more than a small cup of juice each day. Only drink juice at mealtime, not in between.
- Take your child for a dental checkup if your child has not had one yet.

2 Years to 6 Years

- Brush your child's teeth twice a day. Help your child brush. Or repeat the brushing after your child is done. Children this age need to learn to brush, but they can't really do a good job yet.
- Start using a fluoride toothpaste. Teach your child not to swallow it. Use only a pea-sized amount and smear the paste into the bristles. Too much fluoride can make white or brown spots on your child's adult teeth.
- Floss between any teeth that touch each other.
- Take your child for a dental checkup at least once a year.

6 Years and Up

- Have your child brush his or her teeth **twice a day** with fluoride toothpaste.
- Teach your child to floss every night after brushing.
- Take your child for a dental checkup at least once a year.

What Else *You* Can Do

Make sure your child has regular checkups with a dentist. Your child's doctor will also look at your child's teeth and gums during well-child visits and help you find a dentist if the teeth have early tooth decay.

Make sure *you* have healthy teeth and gums. You can pass germs that cause cavities if you share food or drinks with your child.

Don't share food or drinks with your child. If you do you can pass germs that cause cavities and gum disease. You can also pass germs that cause cavities if you lick your child's spoon or pacifier.

Call the dentist if you are worried about tooth decay and other problems. If you don't have a dentist, call your child's doctor to help you find one. Only a dentist can treat tooth decay.

✳ Words to Know

fluoride (FLOR-eyed)—a natural chemical that helps teeth stay strong and helps prevent tooth decay. It hardens the outer coating on the teeth called enamel. Fluoride also helps repair early damage to teeth.

permanent (PUR-muh-nint)—lasting for a lifetime. Permanent teeth replace baby teeth one by one in your child's mouth. If your child loses a permanent tooth, it *won't* grow back.

Continued on back

What Is a Cavity?

An outer coating called enamel protects teeth. **Tooth decay** happens when germs in the mouth mix with sugar in foods and drinks. The germs then make acids that break down the enamel. **Cavities** (KA-vuh-deez) are holes in the enamel caused by tooth decay.

Cavities may look like white or brown spots on the teeth. You might also see white lines on the teeth where they meet the gums.

Tooth decay in your baby's teeth used to be called baby bottle tooth decay, but is now called early childhood caries. **Caries** (KAIR-eez) is another word for tooth decay.

Eating and Tooth Decay

To help prevent tooth decay in your infant or child:

- Don't put your child to bed with a bottle with anything other than water.
- Don't let your child suck on a bottle or sippy cup with anything other than water except at feeding times.
- Don't let your child eat sweet or sticky foods, like candy, cookies, or fruit roll-ups. There is sugar in foods like crackers and chips too. These are especially bad if your child snacks on them a lot. They should only be eaten at mealtime.
- Don't let your child sip drinks that have sugar and acid, like juices, sports drinks, flavored drinks, soda pop, or flavored teas.

How Does My Child Get Fluoride?

Fluoride can be added to drinking water and toothpaste. Your water department can tell you if your tap water has fluoride. If your water comes from a well, get a fluoride water test. If needed, your dentist or child's doctor will give your child fluoride drops or pills to take every day, or may suggest you buy bottled water with fluoride. Your child may also get fluoride treatments (varnish or gel) at a medical or dental visit.

Do Pacifiers or Thumb and Finger Sucking Hurt Teeth?

Sucking a pacifier, thumb, or fingers can affect the shape of the mouth, and how the top and bottom teeth line up. This is called your child's "bite."

It's OK if you give your baby a **pacifier,** but…

- Wait until your baby is 1 month old if you're breastfeeding.
- Do not dip the pacifier in any sweet liquid.
- Wash and replace the pacifier often.

If your child sucks his or her **thumb or fingers…**

- Your child's bite will most likely be OK if he or she stops sucking by 4 or 5 years of age. That's when the **permanent*** teeth start coming in.
- Ask your child's dentist or doctor about how to help your child stop his or her sucking habits.

To learn more, visit the American Academy of Pediatrics (AAP) Web site at www.aap.org or visit the American Academy of Pediatric Dentistry Web site at www.aapd.org.

Your child's doctor or dentist will tell you to do what's best for your child. This information should not take the place of talking with your child's doctor or dentist.

We hope the resources in this handout are helpful. The AAP is not responsible for the information in these resources. We try to keep the information up to date but it may change at any time.

Adaptation of the AAP information in this handout into plain language was supported in part by McNeil Consumer Healthcare.

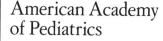

American Academy of Pediatrics

DEDICATED TO THE HEALTH OF ALL CHILDREN™

El cuidado de los dientes de su niño
(Caring for Your Child's Teeth)

En los Estados Unidos, más o menos 1 de cada 4 niños tendrá una **caries** antes de cumplir 4 años. Por eso es importante que los padres sepan cómo cuidar los dientes de sus hijos.

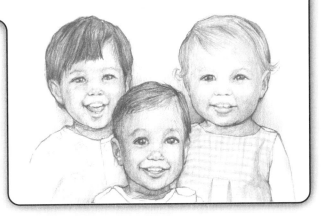

Qué puede hacer para cuidar los dientes de su niño

Desde el nacimiento hasta un año de edad

- Después de las comidas cepille suavemente las encías y cualquier diente de leche con agua y un cepillo de dientes suave para bebé. O use una toallita o gasa limpia.
- Después de que le salga el primer diente, pregúntele al doctor si su niño está tomando suficiente **fluoruro***.
- El doctor le examinará la boca a su bebé en las visitas de seguimiento. Los bebés con un alto riesgo de caries serán enviados a un dentista.

De 1 a 2 años

- Cepille los dientes de su niño dos veces al día con agua y un cepillo de dientes suave para bebé. Es mejor hacerlo después del desayuno y antes de ir a la cama. Comience en cuanto su niño tenga algún diente.
- Asegúrese de que su niño no tome más de una taza pequeña de jugo al día. Sólo debe tomarlo a la hora de comer, no entre comidas.
- Si su niño todavía no ha tenido un chequeo dental, llévelo al dentista.

De 2 a 6 años

- Cepille los dientes de su niño dos veces al día. Ayúdelo a cepillarse. O repita el cepillado después de que él haya terminado. A esta edad, los niños deben aprender a cepillarse pero todavía no lo hacen bien.
- Empiece a usar una pasta con fluoruro. Enséñele a su niño a no tragársela. Use una cantidad similar a la del tamaño de un grano de maíz y úntela en la cerda del cepillo. Demasiado fluoruro puede provocar manchas de color blanco o café en los dientes permanentes de su niño.
- Use hilo dental entre los dientes que no tienen espacio entre sí.
- Lleve a su niño a chequearse los dientes al menos una vez al año.

De 6 años en adelante

- Haga que su niño se lave los dientes **dos veces al día** con una pasta que contenga fluoruro.
- Enséñele a su niño a usar hilo dental todas las noches, después de cepillarse los dientes.
- Lleve a su niño a chequearse los dientes al menos una vez al año.

Qué más puede hacer

Asegúrese de que su niño asista a chequeos regulares con el dentista. El doctor de su niño también le examinará los dientes y las encías durante las visitas de seguimiento. El doctor de su niño le ayudará a encontrar un dentista si los dientes ya tienen caries.

Asegúrese de que usted tenga dientes y encías sanos. Usted puede pasarle a su niño los gérmenes que provocan las caries si comparten comidas y bebidas.

No comparta comidas ni bebidas con su niño. Si lo hace, puede pasarle los gérmenes que provocan las caries y las enfermedades de las encías. También puede pasarle estos gérmenes si usted lame la cuchara o el chupete de su niño.

Comuníquese con el dentista si le preocupan las caries u otros problemas de los dientes. Si no tiene dentista, llame al doctor de su niño para que le recomiende uno. Sólo un dentista puede tratar las caries.

✱ Palabras que debe conocer

fluoruro: Una sustancia química natural que ayuda a que los dientes se mantengan fuertes y a prevenir las caries. Endurece la capa externa de los dientes que se llama esmalte. El fluoruro también ayuda a reparar daños tempranos en los dientes.

dientes permanentes: Que duran toda la vida. Los dientes permanentes reemplazan uno por uno a los dientes de leche. Si su niño pierde un diente permanente, no le volverá a salir.

Continúa atrás

¿Qué es una caries?

Una capa externa que se llama esmalte protege los dientes. La caries se produce cuando los gérmenes de la boca se mezclan con el azúcar de los alimentos y las bebidas. Los gérmenes producen ácidos que destruyen el esmalte. Las caries son **agujeros (hoyos)** en el esmalte.

Pueden verse como manchas color blanco o café en los dientes. También pueden lucir como líneas color blanco donde éstos se unen con las encías.

Las caries en los dientes de su bebé se conocían como caries de biberón, pero ahora se les llama **caries** a edad temprana. **Caries** es sólo otro nombre que se le da a los dientes picados.

La alimentación y las caries

Para ayudar a prevenir las caries en su niño o bebé:

- No deje a su niño en la cama con un biberón con bebidas que no sean agua.

- No permita que su niño tome bebidas que no sean agua en el biberón o vasito infantil, excepto a la hora de las comidas.

- No permita que su niño coma alimentos dulces o pegajosos, como caramelos, galletas dulces o chocolates. Los alimentos como las galletas saladas y las papas fritas también contienen azúcar. Estos alimentos no son buenos si su niño los come mucho. Puede comerlos únicamente a la hora de las comidas.

- No permita que su niño tome por poquitos y durante todo el día bebidas con azúcar y ácido. Por ejemplo: jugos de fruta, bebidas para deportistas, bebidas con sabores, sodas, café o refrescos dulces.

¿De qué forma obtiene mi niño el fluoruro?

El fluoruro se le puede agregar al agua potable y a la pasta de dientes. El departamento de agua puede informarle si el agua del grifo contiene fluoruro. Si su agua proviene de un pozo, haga una prueba para saber si contiene fluoruro. Si fuera necesario, el dentista o el doctor le darán al niño gotas o pastillas de fluoruro para que tome todos los días. También pueden sugerirle que compre agua embotellada con fluoruro. El doctor o el dentista también podrían darle al niño tratamientos con fluoruro (líquido o en jalea).

¿Dañan los dientes los chupetes o chuparse los dedos?

Chupar un chupete o chuparse los dedos puede afectar la forma de la boca y la alineación de los dientes. A esto se le conoce como la "mordida" de su niño.

Está bien que le dé **un chupete** a su bebé, pero…

- Espere hasta que tenga un mes de edad si le da pecho.
- No moje el chupete en ningún líquido dulce.
- Lave y reemplace seguido el chupete.

Si su niño se chupa **uno o varios dedos…**

- La mordida de su niño tendrá más probabilidades de no dañarse si deja de chuparse el dedo a los 4 ó 5 años. A esta edad, los **dientes permanentes*** empiezan a salir.
- Pregúntele al dentista o doctor de su niño sobre cómo ayudar a que su niño deje estos hábitos.

Para aprender más, visite el sitio web de la Academia Americana de Pediatría (AAP) en www.aap.org. o visíte el sitio web de la Academy of Pediatric Dentistry en www.aapd.org
Su pediatra o el dentista le dirán qué es lo mejor para la salud de su hijo.
Esta información no debe usarse en lugar de consultar con su doctor.
Esperamos que la información en este folleto le sea útil. La AAP no es responsable por la información contenida en este folleto. Tratamos de presentar la información más actual pero a veces las recomendaciones cambian.
La adaptación de la información de este folleto de la AAP a lenguaje sencillo se hizo con el apoyo de McNeil Consumer Healthcare. La traducción al español fue patrocinada por Leyendo Juntos (Reach Out and Read), un programa pediátrico de alfabetización.

American Academy of Pediatrics

DEDICATED TO THE HEALTH OF ALL CHILDREN™

Reading

This section focuses on the issue of children learning to read, on the role that the primary care physician can have in helping parents support their young children's emerging literacy skills, and in the provider's continued attention to children's reading skills as they attend the early grades of school.

Reading skills are strongly linked to young children's language skills on entering school and are the best predictor of children's general school success. Reading problems are much more common among children growing up in poverty and can contribute to the perpetuation of poverty; social marginalization; and disparities in health, education, and economic potential. Interventions that support print-rich environments for young children, reading aloud, and other enhanced exposure to language and books offer a way to reduce the language and school-readiness gaps that can leave some children struggling in the early grades of school.

There is strong evidence to show that literacy promotion in primary care, following the Reach Out and Read model, leads to parents' reading aloud more often to young children. It also shows that, at least among children growing up under economically disadvantaged circumstances, literacy promotion in primary care is associated with significant improvements in expressive and receptive language scores by the second year of life.[1,2]

Children are expected to reach fluency and proficiency in reading by the fourth grade; those who struggle with reading in the early grades are at high risk for continued reading difficulties, and may find themselves struggling in school.[3–5]

This is an area in which the families who most need help and support can be the most difficult to reach; the more intimidated a parent feels around issues of literacy and written language, the more

A Patient Story...

Dr Gardner is seeing Jenny Morton, a 5-year-old girl who will be starting kindergarten this year.

As part of the visit, Dr Gardner tries to assess the child's school readiness skills, verifying that she knows the names of colors, asking her to pick out the letter "J" on the page of a book. Ms Morton interrupts hastily to say that Jenny hasn't been to school yet, so she doesn't know any letters.

Dr Gardner tells Ms Morton that children should be recognizing letters before they start kindergarten, and advises her to practice this skill with Jenny whenever she reads to her. He gives Jenny a *Reach Out and Read* book to take home. Ms Morton nods.

Ms Morton hands Dr Gardner the school physical form, which she says she'll come by and pick up later. After the pair leaves, he looks at the form and notes that the part that parents are supposed to complete has been left blank.

- -

Although it was great that Dr Gardner took the time and trouble to ask about Jenny's early reading skills, and wonderful that he had a book to use in the visit, he missed an opportunity to talk with Jenny's mother about all the kinds of reading that can go on outside of school—and perhaps more importantly—to open up the question of her own reading skills, in a supportive and non-judgmental manner.

If Dr Gardner had asked about Ms Morton's school experiences, she might have told him that she was in special education classes all through school, and that she left in the eleventh grade. It might have been an opportunity to ask her whether she has concerns about her own ability to help Jenny learn to read, and to encourage her to look at books together with Jenny, even if they would rather discuss the pictures and make up stories than read.

(continued)

that the parents and child stand to profit from help and advice, and the more complex and delicate it becomes to address the subject.

Parents who have limited literacy skills, or limited English proficiency, may find it difficult or threatening to read to their young children, or simply may not think in terms of reading for pleasure. Other parents may find the idea of reading aloud to a young child unfamiliar, or have no sense of what it looks like or how it is done.

Even if the physician intends to advise reading aloud, this advice may not be easily understood or carried out by a parent in this position. And once a child is in school, parents with limited literacy or limited English proficiency may be less likely to feel comfortable discussing the child's reading progress—or reading problems—with the teacher, and less able to work with the child at home on homework, reading practice, or reading for pleasure.

Addressing this topic with parents and patients clearly, and with sensitivity and solutions, can also have potential benefits to your practice.

- Talking about books and reading aloud from the time that a child is very young allows the pediatrician to reinforce important developmental concepts, including repetition, routine, and the importance of the child's hearing the parent's voice.
- Using books during the health supervision visit allows opportunities for developmental assessment, and also for offering parents an evidence-based tool for helping their children's literacy development—and sometimes their own.
- Discussing the importance of books, reading, and helping children as they learn to read may give parents who would like to improve their own literacy skills the opportunity to connect with adult and family literacy programs.
- Giving children books at regular office visits may lead to improved patient satisfaction and fewer missed appointments.

Ask Me 3

During your patient encounter, you should communicate using plain language and health literacy principles so that by the end of the visit, the parent or child will know the answers to the *Ask Me 3* questions.

Patient: Sylvia, 1½-year-old girl whose mother didn't graduate high school	
Ask Me 3 questions	**What the parent should understand at the end of the visit**
What is my child's main problem?	Sylvia needs to be exposed to books so she'll be ready for kindergarten.
What do I need to do?	I need to look at books with my baby every day. I need to point to the pictures and tell her the names of things. I need to look at a book with her at bedtime.
Why is it important for me to do this?	This will help Sylvia learn more words, get used to books, and enjoy reading and hearing stories. And it's a wonderful way to spend time together.

Patient: Tasha, 4-year-old girl whose mother wants her to be ready for kindergarten	
Ask Me 3 questions	**What the parent should understand at the end of the visit**
What is my child's main problem?	Tasha will start kindergarten in a few months, and I can help her get ready.
What do I need to do?	• I need to look at books with Tasha every day. • I should let her choose the book and take her to the library. • We can look at the pictures and make up a story, or I can read the words to her. • I should ask her questions about the pictures and the story so that she tells me what she thinks will happen next and why. • I can point to letters on the page and she can tell me what they are. • I can also point to letters and words on signs or on packages and ask Tasha to tell me what they are.
Why is it important for me to do this?	• Looking at books with Tasha will help her get used to printed words and comfortable with books. • Tasha will enjoy spending time with me looking at books, and that will help her be ready to learn when she gets to school.

Patient: Billy, 9-year-old boy who is having trouble reading	
Ask Me 3 questions	**What the parent should understand at the end of the visit**
What is my child's main problem?	It is important for Billy to learn to read well enough so he can use reading to learn other subjects and succeed in school.
What do I need to do?	• I need to help him with his reading homework and make sure he does it every day. • I need to help him set up a quiet place, with no TV and no one bothering him, where he can do his homework. • I need to help him with his mistakes and be patient when he tries to read to me, and I need to tell him how well he's doing. • I need to help him find books he will like. I need to take him to the library.
Why is it important for me to do this?	• It is important to help Billy learn to read better, so that he will do well in school—both of which will boost his self-esteem. • It will also help him learn to read for fun.

Confusing Terms and Concepts

With any condition, there are likely to be terms or concepts for which patients and families have a different understanding than a health care professional. These may include preventive strategies, complex disease processes, medication or treatment regimens, abstract laboratory results or measurements, technical terms, or words that have a different meaning in the health care arena than in everyday use. Cultural issues and misconceptions can also contribute to lack of understanding.

Communication Issues

Consider the following communication issues when talking with parents about reading:

- Parents may be embarrassed by seeing a baby or toddler mouth or chew on a book, or handle it roughly, and may feel that such behavior proves that the child is too young for books.

Offer an age-appropriate board book, and explain to parents that mouthing the book is appropriate exploratory behavior for a young child. In fact, if you say this before giving the book to the baby, the parent will often be pleased to see the child perform as predicted.

- Parents may feel it is a waste of time to read to a child who is too young to talk. Discuss this as part of young children's language development, and explain how important it is for them to hear the parent's voice.

Parents may be frustrated by the activity level of a toddler, who is unwilling to sit still and listen to a story.

- Offer them an age-appropriate book with short sentences and rhymes.
- Encourage parents to ask the child questions.
- Assure parents that the activity level is normal, and that reading in short bursts is still a good thing.
- Encourage parents to pick 2 or 3 books to focus on until the child knows them well. This will reinforce the "reading routine" and give the child a sense of accomplishment. Familiarity and repetition are good at this age. They are like practicing to get better and better at something.

Cultural Spotlight

Reading Aloud

Many cultures have strong storytelling traditions. By encouraging parents and grandparents to tell stories, even to young children, and by linking storytelling to books and illustrations, you may be able to help adults who are less familiar with the practice of reading aloud find new ways of enjoying books with their children.

For example, in health centers in Boston that serve a large Haitian community, many parents responded very positively to a beautifully illustrated picture book about a little girl on an island in the Caribbean who goes to market on market day. The book would not have seemed like an ideal choice for parents who didn't speak English as a first language because it existed only in an English edition, and it had dense blocks of text on the page.

However, several Haitian parents pointed out that because the illustrations were so evocative of life in the Caribbean, they could use the book to tell stories about their own childhoods, their families, and in general about a world that they wanted to make real for their children growing up in an American city.

It's important to emphasize to parents that telling stories to their children helps their children learn language, and to encourage parents to tell their stories in the language in which they feel most comfortable.

Parents should understand that books don't need to be read word by word, and that they can make up stories about characters, scenes, animals, or anything at all, and that by linking their storytelling at least some of the time to books, these parents are helping their children grow up enjoying books, and looking at books as sources of pleasure and information.

- Be sensitive to parents and their literacy levels; reading may be a challenge, a reminder of school failure, or simply an activity fraught with difficulty, rather than a pleasure. These are parents who are unlikely to model silent reading and are unlikely to find it easy or obvious to read to their own children, especially as their children grow into the preschool years and may want to hear longer and more complex stories. The children of parents who have difficulty reading are at particularly high risk for reading problems.

Speak positively and encouragingly to parents about their ability to help their children love and enjoy books. Suggest toys in the home that will give children more exposure to the alphabet, such as alphabet blocks and alphabet magnets.

Ask, in a nonjudgmental way, whether the parents would like to improve their own reading skills, and be prepared with a referral for parents who are interested.

- It may be difficult to discuss parents' literacy issues because of the shame and secrecy often associated with poor adult literacy.

As is the case for other uncomfortable topics that physicians are trained to discuss (eg, drug use, sexuality, domestic violence, gun ownership, etc), questions about literacy become easier to ask as the doctor becomes convinced of their worth and develops comfort with broaching the topic over time.

Typically, literacy-related questions fit easily in the context of gathering the social history, especially after the child's school performance or language development, or when handing out educational materials.

- How comfortable are you with your reading?
- Have you ever had difficulty reading?
- Has reading ever been a problem for you?
- If you had the time, would you be interested in a program to help you read better?

To be successful, any attempt to assist patients and families who have inadequate or marginal literacy skills must be accompanied by referrals to appropriate literacy programs. Providers can be of great service in this arena by sensitively making referrals to the most appropriate local literacy resource.

- Parents who struggled in school—or who saw an older child struggle in school—may project low expectations onto their children because of their own experiences.
- As children start school, some parents may be particularly intimidated by the school system and by teacher conferences, unable or reluctant to help with homework assignments that they themselves find difficult.

Some parents will find any discussion of their own school issues brings up bad memories. This underscores the importance of asking about and discussing reading comfort in a sensitive, non-stigmatizing way.

Many schools assign extensive reading homework in the lower grades, expecting parents to read with a child for some period every day, a particularly difficult assignment for parents not confident in their own skills. Continue to ask about reading progress and reading problems after children start school. Encourage parents who are concerned to speak with their children's teachers, and encourage parents to continue looking at books with their children after the children are in school and to let their children read aloud to them at home.

- Reading to children might not be a priority or a concern in a particular family.

- Parents who can decode print, but not fluently, may think of themselves as perfectly adequate readers, but again will be very unlikely to read for pleasure or to read aloud to their children.

- The family may view helping a child learn to read as strictly the job of the school and the teacher. The family may not come from a cultural tradition in which reading to children is common.

- Emphasize to parents that because their children care so much about spending time with them, they can play a very important role in helping a child grow up loving books.

- Talk to parents about incorporating books into the everyday routines of a young child, at bedtime, naptime, and other transition moments. Sharing books together can make these times easier.

- Encourage parents to continue using books in a child's routine even when the child is older and learning to read.

- Remember that there may be home and family issues that make homework problematic, including multiple caregivers, lack of a quiet place for the child to work, and schedule or work issues that make it difficult for the parent to spend time with the child on reading homework at a reasonable hour. Ask parents about their child care arrangements for the end of the day, and encourage them to think about who will be able to help the child with homework, and where that homework should be done.

Behavior Change

Behavior change is a key element in preventing and managing many pediatric conditions. Shifting from paternalistic advice that is either too vague or too complicated to a patient- or family-centered approach that incorporates elements of motivational interviewing and goal-setting, and that makes use of plain language, can be an effective way to empower patients and families to make changes and improve their health.

Help parents see that reading can be a family project—they can improve their own reading skills by reading to and with their children. Older siblings can read to younger siblings and receive praise and attention from their parents. And a child who is learning to read can come home and practice, and feel the family is impressed with his skills.

The more a family can incorporate reading into its routine, the better; if there's always a "book moment" when a parent comes home from work, or at bedtime, children will look forward to it. Suggest strategies to make the home into a more print-rich environment, including toys that help children get familiar with the alphabet; paper and pencils for writing practice; and books, magazines, and newspapers for all. Discuss family trips to the library and games to spot letters and words on the street, in the car, or at the supermarket. Play rhyming games to build phonemic awareness.

Child Involvement

Including the child, to the extent possible, is respectful and patient-centered and can contribute to developing health literacy skills as the child moves toward managing his or her own health as an adolescent and an adult. It can include direct, age-appropriate statements to the child, and also ways for the child to be involved in his or her health.

For example, even preverbal children can understand that a book can be a way of drawing a parent's attention, or it can be a good transitional object at bedtime; certainly 2-year-olds can badger their parents endlessly to have a particular book read aloud over and over. While this doesn't actually constitute understanding the process, in a certain sense—by putting appropriate and appealing books in the child's home environment—we can allow the child to assume some "self-management."

By 4 or 5 years old, children can understand the connection explicitly between looking at books, understanding books, and being ready for school. And as soon as they start school and grasp the importance of reading success, children can understand that practicing reading at home with a parent or older sibling is helpful.

Messages of encouragement (listening to the child read aloud briefly in the examination room, encouraging the child to read to the parent, encouraging the parent to listen and help) should reinforce the idea that learning to read is hard, and that you have to work on it every day. But include praise for the child's efforts, and confidence that they will succeed.

Teach-back

The concept of teaching back entails asking parents or patients to demonstrate understanding *using their own words*, not simply asking whether they have questions or whether they understand, because that may not elicit lack of understanding. Having patients explain in their own words not only assesses their understanding, but it reinforces the information by repeating it, and internalizes it for the patient. When there is a lot of information, go over each concept and elicit a teach-back before moving to the next idea.

When using teach-back, it's important to keep the burden on yourself. Avoid the perception that you are quizzing the parent or patient—emphasize that you want to be sure you've explained things clearly. The practice of using teach-back can be especially important over the phone, because it may be the only way to gauge whether the parent or patient understands fully.

Here are some approaches to using teach-back with respect to reading.

- What do you think you could do this evening to help Mariana enjoy books?
- When are the best times in Sam's day to look at a book with him?
- What kinds of questions could you ask Jackie about a picture like this one?
- Tell me what the reading homework is that Leo's teacher wants him to do (or wants you to do with him)?
- To make sure this plan works for you, who will do the reading homework with Olivia when you're at work?
- What can you do to help Monroe practice reading when you're driving with him or shopping with him?

Key Messages for Use by All Members of the Health Care Team

It is important to reinforce key messages for parents and children so they hear them more than once and recognize them as priorities in managing their health. Your staff can reemphasize the importance of care concepts. In addition, families should not receive conflicting advice about their health and what to do.

Key concepts for reading

- Looking at books with your child is good, important, helpful, and enjoyable.
- Children who grow up with books are more likely to love books and to learn to read without problems.
- Talk to your baby, and look at books with your baby even before your baby can talk.
- Teach your baby the names of all different things; show him pictures in books and point at them and name them.
- Your baby will love books because he will think of your voice, and he loves your voice.

- When your child is learning to read in school, let him practice by reading to you—tell him he's doing a good job, and give him time to figure out the words before you tell him what they are.
- Keep reading to your child even after he can read, and keep talking about the books and the pictures together.

Miscellaneous

These discussions may raise with some parents the often-sensitive issue of their own school problems, reading problems, or literacy limitations. Referral information should be available for adult and family literacy programs, and strong positive encouragement for adults who are thinking of taking this step: "As your reading skills get better, you will be able to help your child more and more."

To find an adult literacy program near you, go to http://www.literacydirectory.org and enter your ZIP code.

References

1. Mendelsohn AL, Mogilner LN, Dreyer BP, et al. The impact of a clinic-based literacy intervention on language development in inner-city preschool children. *Pediatrics.* 2001;107(1):130–134

2. High PC, LaGasse L, Becker S, et al. Literacy promotion in primary care pediatrics: can we make a difference? *Pediatrics.* 2000;105:927–934

3. Francis DJ, Stuebing KK, Shaywitz SS, et al. Developmental lag versus deficit models of reading disability: a longitudinal, individual growth curves analysis. *J Educ Psychol.* 1996;88:3–17

4. Shaywitz BA, Holford TR, Holahan JM, et al. A Matthew effect for IQ but not for reading: results from a longitudinal study. *Read Res Q.* 1995;30(4):894–906

5. Juel C. Learning to read and write: a longitudinal study of 54 children from first through fourth grades. *J Educ Psychol.* 1988;80(4):437-447

Start Reading to Your Child Early

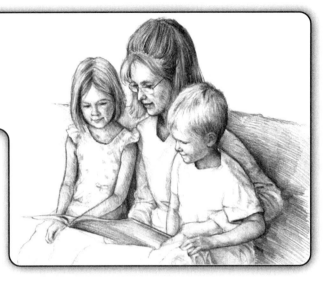

How to Help Your Child Learn to Read

A baby can enjoy books by 6 months of age! Here are things you can do with your child at different ages to help your child learn to love words and books.

Birth to Age 1

- Play with your baby often. Talk, sing, and say rhymes. This helps your baby learn to talk.
- Talk with your baby, making eye contact. Give your baby time to answer in baby talk.
- Give your baby sturdy board books to look at. It's OK for a baby to chew on a book.
- Look at picture books with your baby and name things. Say "See the baby!" or "Look at the puppy!"
- Babies like board books with pictures of babies and everyday objects like balls and blocks.
- Snuggle with your baby on your lap and read aloud. Your baby may not understand the story, but will love the sound of your voice and being close to you.
- Don't let your child watch TV until age 2 or older.

1 to 3 Years of Age

- Read to your child every day. Let your child pick the book, even if it's the same one again and again!
- Younger toddlers (1 to 2 years of age) like board books with pictures of children doing everyday things (like eating and playing). They also like "goodnight" books and books with rhymes. Books should only have a few words on each page.
- Older toddlers (2 to 3 years of age) like board books and books with paper pages. They love books with rhymes and words that are repeated. Books about families, friends, animals, and trucks are also good.
- Let your child "read" to you by naming things in the book or making up a story.
- Take your child to the library. Celebrate your child getting a library card!
- Keep talking, singing, saying rhymes, and playing with your child.
- Don't let your child watch TV until age 2 or older.

Reading Tips

- Set aside time every day to read together. Reading at bedtime is a great way to get ready for sleep.
- Leave books in your children's rooms for them to enjoy on their own. Have a comfortable bed or chair, bookshelf, and reading lamp.
- Read books your child enjoys. Your child may learn the words to a favorite book. Then, let your child complete the sentences, or take turns saying the words.
- Don't drill your child on letters, numbers, colors, shapes, or words. Instead, make a game of it.

Continued on back

3 to 5 Years of Age

- Read ABC books with your child. Point out letters as you read.

- Preschool children like books that tell stories. They also love counting books, alphabet books, and word books. Like toddlers, they love books with rhymes and words they can learn by heart.

- Help your child recognize whole words as well as letters. Point out things like letters on a stop sign or the name on a favorite store.

- Ask your child questions about the pictures and story. Invite him or her to make up a story about what's in the book.

- Some public TV shows, videos, and computer games can help your child learn to read. But you need to be involved too. Watch or play *with* your child and talk about the program. Limit TV time to 1 or 2 hours per day. Avoid violent shows and movies. Try to stick to educational shows.

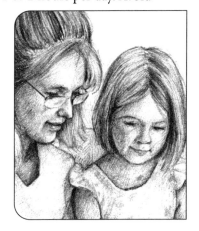

- Give your child lots of chances to use written words. Write shopping lists together. Write letters to friends or family.

Read Aloud With Your Child

Reading aloud is one of the best ways to help your child learn to read. The more excited you act when you read a book, the more your child will enjoy it.

- Use funny voices and animal noises!

- Look at the pictures. Ask your child to name things in the pictures. Talk about how the pictures go with the story. Ask what is happening in the story.

- Invite your child to join in when a line is repeated over and over.

- Show your child how things in the book are like things in your child's life.

- If your child asks a question, stop and answer it. Books can help children express their thoughts and solve problems.

- Keep reading to your child even after he or she learns to read. Children can listen and understand harder stories than they can read on their own.

Listen to Your Child Read Aloud

Once your child starts reading, have him or her read out loud. Take turns reading.

If your child asks for help with a word, give it right away. But let your child sound out words if he or she wants to.

Know when your child has had enough. Stop if your child is tired or frustrated.

Most of all, give lots of praise! You are your child's first, and most important, teacher!

The American Academy of Pediatrics (AAP) is grateful for the Reach Out and Read program's help with this handout. Reach Out and Read works with children's doctors to make promoting literacy and giving out books part of children's basic health care. This program is endorsed by the AAP. To learn more about Reach Out and Read, go to www.reachoutandread.org.

To learn more, visit the American Academy of Pediatrics (AAP) Web site at www.aap.org.

Your child's doctor will tell you to do what's best for your child.
This information should not take the place of talking with your child's doctor.

We hope the resources in this handout are helpful. The AAP is not responsible for the information in these resources. We try to keep the information up to date but it may change at any time.

Adaptation of the AAP information in this handout into plain language was supported in part by McNeil Consumer Healthcare.

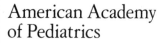

American Academy of Pediatrics

DEDICATED TO THE HEALTH OF ALL CHILDREN™

Léale temprano a su niño
(Start Reading to Your Child Early)

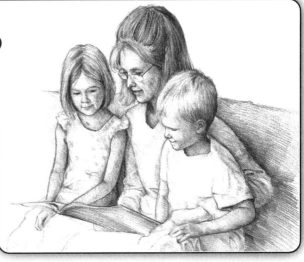

Ayude a su niño a aprender a leer

¡Los bebés pueden disfrutar de los libros desde los seis meses de edad! Leyendo juntos, su niño aprenderá a amar las palabras y los libros.

Desde el nacimiento hasta la edad de un año

- Juegue con su bebé lo más que pueda. Hable, cante con rimas. Esto le ayudará a aprender a hablar.
- Hable con su bebé y mírelo a los ojos. Dele tiempo para responder en su lenguaje de bebé.
- Dele a su bebé libros de cartón grueso para que los mire. No importa si se los mete en la boca.
- Muéstrele a su bebé libros con dibujos. Mencione los nombres de los objetos. Diga, "¡mira el bebé!" o "¡mira el perrito!".
- A los bebés les gustan los libros con fotos de bebés y objetos comunes como los animales y los juguetes.
- Siente a su bebé sobre sus piernas y léale en voz alta. Puede ser que su bebé no entienda la historia. Aún así, le encantará el sonido de su voz y estar cerca de usted.
- No deje que su bebé mire televisión sino hasta que sea mayor de dos años.

De uno a tres años de edad

- Léale a su niño todos los días. Deje que su niño escoja el libro. ¡Incluso, está bien si escoge el mismo libro una y otra vez!
- A los niños pequeños (de uno a dos años) les gustan los libros con fotos de niños haciendo actividades diarias y comunes. (Por ejemplo, niños comiendo y jugando).

  También les gustan los libros para dar las "buenas noches" y los libros con rimas. Los libros deben tener pocas palabras en cada página.

- A los niños más grandes (de dos a tres años) les gustan los libros con páginas de papel. Les encantan los libros con rimas y palabras que se repiten. Los libros sobre familias, amigos, animales y carritos también son buenos.
- Deje que su niño le "lea" nombrando cosas de su libro o inventando su propio cuento.
- Lleve a su niño a la biblioteca. ¡Celebre cuando él reciba su tarjeta de la biblioteca!
- Siga hablándole, cantándole, diciéndole rimas y jugando con él.

Consejos para leer

- Haga tiempo cada día para leer juntos. Leer de noche ayuda al niño a prepararse para dormir.
- Ponga los libros al alcance de su niño para que los disfrute a solas. ¡Sólo necesita una buena luz!
- Lea libros que su niño disfruta. Su niño puede aprenderse las palabras de su libro favorito. Lean las palabras por turnos. También, dejen que su niño termine las frases en cada página.
- No le exija que aprenda letras, números, colores, formas o palabras. Al contrario, haga que todo sea sólo un juego, ¡y verá cómo aprende jugando!

Continúa atrás

Viene de la página anterior

De tres a cinco años de edad

- Lea libros sobre las letras del alfabeto con su niño. Señale las letras a medida que las lee.

- A los niños preescolares les gustan los libros que cuentan historias. También les encantan los libros con números, rimas y palabras que se pueden aprender de memoria.

- Ayude a que su niño también reconozca palabras completas. Muéstrele la señal de pare ("stop") o el letrero del nombre de su tienda favorita.

- Hágale preguntas sobre los dibujos y las historias. Invítelo a inventar un cuento sobre los dibujos del libro.

- Algunos programas públicos de televisión, videos y juegos de computadora pueden ayudar a su niño a aprender a leer. Pero usted también necesita participar. Vean los juegos juntos y hablen sobre ellos. Limite el tiempo de ver televisión a una o dos horas al día. Evite programas o películas de violencia.

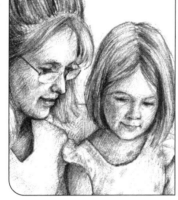

- Intente ver solamente programas educativos.

- Dele a su niño muchas oportunidades para usar palabras escritas. Escriban las listas para las compras. Escriban cartas para los amigos o familiares.

Lea en voz alta con su niño

Leer en voz alta es una de las mejores maneras de ayudar a su niño a aprender a leer. Entre más divertida se muestre usted al leer el libro, más lo disfrutará su niño.

- ¡Haga voces graciosas y sonidos de animales!

- Miren los dibujos. Pida a su niño que le diga los nombres de las cosas en los dibujos.

- Hablen de cómo los dibujos se relacionan con la historia. Pregúntele qué está sucediendo en la historia. Invite a su niño a participar cuando una línea se repita varias veces.

- Platique con su niño sobre cómo lo leído se relaciona con su vida diaria.

- Si su niño le hace una pregunta, deténgase y respóndala. Los libros pueden ayudar a los niños a expresar sus pensamientos y resolver sus problemas.

- Siga leyéndole incluso cuando ya haya aprendido a leer. Los niños pueden escuchar y comprender historias más difíciles de las que pueden leer por sí mismos.

Escuche a su niño leer en voz alta

Después de que su niño empiece a leer, haga que le lea en voz alta. Lean las palabras por turnos.

Si su niño le pide ayuda con una palabra, léala de inmediato. Pero deje que su niño deletree las palabras si desea hacerlo.

Preste atención para darse cuenta de cuando su niño ya leyó lo suficiente. Pare de leer si su niño está cansado o frustrado.

Sobre todo, ¡festéjelo mucho! ¡Usted es la primera maestra de su niño y quizás la más importante!

La "American Academy of Pediatrics (AAP)" agradece la ayuda del programa *Leyendo Juntos* ("Reach Out and Read") para la elaboración de este folleto. "Reach Out and Read" trabaja con los doctores de los niños para ayudar a promover el alfabetismo y distribuir libros como parte del cuidado de salud básico para los niños.

Este programa está apoyado por la AAP. Para conocer más acerca de "Reach Out and Read", visite la página en el Internet www.reachoutandread.org

Para aprender más, visite el sitio de la Academia Americana de Pediatría (AAP) en www.aap.org. Su pediatra le dirá qué es lo mejor para la salud de su hijo.

Esta información no debe usarse en lugar de consultar con su doctor.

Esperamos que la información en este folleto le sea útil. La AAP no es responsable por la información contenida en este folleto. Tratamos de presentar la información más actual pero a veces las recomendaciones cambian.

La adaptación de la información de este folleto de la AAP a lenguaje sencillo se hizo con el apoyo de McNeil Consumer Healthcare. La traducción al español fue patrocinada por Leyendo Juntos (Reach Out and Read), un programa pediátrico de alfabetización.

American Academy of Pediatrics

DEDICATED TO THE HEALTH OF ALL CHILDREN™

Temper Tantrums

Temper tantrums—a common behavioral concern of toddlers and young children—are the major reason for the phrase "the terrible twos." Some 50% to 80% of 2- and 3-year-old children have temper tantrums at least weekly, and 20% at least once a day.[1]

There are many opportunities for misunderstanding the health care professional's directions for managing and preventing temper tantrums. If tantrums are not managed appropriately, they can lead to loss of self-esteem in the child, inappropriate punishments or bribery to get the child to stop, and even child abuse. If caretakers give in to a child during a tantrum, the child may act out even longer the next time she has a temper tantrum, exacerbating the underlying behavior.

Common areas for miscommunication may include

- Expectations and fears by the caretakers
- Prevention and health promotion strategies
- Management and treatment
- Indicators that the tantrums are not within the spectrum of normal, age-related behavior and need further attention

Ask Me 3

During your patient encounter, you should communicate using plain language and health literacy principles so that by the end of the visit, the parent or child will know the answers to the *Ask Me 3* questions.

A Patient Story. . .

Chris is a 3-year-old healthy male who has an appointment with Dr Snyder for a routine health supervision visit. The schedule for today is very tight due to widespread influenza activity.

When Dr Snyder asks what concerns Chris' mother has about her son, she says, "I am afraid he is going to hurt himself one day when he has one of his fits."

Thinking that "fit" meant seizure, Dr Snyder asked the mother a number of questions to help diagnose the reason Chris was having "fits."

Finally the physician asked the mother to describe what Chris does during a typical "fit."

"Well, it looks just like what happens when his other friends don't get what they want. He throws himself on the ground, kicking and screaming for about 30 minutes."

At this point, the doctor realized that Chris was most likely having temper tantrums and not seizures.

Dr Snyder spent precious minutes out of an already hectic day related to a miscommunication, and he still needs to address the mother's concerns, and counsel her on behavioral management of the tantrums.

· ·

In this case, the physician did not initially understand what the mother meant by "fits," and assumed she was describing a seizure.

Communication is at the core of the patient-physician relationship, and represents a bidirectional discussion that requires each party's understanding.

Sometimes, one's understanding of what a word means can either interfere with communication, or at least take one off the right diagnostic track when talking with families.

Dr Snyder could have enhanced communication and efficiency by asking questions to clarify the problem first, prior to jumping directly to diagnostic or management discussions based on assumptions.

Patient: Arturo, a 4-year-old who has frequent temper tantrums	
Ask Me 3 questions	**What the parent should understand at the end of the visit**
What is my child's main problem?	It is hard for Arturo to hold strong feelings inside, so he acts out his feelings instead of saying what he feels.
What do I need to do (to prevent a tantrum)?	• I must create a daily routine for Arturo. He should get up, eat, and go to bed at the same time each day. • I need to childproof the house to make it hard for Arturo to hurt himself and to decrease the number of times I have to say "no." • I need to give Arturo choices, when possible, like letting him choose what color shirt to wear. • I need to set a good example when I am angry. • When I say "no," I mean "no." I must not change my mind from minute to minute or day to day. • I will pay attention to Arturo when he is being good. When I see him playing nicely, I will tell him what a good boy he is and sit down and play with him.
What do I need to do (when my child has a tantrum)?	• I need to distract him by saying something like: "Look at the funny kitty," "Did you notice that big hat?" • I must stay calm, even if he is screaming at the top of his lungs. If I feel that I am about to scream, I must make sure he is safe and leave the room. • I need to ignore his crying, screaming, and kicking, even if other people are staring at us.
Why is it important for me to do this?	Doing this will reward Arturo's good behavior, not his tantrums, with my attention. That will help Arturo learn how to act and better control his feelings.

Medical Terms and Plain Language Alternatives

Many of the medical terms we use every day don't mean much to many parents. Below is a list of medical terms that may be confusing or difficult to explain and suggestions for plain language alternatives.

Medical Terms	Plain Language Alternatives
Confident	Sure, certain
Consequences	Something that happens because of a tantrum
Corporal punishment	Spanking, paddling
Developmental	Growing and learning
Discipline	To correct; to teach; using ways to set limits on how a child acts, like putting a child in time-out
Distract	Point out something else, sidetrack

Precipitants	Things that happen before a tantrum and lead to it
Reinforce	Things you do that cause something (good or bad) to happen again
Supportive	Caring, loving, helpful
Temper tantrum	Make a scene, throw a fit, melt down, scream, cry and kick
Time out	The time you take a child out of an activity to allow her to cool down. Try 1 minute of time-out for every year of your child's age.
Verbalize	Use words

Confusing Terms and Concepts

With any condition, there are likely to be terms or concepts for which patients and families have a different understanding than a health care professional. These may include preventive strategies, complex disease processes, medication or treatment regimens, abstract laboratory results or measurements, technical terms, or words that have a different meaning in the health care arena than in everyday use. Cultural issues and misconceptions can also contribute to lack of understanding.

Consider the following when talking with parents about temper tantrums:

Prevention and Health Promotion

Parents are the experts on their children. Help them identify ways to stop a tantrum before it occurs. Teach parents about "time-in," and help them practice catching their child being good. Ask parents to identify times when they could let their child make choices. Advise parents to childproof their home as much as possible, thereby decreasing their need to say "no."

Diagnosis

Parents may not understand their child's behavior and may also have unrealistic expectations and fears about the problem. Empathize with the parents' feelings of frustration.

Emphasize that temper tantrums are very common: 50% to 80% of 2- and 3-year-old children have temper tantrums at least weekly, and 20% at least once a day.[1]

Empower the caretaker to identify situations that trigger tantrums, such as lack of sleep, hunger, and developmental frustrations. Have caretakers keep a tantrum log that notes time, duration, precipitants, and consequences of the child's tantrums.

Symptoms

Although tantrums are common, outline those symptoms that may indicate a more severe problem.

- Typical symptoms of temper tantrums include displays of anger (yelling, screaming, kicking, hitting, dropping to the floor, and throwing things) that progress to crying and signs of distress.
- Breath-holding spells may sometimes occur with a tantrum.
- Tantrums that occur 3 or more times a day or last longer than 15 minutes should be brought to a doctor's attention because frequent and prolonged episodes may indicate a serious emotional problem.
- Contact the doctor if the child attacks others, breaks valuable items on purpose, or demonstrates behavior that could hurt himself or herself.

Management and Treatment

Some parents may want to punish a child for having a tantrum.

- Punishing a child may cause the child to keep his or her feelings inside, which is actually worse in the long run than having a tantrum.
- Spanking a child will only cause the child to scream louder, and it will teach the child that hitting others is OK.

Some parents have been told to ignore all behaviors during a tantrum.

- There are exceptions: A child should never be ignored for hitting, kicking, spitting, pinching, or throwing things at another person during a tantrum. These behaviors cannot be ignored.

Some parents may want to yell at their child or try to reason with him or her during a tantrum.

- You cannot reason with a screaming child, and yelling may only make things worse. The more attention you give a child during a temper tantrum the more likely it is to happen again.
- It is hard to stay calm. If you start to feel angry, you should put your child in a safe place and leave the room for a minute or two, and then come back.

Some parents may give in to the child's demands just to stop a tantrum, especially if it is in public.

- The best way to stop a "public" tantrum is to take your child home or to the car.
- If you give in, that will only teach the child that a temper tantrum will help him get his way.

Cultural Beliefs

Parents tend to discipline their children in the same manner they were disciplined. Because difficulties can arise with differing parenting styles of multiple caregivers, talk to parents about coming up with a plan so that everyone who cares for the child delivers the same discipline.

One study found that a family's disagreement about child-rearing practices can pose an independent risk for behavioral problems.[2]

In addition to differing child-rearing styles, parental perceptions (or other caretakers' perceptions) of the behavior problem can have an impact on communication between families and physicians.

There are cross-cultural differences in parenting styles and intolerance of temper tantrums.[3] Some of the differences associated with severe temper tantrums include use of corporal punishment, marital stress, and child care provided exclusively by the mother.[4] In counseling, it is important to remember that the frequency of tantrums is not related to gender or social class.

Extended family members may play an important role in decision-making and management, which can result in further confusion or lack of adherence to suggested management. Explore all of these issues by asking the parent what they think is causing the tantrums and what they think will make them better. This will increase your understanding of their culture while uncovering possible roadblocks or cultural issues with treatment before they arise. In addition, ask what other members of the family believe is the cause.

Worsening Condition

Parents may not know what to look for when determining whether their child's tantrums are a problem or not. Explain to a parent that tantrums are a problem if the parent or other caretaker believes that they are a problem. Tell parents to inform you of the following:

- If tantrums occur 3 times a day or last more than 15 minutes apiece
- If tantrums continue after the child is 4 years old

- If the child intentionally breaks valuable objects, attacks others, or exhibits self-injurious behavior
- If the child has other behavioral problems (disturbed sleep, aggressive behaviors, or an explosive temper)

Behavior Change

Behavior change is a key element in preventing and managing many pediatric conditions. Shifting from paternalistic advice that is either too vague or too complicated to a patient- or family-centered approach that incorporates elements of motivational interviewing and goal-setting, and that makes use of plain language, can be an effective way to empower patients and families to make changes and improve their health.

When seeing a family with behavioral concerns, it is important to address the family's motivation and confidence in creating change. Some questions you might ask a family whose child engages in temper tantrums would include

- How sure are you that you can prevent some of these tantrums?
- How certain are you that you will not give in the next time your child has a tantrum? What if he or she cries for an hour? What if he or she has the tantrum in public?
- Do you believe "time out" will work with your child?
- How confident do you feel in teaching others who help take care of your child about preventing and handling the tantrum?
- Can you go over what you will tell Frankie's father about managing his temper tantrums?

Child Involvement

Temper tantrums are a child's physical expression of what he or she is feeling inside. A young child or one who has a speech or language delay cannot express with words what he is thinking. As the number of words a child can say increases, temper tantrums occur less often. By the time the child is 3, parents can begin to teach their children to verbalize their feelings. Adults, or even older siblings, can suggest words or phrases that would help the toddler such as, "You look really mad."

It is also important to teach a child what to *do* when she is angry, like going outside and running around or going into the bedroom and hitting a pillow or a punching bag. Make sure that whatever is chosen is not going to disturb or hurt other people and that nothing is damaged or destroyed.

Another method that can be used with a child is to read books. There are numerous books that describe what happens when a child

Did You Know...?

One study found that parents want more information on common pediatric topics such as discipline. Parents who had discussed more topics with their physicians were more likely to report excellent health care. Parents who reported they could use more information on a larger number of topics were also much more willing to pay for additional care.

Source: Regalado M, Klein DJ. Anticipatory guidance: what information do parents receive? What information do they want? *Arch Pediatr Adolesc Med.* 2000;154(12):1191–1198.

is angry, sad, or frustrated, such as *Andrew's Angry Words* by Dorothea Lachner and *Don't Rant and Rave on Wednesdays!* by Adolph Moser and David Melton. Scholastic has a book series titled *Help Me Be Good*, which includes a book by Joy Berry on *Throwing Tantrums*. The book *Alexander and the Terrible, Horrible, No Good, Very Bad Day* by Judith Viorst and Ray Cruz is available both in English and Spanish. Reading with a child can not only help the child learn to deal with feelings, but also can bring a family together for quality time and enhance the role of reading in a child's life.

Teach-back

The concept of teaching back entails asking parents or patients to demonstrate understanding *using their own words,* not simply asking whether they have questions or whether they understand, because that may not elicit lack of understanding. Having patients explain in their own words not only assesses their understanding, but it reinforces the information by repeating it and internalizes it for the patient. When there is a lot of information, go over each concept and elicit a teach-back before moving to the next idea.

When using teach-back, it's important to keep the burden on yourself. Avoid the perception that you are quizzing the parent or patient— emphasize that you want to be sure you've explained things clearly.

The practice of using teach-back can be especially important over the phone, because it may be the only way to gauge whether the parent or patient understands.

Here are some approaches to using teach-back when talking about temper tantrums.

- What will you tell your (mother, babysitter) about why Tenecia has tantrums?
- To make sure that I've explained things clearly, can you tell me what you will do when Tenecia throws her next fit in the grocery store?
- What would you tell another parent about how to prevent tantrums?

Key Messages for Use by All Members of the Health Care Team

It is important to reinforce key messages for parents and children so they hear them more than once and recognize them as priorities in managing their health. In addition, families should not receive conflicting advice about their health and what to do.

First, make sure everyone on your staff is equipped to deal appropriately with the inevitable tantrum that will occur in your office.

- Have staff provide choices for children where applicable: "Would you like the yellow or the blue bandage?"
- Childproof the office, including keeping equipment and supplies out of a young child's reach.
- Encourage all staff members to help the child to use words instead of actions such as, "I can see that you are scared."
- Provide distractions for a child while he is in the office, like pages to color or draw on, having someone blow bubbles when the child is getting a shot, and having the child blow on a pinwheel when he is getting his lungs examined.
- Encourage a child to bring her favorite stuffed animal or doll with her to the visit.
- Keep Cheerios, crackers, and drinks available in the office for a child who might have a meltdown in the office when she is hungry and has waited a long time.
- When a child throws a tantrum in the office, be supportive and reinforce what the caretaker is doing right. Use it as a teaching opportunity for other parents who are in the office at the same time who have children around the same age.
- Loan or provide reading materials, audiotapes, or even videotapes on temper tantrums for other people who help take care of the child but are not at the visit. Videotapes can also be shown while families are waiting in the waiting room or examination room.

Then, when talking with parents and caregivers about tantrums, make sure the whole staff remembers these key concepts.

- It is hard for children to hold strong feelings inside or to express what they are feeling, so they act out their feelings instead.
- Routines allow children to feel comfortable.
- Childproofing the home not only makes it more difficult for children to hurt themselves, but it also decreases the number of times you have to say "no."
- Give the child choices.
- Set a good example when you are angry by staying calm, even if she is screaming at the top of her lungs. If you feel that you are about to scream, make sure the child is safe and leave the room.
- When you say "no," mean "no," and keep rules consistent.
- One technique for bringing a child out of a tantrum is to distract him.

- Ignore his crying, screaming, and kicking, even if other people are staring at you.

- Reward good behavior—not tantrums—with attention and verbal praise to show the child how to act and better control her feelings. In other words, catch your child being good. Use "time-in" more than "time-out."

Miscellaneous

If you teach a family how to help one child, what they have learned can be translated to future children and even grandchildren. If you have group visits for well-child care visits, parents can teach other parents. Parents are even more powerful in their ability to teach than the physician or staff, because other parents realize that they understand what they are going through. Teaching families what they are doing right empowers them and accentuates the positives. In addition, teaching about how to prevent temper tantrums can provide an opportunity to encourage reading in the home.

References

1. Needlman R. Temper tantrums. In: Parker S, Zuckerman B, Augustyn M, eds. *Behavioral and Developmental Pediatrics: A Handbook for Primary Care.* 2nd ed. Philadelphia, PA: Lippincott Williams & Wilkins; 2005

2. Li Y, Shi A, Wan Y, Hotta M, Ushijima H. Child behavior problems: prevalence and correlates in rural minority areas of China. *Pediatr Int.* 2001;43(6):651–661

3. Javo C, Ronning JA, Heyerdahl S. Child-rearing in an indigenous Sami population in Norway: a cross-cultural comparison of parental attitudes and expectations. *Scand J Psychol.* 2004;45(1):67–78

4. Needlman R, Stevenson J, Zuckerman B. Psychosocial correlates of severe temper tantrums. *J Dev Behav Pediatr.* 1991;12(2):77–83

Temper Tantrums

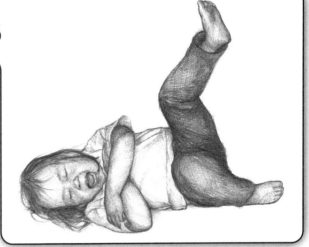

It's hard for a young child to hold strong feelings inside. Young children often cry, scream, or stomp up and down when they are upset. As a parent, you may feel angry, helpless, or ashamed.

Temper tantrums are normal. They are one way a child learns self-control. Almost all children have tantrums between the ages of 1 and 3. By age 4, they usually stop.

What to Do for a Temper Tantrum

Try these tips when your child has a temper tantrum:

- **Try to stay calm.** *If you can't stay calm, leave the room.* Wait a minute or two before coming back, or wait until the crying stops.
- **Distract your child.** Point out something else to do, like read a book or play with a toy. Say something like, "Look at what the kitty is doing."
- **Let your child cool off or have a "time-out."** Take your child away from the problem. Give your child some time alone to calm down. Try 1 minute of time-out for every year of your child's age. (For example, a 4-year-old would get a 4-minute time-out.) Don't use time-out too much or it won't work.
- **Be ready to take your child home if your child has a "public" tantrum.** The best way of stopping "public" tantrums is to take your child home or to the car.
- **Ignore your child's crying, screaming, or kicking if you can.** Stand nearby or hold your child without talking until your child calms down. The more attention you give a tantrum, the more likely it is to happen again.

The following things are *not* OK. Don't ignore these actions:

- Hitting or kicking people
- Throwing things that might hurt someone or break something
- Yelling for a long time

If your child does these things, take him or her away from the problem. Hold your child. Say firmly, "No hitting" or "No throwing" to make sure your child knows what behavior is not OK.

What *Not* to Do

Never punish your child for temper tantrums. Your child may start to keep feelings inside, which is worse.

Don't give in to your child's demands just to stop a tantrum. This teaches that a temper tantrum will help your child get his or her way. Tantrums are more likely to stop if your child doesn't gain anything from them.

Don't talk too much to your child during the tantrum. It is hard to reason with a screaming child. When your child calms down, talk about better ways to deal with anger and frustration.

What to Expect

Your child should have fewer temper tantrums by age 3 1/2. Between tantrums, he or she should seem normal and healthy. Every child grows and learns at his or her own pace. It may take time to learn how to control his or her temper.

Continued on back

Continued from front

A Word About Safety

Sometimes you have to say "no" to protect your child from harm. This is a common cause of a tantrum. So, what can you do?

- Childproof your home as much as you can.
- Make dangerous places and things off-limits.
- Keep an eye on your child at all times. Never leave small children alone, especially if there may be danger.
- Take away anything dangerous right away. Give your child something safe in its place.
- Be clear and firm about safety rules.

Call the Doctor If...

...your child shows any of these signs:

- Hurts himself or herself or others during tantrums
- Holds his or her breath and faints
- The tantrums get worse after age 4
- Has lots of other behavior problems

When tantrums are bad or happen often, they may be a sign of emotional problems. Your child's doctor can help you find out what is behind the tantrums. The doctor can also give you advice on dealing with them.

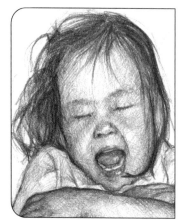

How to Help Prevent Temper Tantrums

You can't prevent *all* tantrums, but these ideas may help:

- **Make sure you give your child enough attention.** Children try to get attention in many ways. If being good doesn't do it, they may try being bad. To children, even "negative" attention (when you are upset) is better than none at all. So notice your child being good and reward the behavior.

- **Set limits that make sense.** Give simple reasons for the rules you set, and don't change the rules.

- **Keep a daily routine** as much as you can. This helps your child know what to expect.

- **Let your child make choices whenever you can.** For example, "Do you want apple juice or orange juice?" Or let's say your child doesn't want to take a bath. Make it clear that he or she will be taking a bath. But offer a real choice he or she can make. Try saying, "It's time for your bath. Would you like to walk or have me carry you?"

- **Try not to say "no" too much.** Choose your battles. Children need to have some feeling of control.

- **Give your child a few minutes' warning before changing activities.** This helps children get ready for a change.

- **Ask your child to use words to tell you how he or she is feeling.** Suggest words he or she can use to describe those feelings. For example, "I'm really mad."

- **Be ready with healthy snacks when your child gets hungry.**

- **Make sure your child gets enough rest.**

- **Set a good example.** Try not to argue or yell in front of your child.

To learn more, visit the American Academy of Pediatrics (AAP) Web site at www.aap.org.

Your child's doctor will tell you to do what's best for your child.
This information should not take the place of talking with your child's doctor.

Adaptation of the AAP information in this handout into plain language was supported in part by McNeil Consumer Healthcare.

American Academy of Pediatrics

DEDICATED TO THE HEALTH OF ALL CHILDREN™

Las rabietas o berrinches

(Temper Tantrums)

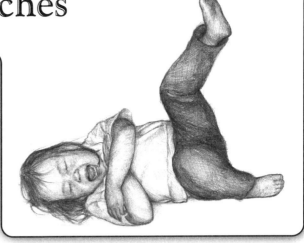

Es difícil para los pequeños contener la expresión de sus sentimientos fuertes dentro de sí mismos. Los niños pequeños con frecuencia lloran, gritan o patean cuando están enojados. Como padre, usted puede sentirse enojado, impotente o avergonzado.

Las rabietas o berrinches son normales. Son una manera en que el niño aprende el autocontrol. Casi todos los niños hacen berrinches entre las edades de 1 a 3 años. Normalmente terminan a los cuatro años de edad.

Qué hacer con las rabietas

Practique estos consejos cuando a su niño le dé una rabieta:

- **Trate de mantener la calma.** *Si usted no puede mantener la calma, salga de la habitación.* Espere uno o dos minutos antes de regresar o espere hasta que su niño deje de llorar.
- **Distraiga a su niño.** Enséñele algo diferente que él pueda hacer, como leer un libro o jugar con un juguete. Dígale algo como, "mira lo que está haciendo el gatito".
- **Deje que su niño se calme o póngalo en un "tiempo a solas".** Aleje a su niño del problema. Déjelo un tiempo solo para que se calme. Intente darle un minuto de "tiempo a solas" por cada año de la edad de su niño. (Por ejemplo, a un niño de cuatro años se le darían cuatro minutos de "tiempo a solas"). No utilice mucho el "tiempo a solas" o ya no funcionará.
- **Esté listo para llevarse a su niño a casa si le da una rabieta "en público".** La mejor manera de detener los berrinches en público es llevarse al niño a la casa o al automóvil.
- **Si puede, ignore el llanto, los gritos o las patadas de su niño.** Manténgase de pie cerca de su niño o sosténgalo sin hablarle hasta que se calme. Entre más atención le ponga a los berrinches del niño, más los repetirá.

No deje que su niño:

- Pegue o patee a la gente.
- Tire cosas que pueden herir a alguien o romper algo.
- Grite por mucho tiempo.

Si su niño hace estas cosas, aléjelo del problema. Sosténgalo y dígale firmemente, "no pegues" o "no empujes" para que aprenda que tal conducta no está bien.

Qué cosas *no* debe hacer

No castigue a su niño por hacer una rabieta.

No acceda a las peticiones de su niño sólo para detener la rabieta. Esto le enseñará que hacer una rabieta le ayudará a obtener lo que desea. Es más probable que las rabietas paren si su niño no obtiene nada de ellas.

No le hable mucho durante una rabieta. Es difícil razonar con un niño que grita. Cuando su niño se calme, háblele sobre las mejores maneras para expresar el enojo y la frustración.

Qué puede esperar

Su niño debe tener menos rabietas después de los tres años y medio. Entre rabietas, el niño debe parecer normal y sano. Cada niño crece y aprende a su propio ritmo. Quizás le tome algún tiempo aprender cómo controlar su temperamento.

Continúa atrás

Unas palabras sobre la seguridad

A veces usted tiene que decir "no" para proteger a su niño de algún peligro. Esta es una de las razones comunes que causan las rabietas en el niño. Entonces, ¿qué puede hacer?

- Instale medidas de seguridad para niños en su casa.
- Haga que los lugares y las cosas peligrosas estén fuera del alcance del niño.
- Vigile a su niño en todo momento. Nunca deje solos a los niños pequeños, en especial si hay algún peligro.
- Quítele todas las cosas peligrosas de inmediato. En su lugar, dele algo que no sea peligroso.
- Sea claro y firme al explicar las reglas de seguridad.

Llame al doctor si…

…su niño muestra cualquiera de estas señales:

- Se lastima a sí mismo o a otros durante las rabietas.
- Retiene la respiración y se desmaya.
- Las rabietas empeoran después de los cuatro años.
- Tiene muchos problemas de conducta.

Cuando las rabietas son severas o suceden con frecuencia, pueden ser una señal de problemas emocionales. El doctor de su niño puede ayudarle a descubrir por qué el niño tiene rabietas. También puede darle consejos sobre cómo tratar las rabietas.

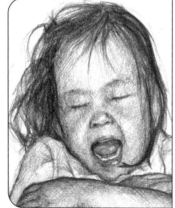

Cómo prevenir las rabietas

Las rabietas no se pueden prevenir por *completo*. Las siguientes ideas pueden ayudar:

- **Asegúrese de ponerle suficiente atención al niño.** Los niños tratan de llamar la atención de muchas maneras. Si ser buenos no es suficiente, pueden intentarlo portándose mal. Para los niños, incluso la atención "negativa" (cuando usted está enojado) es mejor que no tener nada de atención. Así que ponga atención cuando su niño es bueno y recompense esa conducta.
- **Establezca límites que tengan sentido.** Dé razones sencillas para las reglas que ponga y no cambie las reglas.
- **Mantenga una rutina diaria** lo más que pueda. Esto ayudará a que su niño sepa qué puede esperar.
- **Deje que su niño tome decisiones cuando pueda.** Por ejemplo, "¿quieres jugo de manzana o de naranja?" Digamos que a su niño no le gusta bañarse. Dígale bien claro al niño que se tiene que dar un baño. Pero ofrézcale opciones para que pueda tomar una decisión. Trate de decirle, "Es hora del baño". "¿Quieres caminar o que te lleve cargado?"
- **Trate de no decir "no" demasiadas veces.** Escoja qué batallas quiere pelear. Los niños necesitan tener cierta sensación de control.
- **Avísele unos minutos antes de cambiar las actividades.** Esto ayuda a que los niños se preparen para el cambio.
- **Pídale que use palabras para describir cómo se está sintiendo.** Sugiera las palabras que puede usar para describir esos sentimientos. Por ejemplo, le puede decir "veo que estas enojado….."
- **Prepare bocadillos saludables para tenerlos listos cuando le dé hambre.** Cuando los niños tienen hambre o están cansados, tienen más berrinches.
- **Asegúrese de que su niño descanse lo suficiente.**
- **Dé un buen ejemplo.** Trate de no discutir o gritar frente a su niño.

American Academy of Pediatrics

DEDICATED TO THE HEALTH OF ALL CHILDREN™

Tobacco
Secondhand Smoke Exposure

This section focuses on children's exposure to tobacco use and secondhand smoke. In the United States, 21 million children (35%) live in homes where residents or visitors smoke on a regular basis.[1] And approximately 50% to 75% of US children have detectable levels of cotinine, the breakdown product of nicotine in the blood.[1]

Based on the following American Lung Association statistics,[1] secondhand smoke is especially harmful to young children:

- Secondhand smoke is believed to be responsible for between 150,000 and 300,000 lower respiratory tract infections in infants and children younger than 18 months, resulting in between 7,500 and 15,000 hospitalizations each year.

- Secondhand smoke is blamed for 430 deaths from sudden infant death syndrome (SIDS) in the United States every year.

- Secondhand smoke exposure may cause buildup of fluid in the middle ear, resulting in 790,000 physician office visits per year.

- Secondhand smoke can also aggravate symptoms in 400,000 to 1 million children with asthma.

Each one of these contacts between physician and parent or patient is an opportunity for miscommunication, which can lead to prolonged or increasingly severe symptoms and ailments. Each is also an opportunity to communicate about the importance of avoiding all tobacco exposure.

Because smoking is a personal choice for adults, it can be a touchy subject to approach. More than 38 million people in the United States have successfully quit smoking, but there are still around 50 million Americans who smoke. Most say they would like to quit.[2] Tobacco is believed to have an

A Patient Story. . .

Jana is a healthy 2-year-old girl whose mother is concerned because Jana seems to have "constant colds." Jana has been seen in her pediatrician's office 6 times over the past 3 months for cough and congestion, but otherwise has had no health problems.

Mrs Miller has grown increasingly frustrated that "nothing is being done about Jana's bad immune system."

Jana's dad smokes, and the pediatrician, Dr Smythe, has explained that secondhand smoke is harmful to Jana's lungs. Mrs Miller insists that she and her husband know about secondhand smoke, and she adds, "He doesn't smoke in the house or car when Jana is around, so it's not a problem."

Dr Smythe tells Mrs Miller that Jana's symptoms do not warrant antibiotics. She counsels Mrs Miller that Jana's symptoms are partly related to tobacco smoke exposure, and she recommends symptomatic treatment for Jana's cold symptoms.

Dr Smythe also tells Mrs Miller to monitor Jana for fever or other new symptoms, and again admonishes her to keep Jana away from tobacco smoke.

....

Mrs Miller assumes that because Jana's father doesn't smoke "when Jana is around," they are keeping her safe from secondhand smoke exposure. It wasn't made clear to the family that tobacco smoke gets into the fabrics of the home and car, and into clothes, hair, and skin.

Dr Smythe could have been clearer that recurrent upper respiratory infections are common at Jana's age and do not signal immune problems. This would also have been an excellent opportunity to review more specifics about the health risks of tobacco smoke exposure, including risks of more frequent respiratory problems.

In admonishing Mrs Miller, Dr Smythe decreased the chances of partnering with the parents to improve Jana's health. Mrs Miller needs the pediatrician's support because Mr Miller's smoking may be a point of conflict within the family.

(continued)

A Patient Story. . .

(continued from previous page)

It would be more helpful to review ways to limit Jana's secondhand smoke exposure, discuss ways for Mrs Miller to educate her husband about dangers to Jana's health, and encourage Mrs Miller to explore her husband's willingness to consider smoking cessation.

addictive potential comparable to alcohol, cocaine, and morphine.[2] So remember to be sensitive to the parent's feelings on the subject—as well as to the difficulty of quitting—or your message about the child's health may get lost.

Ask Me 3

During your patient encounter, you should communicate using plain language and health literacy principles so that by the end of the visit, the parent or child will know the answers to the *Ask Me 3* questions.

Patient: Jessica, a 4-year-old with a cough. Both of her parents smoke.	
Ask Me 3 questions	**What the parent should understand at the end of the visit**
What is my child's main problem?	Jessica is being exposed to secondhand smoke. That means she is more likely to have colds, ear infections, throat infections, lung infections, and even cavities in her teeth.
What do I need to do?	• I have to keep Jessica away from smoke, and that means not smoking or letting anyone else smoke in the home or car—even when Jessica isn't there. • I must immediately talk with my own doctor about quitting smoking. • Quitting smoking isn't just something I should do for me—it is one of the ways I can help Jessica feel better and stay healthy.
Why is it important for me to do this?	It's one way to help make sure Jessica has a healthy childhood. She will have fewer colds, ear infections, throat infections, and lung infections. It may help her as an adult because the effects of secondhand smoke exposure can lead to lung cancer or heart disease, and it will make it less likely she will smoke when she's older.

Medical Terms and Plain Language Alternatives

Many of the medical terms we use every day don't mean much to many parents. Below is a list of medical terms that may be confusing or difficult to explain and suggestions for plain language alternatives.

Medical Terms	Plain Language Alternatives
Asthma	A disease that makes it hard to breathe because the tubes that carry air to the lungs get narrow and tight. There is no cure for asthma.
Bronchitis/bronchiolitis	An infection of the tubes that carry air into the lungs

Pneumonia	A lung infection
Secondhand smoke or environmental tobacco smoke (ETS)	The smoke that a person breathes out or that comes from burning tobacco in a cigar, pipe, cigarette, etc
Sudden infant death syndrome (SIDS)	When a baby younger than 1 year dies during sleep and doctors can't figure out why. Babies are at higher risk for SIDS if they breathe in secondhand smoke.
Wheeze	A whistling sound the lungs make when breathing

Confusing Terms and Concepts

With any condition, there are likely to be terms or concepts for which patients and families have a different understanding than a health care professional. These may include preventive strategies, complex disease processes, medication or treatment regimens, abstract laboratory results or measurements, technical terms, or words that have a different meaning in the health care arena than in everyday use. Cultural issues and misconceptions can also contribute to lack of understanding.

Consider the following when talking with parents about tobacco and secondhand smoke exposure:

Communication Issues

Parents who smoke may not understand or accept their responsibility for and role in the child's health problems. This is a tough concept and must be treated with sensitivity so the parent isn't blamed or made to feel ashamed, guilty, or defensive.

Use common examples to explain secondhand smoke exposure, for example: "Smoking makes the people around you breathe in the smoke too—just like you breathe in car exhaust and fumes when you're standing beside a busy street."

Explain that most of the chemicals in tobacco smoke stay in the parents' clothes, hair, and skin and can still be harmful, even if the parent is not actually smoking in front of the child. When the parent hugs the child, for example, the child may breathe in deadly chemicals from the tobacco smoke.

Breathing in secondhand smoke can have a variety of health implications (with a variety of symptoms) that may not be obvious to the parent.

In addition to explaining the causes and symptoms of the child's immediate illness (the illness that prompted the visit), explain that children who breathe in secondhand smoke can have more ear infections; more nose, throat, and sinus infections; more lung infections (such as pneumonia and bronchitis); and more tooth decay and cavities than children who don't breathe in secondhand smoke. Babies who breathe secondhand smoke are also at higher risk for SIDS.

Did You Know...?

Secondhand smoke causes approximately 3,400 lung cancer deaths and 46,000 heart disease deaths in adult nonsmokers in the United States each year.

Source: American Lung Association. Secondhand smoke fact sheet. http://www.lungusa.org/site/pp.asp?c=dvLUK9O0E&b=35422. Accessed March 31, 2008.

Explain that because it is likely we will discover more bad effects of secondhand smoke exposure in children, it's best not to expose the child to secondhand smoke at all.

Behavior Change

Behavior change is a key element in preventing and managing many pediatric conditions. Shifting from paternalistic advice that is either too vague or too complicated to a patient- or family-centered approach that incorporates elements of motivational interviewing and goal-setting, and that makes use of plain language, can be an effective way to empower patients and families to make changes and improve their health.

With smoking, the top priority is simply to get the child away from the smoke. But to do that, the health care provider must first gain the support and cooperation of the parents, who are in the best position to effect change.

Smoking is a family problem. Parental behaviors influence children's behaviors. But quitting smoking is a difficult change—not only because of addiction to nicotine, but also because the act of smoking is a habit. Providers may want to use principles from the stages of change model to help motivate changes in behavior, moving patients from pre-contemplation to contemplation to action.[3]

Also, when dealing with behavior change, it's important to have the patient and/or parent identify what they think will work best for them, set small goals that they believe are achievable, and identify ways to help them succeed. Motivational interviewing techniques can be used to help them build conviction (the belief that "this is important" so they know why they should change) and confidence (the belief that they can actually carry it out successfully)[4] to make sustained behavior changes in their smoking.

If the parents are smokers, they may have feelings of guilt or may feel they are being blamed for the child's illness or condition.

- Acknowledge the difficulty of smoking cessation.
- Acknowledge and congratulate parents for any steps already taken to decrease the child's tobacco smoke exposure.

Cultural Spotlight

Tobacco and Native Americans

Native Americans have the highest smoking rate of all major racial/ethnic groups in the United States, despite significant variation across tribes and regions of the country.

The influence of family on tobacco use may be especially complex in Native American culture. The extended family plays a dominant role, with a typical Native American family, including extended family members living within a single residence, so investigations of family influences in tobacco use must pay attention to the entire family and not focus exclusively on parents.

Another layer of complexity is added by the traditional uses of tobacco in Native American culture. Tobacco is viewed as a gift from the creator.

Because of the sacred nature of tobacco and its deep roots in Native American culture, conventional tobacco control messages that portray tobacco as entirely negative may be ineffective, as well as culturally insensitive.

Source: *Health Education Research.* 2000;15(5):547–557.

- Have information about smoking cessation available to offer.
- Give them the number for the Smoking Quitline (800/784-8669; http://www.naquitline.org) and other resources listed in the handout "Teens and Tobacco" on page 309.

Parents may not have a full understanding of the many sources of secondhand smoke exposure.

- Be clear about where smoke can "hide," including in hair, clothing, home fabrics (rugs, upholstery, curtains), and car fabrics.
- Ask if the child spends time in another home or car, and discuss the need to ensure safety from secondhand smoke exposure there as well.

Parents may not know where to start to create a safer environment.

- Offer concrete strategies, such as keeping a "smoking jacket" on a convenient hook outside the house's exit door and washing hands after smoking.

If the source of the tobacco smoke is not the parent, but rather someone on whom the parent depends for child care, the parent may be reluctant to confront that person.

- Acknowledge the parent's dilemma and support their need to compromise.
- Offer realistic suggestions for limiting the child's smoke exposure in the context of the child care situation (eg, negotiate with the smoker not to smoke in the house or car when the child is present and to wash hands before handling the child).

Child Involvement

Including the child, to the extent possible, is respectful and patient-centered and can contribute to developing health literacy skills as the child moves toward managing his or her own health as an adolescent and an adult. It can include direct, age-appropriate statements to the child, and also ways for the child to be involved in his or her health.

School-aged children—especially those who have health class—may well be taught that "smoking isn't good for you," and know they shouldn't be around cigarette smoke. We all are familiar with 5- and 6-year-olds who badger their parents about smoking in the home or car. Older children may be brought into the discussion and identified as "motivational forces" for parents who are trying to quit smoking.

And we can work with older children and teens to build self-efficacy in resisting peer pressure to smoke.

Teach-back

The concept of teaching back entails asking parents or patients to demonstrate understanding *using their own words*, not simply asking whether they have questions or whether they understand, because that may not elicit lack of understanding. Having patients explain in their own words not only assesses their understanding, but it reinforces the information by repeating it and internalizes it for the patient. When there is a lot of information, go over each concept and elicit a teach-back before moving to the next idea.

When using teach-back, it's important to keep the burden on yourself. Avoid the perception that you are quizzing the parent or patient—emphasize that you want to be sure you've explained things clearly.

The practice of using teach-back can be especially important over the phone, because it may be the only way to gauge whether the parent or patient understands fully.

Here are some approaches to using teach-back and motivational interviewing when talking about secondhand smoke.

- To make sure that I've explained things well, can you tell me how Samuel might get exposed to secondhand smoke?
- What will you tell your husband/wife/mother (the smoker) about how his/her smoking is affecting Katie?
- What can you do to make sure Nicholas doesn't get exposed to secondhand smoke?
- On a scale of 1 to 10, how convinced are you that it's important to keep David away from cigarette smoke?
- How confident are you that you can get Kari's father to smoke outside?

Key Messages for Use by All Members of the Health Care Team

It is important to reinforce key messages for parents and children so they hear them more than once and recognize them as priorities in managing their health. In addition, families should not receive conflicting advice about their health and what to do.

Key concepts for smoke exposure are

- If you smoke, quit! I know it's very difficult, but there are a lot of resources to help you.
- Minimize the child's exposure to the chemicals in tobacco smoke by not smoking or letting other people smoke around her, or in the home or car (even when the child isn't there).

- Quitting smoking will not only improve your health, but it will lessen the number of colds, ear infections, and other health problems that the child suffers.

Miscellaneous

Some health information is complicated but important. For example, if a parent is interested in quitting smoking, you may need to offer more concrete advice, printed information, and referrals to resources and programs to help them. You may want to explain what options they have. You can always explain more to parents if they are asking questions or you can ask them if there are other questions that they have. But it is essential that all parents leave the office with the key concepts as noted above.

References

1. American Lung Association. Secondhand smoke fact sheet. http://www.lungusa.org/site/pp.asp?c=dvLUK9O0E&b=35422. Accessed March 31, 2008

2. National Institutes of Health. Medline Plus: smoke and smokeless tobacco. http://www.nlm.nih.gov/medlineplus/ency/article/002032.htm. Accessed June 2, 2008

3. DiClemente CC, Prochaska J. Toward a comprehensive, transtheoretical model of change: stages of change and addictive behaviors. In: Miller WR, Heath N, eds. *Treating Addictive Behaviors.* 2nd ed. New York, NY: Plenum; 1998

4. Rollnick S, Mason P, Butler C. *Health Behavior Change: A Guide for Practitioners.* London, UK: Churchill Livingstone; 1999

Secondhand Smoke

Secondhand smoke comes from 2 places:

1) Smokers

2) Burning cigarettes, pipes, and cigars

Even if *you* don't smoke, breathing in someone else's smoke can kill you.

Secondhand smoke has about 4,000 chemicals in it. More than 50 of them cause cancer.

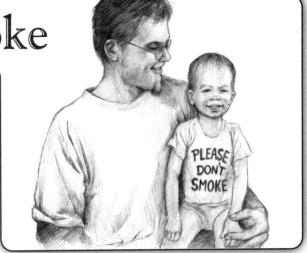

In the United States each year, thousands of **non**smokers die from secondhand smoke.

- About 3,000 die from **lung cancer.**
- More than 20,000 die from **heart disease.**

Secondhand Smoke and Your Young Child

Millions of children breathe in secondhand smoke at *home*. Secondhand smoke is especially bad for children because their lungs are still growing.

Babies have a higher risk of **SIDS*** (sudden infant death syndrome) if they breathe in secondhand smoke.

Children have a higher risk of serious health problems if they breathe in secondhand smoke. For example, children who breathe secondhand smoke can have:

- More ear infections.
- More nose, throat, and sinus (SYE-nis) infections.
- More lung infections like **bronchitis*** and **pneumonia***.
- More tooth decay (cavities, also called caries).
- More learning problems in school.

✳ Words to Know

bronchitis (brahn-KYE-tis)—an infection of the tubes that carry air into the lungs.

pneumonia (nuh-MOH-nyuh)—an infection of the lungs.

SIDS—short for sudden infant death syndrome. It's when a baby younger than 1 year dies during sleep and doctors can't figure out why.

wheeze (weez) or **wheezing** (weez-ing)—high-pitched whistling sound when breathing.

Children who breathe secondhand smoke cough and wheeze* more. They have a harder time with colds, stuffy noses, headaches, sore throats, itchy eyes, and hoarseness.

Secondhand smoke can make bad health problems even worse. **Secondhand smoke is *especially* bad for children with asthma.** It may cause more asthma attacks. And the attacks may be worse, leading to trips to the hospital.

Secondhand Smoke and Your Child Over Time

Secondhand smoke can cause problems for children later in life, such as:

- Lung cancer.
- Heart disease.
- Cataracts (an eye disease).

Children who grow up with parents who smoke are more likely to smoke too. Children and teens who smoke have the same health problems as adults.

How to Protect Your Child From Secondhand Smoke

- **Make your home smoke-free.** Smoke travels everywhere, from room to room, upstairs and downstairs. It gets into furniture and rugs. Ask people not to smoke in your home. Don't put out any ashtrays. Don't smoke inside your home.
- **Make your car smoke-free.** Opening windows isn't enough to clear the air. Don't smoke in your car or let other people smoke in your car.

Continued on back

- **Keep your children away from places where there are smokers.** Sit in "no smoking" parts of public places. Eat at smoke-free restaurants.
- **Choose a babysitter who doesn't smoke.** Smoke can "hide" in hair and clothes. Make sure your babysitter knows that nobody can smoke around your children! Think about changing babysitters if your babysitter smokes.
- **Encourage smoke-free child care and schools.** Help your children's school or child care become smoke-free. That includes outdoor areas and teachers' lounges. Get your children involved to make schools smoke-free!

Secondhand Smoke and Your Unborn Baby

When you're pregnant, your baby shares your blood. When you breathe in smoke, the smoke gets into your bloodstream, and gets to your baby.

If *you* **smoke** when you're pregnant, your baby "smokes" with you. This can lead to:

- **Miscarriage** (losing the baby)
- **Premature birth** ("preemies"—born early and not fully developed)
- **Low birth weight** (which can mean a less healthy baby)

The health risks to your baby go up the longer you smoke and the more you smoke. Quitting during pregnancy helps your baby. The sooner you quit, the better!

Even if *you* don't smoke, breathing in secondhand smoke can hurt your baby. All pregnant women should stay away from secondhand smoke. Ask smokers not to smoke around you.

Choosing to Quit
Why?

Quitting smoking is one of the most important things you can do for your own health. It is also the best way to protect your children from secondhand smoke.

Set an example. If you smoke, quit now! Children are more likely to try smoking if you are a smoker.

How?

- Talk with your doctor to get help. There are medicines that can help you quit.
- You may want to join a stop-smoking class.
- Ask a friend to join you in your fight to quit.
- Call 1-800-784-8669 (1-800-QUIT-NOW) to reach the Telephone Smoking Quitline in your state. Go to www.naquitline.org to learn more.
- Contact the American Lung Association (www.lungusa.org), American Heart Association (www.americanheart.org), or American Cancer Society (www.cancer.org) to learn about support groups where you live.

Fire Safety

Children can get burned playing with lit cigarettes, lighters, or matches. Even children younger than 5 years can start a fire. Lighters are especially dangerous. Some lighters are "child-resistant." But that does *not* mean they are child*proof*. They are just harder for children to use.

- Never let anyone smoke while holding your child. Your child may get burned.
- Never leave a lit cigarette, cigar, or pipe alone. Your child may play with it.
- Keep matches and lighters out of your child's reach.

To learn more, visit the American Academy of Pediatrics (AAP) Web site at www.aap.org.
Your child's doctor will tell you to do what's best for your child.
This information should not take the place of talking with your child's doctor.

We hope the resources in this handout are helpful. The AAP is not responsible for the information in these resources. We try to keep the information up to date but it may change at any time.

Adaptation of the AAP information in this handout into plain language was supported in part by McNeil Consumer Healthcare.

© 2008 American Academy of Pediatrics

American Academy of Pediatrics
DEDICATED TO THE HEALTH OF ALL CHILDREN™

Humo de segunda mano
(Secondhand Smoke)

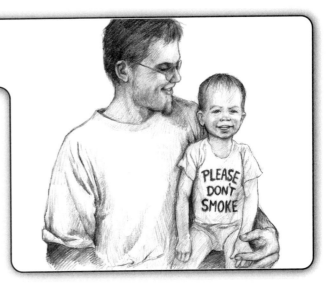

El humo de segunda mano proviene de 2 lugares:

1) Fumadores

2) Cigarrillos, pipas y cigarros encendidos

Aunque *usted* no fume, respirar el humo de alguien más puede matarlo.

El humo de segunda mano contiene más o menos 4,000 compuestos químicos. Más de 50 de estos causan cáncer.

Cada año, en los Estados Unidos, millares de *no fumadores* mueren a causa del humo de segunda mano.

- Más o menos 3,000 mueren de **cáncer de pulmón.**
- Más de 20,000 mueren de **enfermedades del corazón.**

El humo de segunda mano y su niño

Millones de niños respiran el humo de segunda mano en la *casa*. Este humo es aún más dañino en niños porque sus pulmones todavía están creciendo.

Los bebés corren mayor riesgo de sufrir el Síndrome de Muerte Súbita Infantil (**SMSI***) si respiran el humo de segunda mano.

Los niños corren mayor riesgo de tener problemas serios de salud, si respiran el humo de segunda mano. Por ejemplo, los niños pueden desarrollar:

- Más infecciones de oído.
- Más infecciones de nariz, garganta y sinusitis.
- Más infecciones como **bronquitis*** **y neumonía***.
- Más caries en los dientes.
- Más problemas para aprender y estudiar en la escuela.

✳ *Palabras que debe conocer*

Bronquitis: Infección de las vías que conducen el aire hacia los pulmones.

Neumonía: Infección de los pulmones.

SMSI: Forma de abreviar el nombre del Síndrome de Muerte Súbita Infantil. Sucede cuando un bebé menor de 1 año muere mientras duerme y los médicos no pueden explicar la razón.

Respiración sibilante: Respiración fuerte y ruidosa.

Los niños que respiran el humo de segunda mano tosen más y padecen más de la respiración sibilante*. Además sufren de resfriados, nariz tapada, dolores de cabeza, dolor de garganta, picazón en los ojos y ronquera.

El humo de segunda mano puede empeorar los problemas serios de salud. **En especial, a los niños con asma les puede provocar más ataques de asma.** Este humo puede causar peores ataques en estos niños y hasta mandarlos al hospital.

El humo de segunda mano y el futuro de su niño

El humo de segunda mano puede provocarles problemas a los niños en el futuro, tales como:

- Cáncer de pulmón.
- Enfermedades del corazón.
- Cataratas (enfermedad de los ojos).

Los niños que crecen con padres que fuman son más propensos a fumar también. Los niños y adolescentes que respiran el humo tienen los mismos problemas de salud que los adultos.

Cómo proteger a su niño del humo de segunda mano

- **No permita que fumen en su casa.** El humo viaja por todos lados, de habitación en habitación, al piso de arriba y al de abajo. Penetra en los muebles y las alfombras. Pídales a los fumadores que no fumen en su casa. No tenga ningún cenicero en la casa. No fume adentro de su casa.

- **No permita que fumen en su automóvil.** No es suficiente con abrir las ventanas para limpiar el aire. No fume en su automóvil ni permita que otras personas lo hagan.

Continúa atrás

Viene de la página anterior

- **Aleje a su bebé de lugares donde hay fumadores.** Siéntese en las áreas de "no fumadores" cuando esté en lugares públicos. Coma en restaurantes donde se prohíbe fumar.

- **Escoja una niñera que no fume.** El humo se "esconde" en el cabello y la ropa. Asegúrese de que la niñera sepa que nadie debe fumar cerca de sus hijos. Si la niñera fuma, piense en cambiarla.

- **Promueva que en los centros donde cuidan a los niños y las escuelas no se fume.** Ayude a que en la escuela o centros donde cuidan a sus hijos se prohíba fumar. Incluya las áreas al aire libre y los salones de los maestros. ¡Involucre a los niños para que ayuden a tener escuelas libres de humo de cigarrillos!

El humo de segunda mano y su bebé que no ha nacido

Cuando está embarazada, el bebé comparte su sangre. Cuando usted respira humo, este entra en su sangre y llega hasta su bebé.

Si *usted* fuma cuando está embarazada, su bebé "fuma" con usted. Esto puede provocar:

- **Abortos** (la pérdida de su bebé).
- **Nacimiento prematuro** ("bebés prematuros"— que nacen antes de tiempo sin haberse desarrollado por completo).
- **Peso bajo al nacer** (lo que puede significar un bebé no muy sano).

Los riesgos de salud de su bebé aumentan mientras más tiempo y mayor cantidad fume usted. Si deja de fumar durante el embarazo, ayudará a su bebé. ¡Mientras más rápido lo haga, mejor!

Aunque usted no fume, respirar el humo de segunda mano puede dañar a su bebé. Todas las mujeres embarazadas deben alejarse del humo de segunda mano. Pídale a los fumadores que no fumen cerca de usted.

Tome la decisión de dejar de fumar

¿Por qué?

Dejar de fumar es una de las cosas mas importantes que usted puede hacer para mejorar su salud. También es la mejor forma de proteger a sus hijos del humo de segunda mano.

Dé el ejemplo. Si usted fuma, ¡déje de hacerlo! Los niños son más propensos a fumar si usted lo hace.

¿Cómo?

- Hable con su doctor para recibir ayuda. Hay medicinas que pueden ayudarle a dejar de fumar.
- Únase a una clase para dejar de fumar.
- Pídale a un amigo que se una a usted en su lucha por dejar de fumar.
- Llame al 1-800-784-8669 (1-800-QUIT-NOW.) Este es el teléfono de "Telephone Smoking Quitline" en su estado.
- Para más información sobre los grupos de apoyo cerca de donde usted vive, comuníquese con:
  - American Lung Association (www.lungusa.org)
  - American Heart Association (www.americanheart.org)
  - American Cancer Society (www.cancer.org)

Seguridad contra el fuego

Los niños pueden quemarse si juegan con cigarrillos, encendedores o fósforos encendidos. Incluso los niños menores de 5 años pueden empezar un incendio. Los más peligrosos son los encendedores. Algunos son "seguros" para los niños. Pero no quiere decir que sean a prueba de niños. Sólo son más difíciles de usar.

- Nunca permita que alguien fume mientras carga a su bebé. Puede quemarlo.
- Nunca deje sin supervisión una pipa, un cigarrillo o un cigarro encendido.
- Mantenga los fósforos y los encendedores lejos del alcance de los niños.

Para aprender más, visite el sitio de la Academia Americana de Pediatría (AAP) en www.aap.org. Su pediatra le dirá qué es lo mejor para la salud de su hijo.
Esta información no debe usarse en lugar de consultar con su doctor.
Esperamos que la información en este folleto le sea útil. La AAP no es responsable por la información contenida en este folleto. Tratamos de presentar la información más actual pero a veces las recomendaciones cambian.
La adaptación de la información de este folleto de la AAP a lenguaje sencillo se hizo con el apoyo de McNeil Consumer Healthcare. La traducción al español fue patrocinada por Leyendo Juntos (Reach Out and Read), un programa pediátrico de alfabetización.

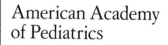

American Academy of Pediatrics
DEDICATED TO THE HEALTH OF ALL CHILDREN™

Teens and Tobacco

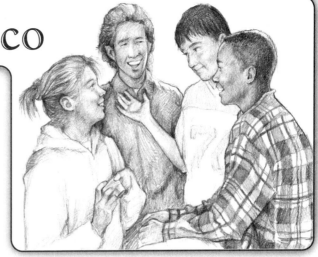

The Dirty Truth:
Tobacco Companies Want *You*

- Tobacco companies need *3,000 new smokers every day.* Why? Because 400,000 "customers" die each year from diseases linked to tobacco.
- Tobacco companies spend billions of advertising dollars every year on TV, movies, magazines, billboards, and sporting events. Teens are the main targets of many of these ads.

The Ugly Truth:
Smoking Stinks

- Smoking causes bad breath and stained teeth. Some teens say that kissing a smoker is like licking an ashtray.
- You may not smell smoke on you, but other people do. Smoking often makes people not want to be near you.
- Studies show that most teens would rather date someone who doesn't smoke.

The Costly Truth:
Smoking Costs $$$

YOU do the math*!!*

Average cost of one pack of cigarettes per day	$ 5.00
Multiplied by the days in a year	x 365
Yearly cost for cigarettes	$ 1,825

That's almost **$2,000** a year! You *could* be spending that on music, clothes, a car, college…whatever.

The Deadly Truth:
Smoking Can Kill

One-third of all new smokers will die from diseases linked to smoking. And nearly 90% of all smokers started when they were teens.

This is what smoking does to your body:

- It sucks oxygen (air) from your body.
- It makes your lungs turn gray and disgusting.
- Nicotine can make your heart beat faster and not work as well.

The earlier you start smoking, the greater your risk of:

- Cancer.
- Heart disease.
- Chronic bronchitis (KRAH-nik brahn-KYE-tus)— a serious disease of the airways to the lung.
- Emphysema (em-fuh-ZEE-muh)—a deadly lung disease.

You breathe in 400 different poisons with every puff. These poisons include:

- Nicotine (pure nicotine can kill).
- Cyanide (a poison).
- Benzene (used in making paints, dyes, and plastics).
- Formaldehyde (used to preserve dead bodies).
- Acetylene (fuel used in torches).
- Ammonia (used in fertilizers).
- Carbon monoxide (the gas in car exhaust).

Chewing tobacco and snuff ("dip") aren't safe either.

Smokeless tobacco raises your risk for mouth problems like gum disease and cancer. You could lose some of your teeth. And you probably won't be able to taste or smell things as well as before.

Smoking and Sports

Athletes who smoke can't run or swim as well as nonsmoking athletes because their bodies get less oxygen. That's why coaches tell athletes never to smoke.

Continued on back

Continued from front

Are You "Hooked"?

People get hooked on cigarettes very soon after they start smoking. You'll know you're addicted when:

- You crave cigarettes.
- You feel nervous without cigarettes.
- You try to quit smoking and have trouble doing it.

Quitting can be hard, and it can take a long time. The longer you smoke, the harder it is to stop.

Myth:

"I won't smoke forever and I can quit any time."

Fact:

Many ex-smokers say, "Quitting tobacco was the hardest thing I've ever done!"

The Happy Truth: It's Not Too Late

- Most teens don't smoke. About 80% of teens in the United States don't smoke. They've made a healthy choice.
- If you do smoke, you *can* quit. It's up to you. Quitting is the best thing you can do for yourself, your friends, and your family.
- Many people who try to quit don't succeed the first time. If you don't succeed the first time, keep trying. It may take several tries to quit for good. Get support from your friends and family. Ask for help from your doctor or school health office.

- Your body starts healing as soon as you quit:
  - *After the first day,* …your sense of taste and smell begin coming back. And your skin starts to look better.
  - *Within a year,* …your risk of heart disease drops by half.
  - *In 10 years,* …your risk of lung cancer drops by half.
  - *After 15 smoke-free years,* …your odds of living a long and healthy life are almost as good as if you never smoked at all.

For More Information

- Campaign for Tobacco-Free Kids
  1-800-803-7178
  www.tobaccofreekids.org
- Telephone Smoking Quitline
  1-800-QUIT-NOW
  (1-800-784-8669)
  www.naquitline.org
- American Cancer Society
  1-800-ACS-2345 (1-800-227-2345)
  www.cancer.com
- American Heart Association
  1-800-242-8721
  www.americanheart.org
- American Lung Association
  1-800-586-4872
  www.lungusa.org

To learn more, visit the American Academy of Pediatrics (AAP) Web site at www.aap.org.

Your doctor will tell you to do what's best for you. This information should not take the place of talking with your doctor.

We hope the resources in this handout are helpful. The AAP is not responsible for the information in these resources. We try to keep the information up to date but it may change at any time.

Adaptation of the AAP information in this handout into plain language was supported in part by McNeil Consumer Healthcare.

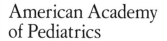
American Academy of Pediatrics

DEDICATED TO THE HEALTH OF ALL CHILDREN™

Los adolescentes y el tabaco

(Teens and Tobacco)

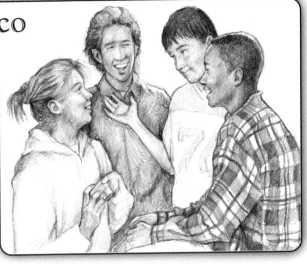

La cruda realidad: Lo que las compañías de tabaco necesitan de ti

- Las compañías de tabaco necesitan 3,000 *nuevos fumadores todos los días.* ¿Por qué? Porque 400,000 "clientes" mueren todos los años de enfermedades relacionadas con el tabaco.
- Todos los años, las compañías de tabaco gastan billones de dólares en anuncios de TV, cine, revistas, carteles publicitarios y eventos deportivos. Los adolescentes son el objetivo principal de muchos de estos anuncios.

La verdad no es muy agradable: Fumar causa mal olor

- Fumar causa mal aliento y manchas en los dientes. Algunos adolescentes dicen que besar a un fumador es como besar a un cenicero.
- Tal vez no sientas el olor a humo propio, pero otros sí lo sienten. A menudo fumar hace que las personas no deseen estar cerca de ti.
- Los estudios demuestran que la mayoría de adolescentes prefieren salir con alguien que no fuma.

Una costosa realidad: Fumar cuesta mucho dinero $$$

¡Haz las cuentas!

El precio promedio de un paquete de cigarrillos al día	$5.00
Multiplicado por los días del año	x 365
Precio por año	$1,825

¡Casi **$2,000** por año! *Podrías* gastar esta cantidad en música, ropa, un automóvil, la universidad… en muchas cosas.

La realidad es mortal: Fumar puede matarte

Un tercio de todos los fumadores morirán por enfermedades relacionadas con este hábito. Es más, cerca del 90% de todos los fumadores empezaron cuando eran adolescentes.

Lo que el fumar provoca en tu cuerpo:

- Disminuye el oxígeno (aire) en tu cuerpo.

- Tus pulmones se vuelven de color gris sucio.
- La nicotina puede hacer que tus latidos se aceleren y que tu corazón no funcione muy bien.

Mientras más temprano comiences a fumar, mayor es tu riesgo de tener:

- Cáncer.
- Enfermedad del corazón.
- Bronquitis crónica – enfermedad seria de los tubos respiratorios.
- Enfisema – enfermedad mortal de los pulmones.

Respiras 400 venenos diferentes con cada aspirada de humo. Estos venenos incluyen:

- Nicotina (la nicotina pura puede causarte la muerte).
- Cianuro (un veneno).
- Benceno (se usa para hacer pinturas, tinturas y plásticos).
- Formaldehído (se usa para preservar cadáveres).
- Acetileno (combustible que se usa en el alumbrado).
- Amoníaco (se usa en fertilizantes).
- Monóxido de carbono (el gas del escape del automóvil).

Masticar tabaco y tabaco en polvo ("rallado")

El tabaco que no produce humo eleva tu riesgo de desarrollar problemas en la boca, como enfermedades en las encías y cáncer. Además, probablemente no podrás sentir el sabor ni el olor de las cosas igual que antes.

Fumar y los deportes

Los atletas que fuman no pueden correr o nadar como los atletas que no fuman, debido a que sus cuerpos reciben menos oxígeno. Por eso es que los entrenadores le dicen a los atletas que nunca fumen.

Continúa atrás

¿Estás "enviciado"?

Las personas se envician muy pronto con los cigarrillos. Tú sabrás si eres adicto cuando:

- Sientas ansias por causa de los cigarrillos.
- Te sientas nervioso sin los cigarrillos.
- Trates de dejar de fumar y tengas problemas para hacerlo.

Dejar de fumar es difícil y puede tomarte bastante tiempo. Mientras más tiempo fumes, más difícil será dejarlo.

> **Mito:**
> "No fumaré para siempre y puedo dejarlo en cualquier momento."
>
> **Realidad:**
> Muchos ex-fumadores dicen: "¡dejar de fumar fue lo más difícil que he hecho!"

La feliz realidad: No es demasiado tarde

- La mayoría de los adolescentes no fuman. Cerca del 80% de los adolescentes en los Estados Unidos no fuman. Han tomado una decisión saludable.
- Si tú fumas, puedes dejar de hacerlo. Todo depende de ti. Dejarlo es lo mejor que puedes hacer por ti mismo, tu familia y tus amigos.
- Muchas personas que tratan de dejar de fumar no tienen éxito la primera vez. Si te sucediera a ti, sigue tratando. Puede tomar varios intentos hasta dejarlo para siempre. Busca el apoyo de la familia y los amigos. Pide la ayuda de tu doctor o de la clínica de salud de la escuela.

- Tu cuerpo empieza a sentirse mejor tan pronto como dejas de fumar:
  - *Después del primer día,*
    …tus sentidos del gusto y el olor comienzan a volver. Además tu piel empieza a lucir mejor.
  - *En un año,*
    …tu riesgo de tener enfermedades del corazón disminuye a la mitad.
  - *En 10 años,*
    …tu riesgo de tener cáncer de pulmón disminuye a la mitad.
  - *Después de 15 años sin fumar,*
    … tus probabilidades de vivir una vida larga y sana son casi tan buenas como si nunca hubieras fumado.

Para más información

- Campaign for Tobacco-Free Kids (Campaña para librar a los niños del tabaco)
  1-800-803-7178
  www.tobaccofreekids.org
- Telephone Smoking Quitline (Teléfono para pedir ayuda para dejar de fumar)
  1-800-QUIT-NOW
  (1-800-784-8669)
  www.naquitline.org
- American Cancer Society (Sociedad Americana del Cáncer)
  1-800-ACS-2345 (1-800-227-2345)
  www.cancer.com
- American Heart Association (Asociación Americana del Corazón)
  1-800-242-8721
  www.americanheart.org
- American Lung Association (Asociación Americana del Pulmón)
  1-800-586-4872
  www.lungusa.org

Para aprender más, visite el sitio de la Academia Americana de Pediatría (AAP) en www.aap.org.
Su pediatra le dirá qué es lo mejor para la salud de su hijo.
Esta información no debe usarse en lugar de consultar con su doctor.
Esperamos que la información en este folleto le sea útil. La AAP no es responsable por la información contenida en este folleto. Tratamos de presentar la información más actual pero a veces las recomendaciones cambian.
La adaptación de la información de este folleto de la AAP a lenguaje sencillo se hizo con el apoyo de McNeil Consumer Healthcare. La traducción al español fue patrocinada por Leyendo Juntos (Reach Out and Read), un programa pediátrico de alfabetización.

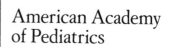
American Academy of Pediatrics

DEDICATED TO THE HEALTH OF ALL CHILDREN™

Medical Terms and Plain Language Alternatives

Medical Terms and Plain Language Alternatives

2 puffs twice a day 2 puffs in the morning and 2 puffs in the evening, so 4 puffs total.

Acetaminophen A medicine for pain and fever. Tylenol is one brand of acetaminophen.

Acute episode/asthma attack When the child has severe difficulty breathing because the air tubes have become swollen.

Adequate calcium intake Getting enough calcium through food and drinks.

Advance Gradually increase or slowly go back to normal.

Albuterol The most common format of quick-relief medicine for asthma.

Allergens Things your child may be allergic to.

Allergic To have a bad reaction to something that doesn't bother most people. For example, some people may get hives if they are stung by a bee.

Anorexia or loss of appetite Not hungry, poor feeding, or doesn't want to eat.

Antibiotic Medicine to get rid of the germs, called "bacteria," that cause infections. Antibiotics don't work against viruses.

Antiviral drug A medicine that can kill some flu viruses if the child is seen in the first 2 days and is older than 1 year.

Anus Bottom, butt, rear; where the poop comes out.

Apnea Stop breathing.

Asthma A disease that makes it hard to breathe because the tubes that carry air to the lungs get narrow and tight. There is no cure for asthma.

Asthma action plan A plan you write with your child's doctor. It lists the medicines your child takes. It also tells what to do if your child has an asthma attack.

Attention-deficit/hyperactivity disorder (ADHD) ADHD makes it hard to sit still, pay attention, take turns, and finish things. It is one of the most common chronic (long-term) problems of childhood.

Autism A long-term problem in the brain and nerves. Many people with autism have trouble understanding others and being understood. They often have trouble making friends. They may like to do one thing over and over again.

Bedwetting alarm An alarm that attaches to your child's pajamas or underwear and goes off when it gets wet, which happens when the child wets the bed.

Behavior How a person acts.

Behavior therapy Tools to help the grown-ups around the child (like parents and teachers) relate to the child with ADHD. Behavior therapy teaches grown-ups how to set and keep rules that can help the child learn and act better.

Beta agonist Rescue medication/quick-relief medicine for asthma.

Bladder A hollow organ, like a balloon, that holds urine in the body until you go to the toilet.

Bone density test The way we measure how strong a person's bones are.

Bone mass accrual How bones store calcium for the rest of the body, like a bank keeps money for when you need it.

Bowel movement When stool passes out of your child's body. Also called a BM, stool, poop, number 2.

Bronchiolitis An infection that makes the breathing tubes of the lungs swell. The swelling blocks airflow through the lungs, making it hard to breathe.

Bronchitis An infection that makes the lining of small breathing tubes of the lungs swell. The swelling blocks airflow, making it hard to breathe.

Bronchoconstriction Breathing tubes getting tight/narrow.

Bronchodilators Medicines that open up the breathing tubes in the lungs.

"C" stands for Centigrade A different scale of numbers to show temperature. Used mostly outside the United States.

Calcium A mineral that the body needs to build strong bones and teeth.

Cataract Clouding of the lens of the eye that causes difficulty in seeing or blindness.

Cavity; tooth decay Tooth decay (rotting teeth) happens when germs in the mouth mix with the sugar in foods and drinks. The germs then make acids that break down the enamel. Cavities are the holes in the enamel caused by tooth decay.

Chewable tablet A flavored pill that a child can chew instead of drinking liquid or swallowing an adult pill.

Chronic Long term.

Chronic bronchitis A serious disease of the airways to the lung.

Comorbid disorder A problem that often occurs with ADHD, but is a separate problem and is not caused by ADHD or part of ADHD; examples are learning problems, anxiety, and depression.

Complete full course Give it for the whole [10] days, that means [30] times, even if your child is feeling better.

Confident Sure, certain.

Congestion Stopped up or stuffy nose.

Consequences Something that happens because of a tantrum.

Constipation Stopped up; poop that is so hard it causes pain in your belly or hurts when you go to the bathroom.

Controller A medicine taken or used every day to keep the breathing tubes healthy and keep an asthma attack from happening.

Copious Large amount; a lot.

Corporal punishment Spanking, paddling.

Cromolyn An inhaled medicine that cuts down inflammation.

Croup An infection that makes the inside of your child's throat swell up.

Croupy cough A loud cough that sounds like a seal barking.

Cyanosis Blue color of the tongue, lips, or body.

Dairy products Foods and drinks that come from milk and have a lot of calcium in them.

Day 24 hours or daytime versus nighttime.

DDAVP A medicine that can be taken as a pill or sprayed in the nose. It works by helping the child make less urine during the night, and can be helpful for older children when they have a sleepover or go away to camp.

Dehumidifier A machine that takes dampness out of the air.

Dehydrated Dry; dried out. The body needs water and other liquids to stay healthy; when it doesn't have enough, it dries out, or gets "dehydrated," which can be dangerous.

Dental Of the teeth.

Dental caries Tooth decay; rotting teeth; cavities.

Development; maturity Growth; growing up.

Developmental Growing and learning.

Developmental-behavioral specialist An expert in the ways children learn and develop.

Developmental delay When a child is behind other children his age; he is unable to do the things that most other children his age can do.

Diarrhea Passing loose, watery stools.

Diet A general word for what a person usually eats. It can also be used to describe special ways to eat that help you be healthy (like a high-calcium diet or a low-salt diet). "Diet" doesn't always mean limiting what you eat to help you lose weight.

Discipline To correct; to teach; using ways to set limits on how a child acts, like putting a child in time-out.

Disinfectant A cleaner that kills germs.

Distract Point out something else, sidetrack.

Dose The amount of medicine you give your child (each time you are supposed to give it).

Early Intervention A program for children younger than 3 years that helps them with talking and other parts of growing and learning.

Electrolyte drink A special sugar and salt drink you can buy in a bottle. These drinks are very helpful for diarrhea. Pedialyte is one brand made for children.

Emphysema A crippling lung disease.

Enamel The hard outer coating that protects the tooth.

Encopresis When poop gets so hard and big that it can barely come out, and some watery poop leaks out around the hard parts.

Enema A liquid put into a person's bottom to make him or her pass stool.

Eruption Teething; teeth coming in.

"F" stands for Fahrenheit A scale of numbers to show temperature. Used mostly in the United States.

Fever See *Temperature.*

Fiber Fiber comes from certain foods, including vegetables, fruits, and grains. It helps absorb water like a sponge, so your stool gets softer and easier to pass.

Fluids Liquids or things to drink or swallow without chewing (like soup).

Fluoride A natural chemical that helps teeth stay strong and helps prevent tooth decay. It hardens the outer coating on the teeth, called enamel. Fluoride also helps repair early damage to teeth.

Fracture Broken bone.

Gastroenteritis Stomach infection, or stomach "flu," that causes you to throw up and have diarrhea. This is different from influenza.

Hand hygiene Keeping hands clean by washing them with soap and water.

Hematochezia Bright red blood in the poop (stool).

HEPA air filter A special kind of filter that cleans the air. You can buy one at some drugstores.

Humidifier Machine that puts water into the air to help clear your child's stuffy nose.

Hyperactivity Moves around a lot; trouble sitting still; squirms; talks too much.

Hypoxia Low oxygen or air in the body.

Ibuprofen A medicine for pain and fever. Advil and Motrin are brands of ibuprofen.

Impulsivity Acts and talks without thinking; has trouble taking turns and interrupts a lot.

Inattention Can't pay attention; can't focus; daydreams; can't get organized and forgets things.

Influenza Flu; a virus that causes high fever, aches, cough, runny nose, and sometimes other symptoms; it's different from the stomach flu that makes you throw up and have diarrhea.

Inhale/exhale Breathe in/breathe out.

Insomnia Trouble sleeping; can't sleep; wakes up a lot in the night.

Intestine Gut; the part of your body that food goes through after you eat it; the healthy parts of the food get absorbed into your body and the leftover parts get made into poop.

Lactose intolerance When a person gets a stomachache or a lot of gas from eating or drinking things that have milk in them.

Larynx Voice box.

Laxative A medicine to make stools softer and makes you poop more.

Lethargic Tired, sleepy, weak.

Leukotriene receptor antagonist A kind of pill you take to prevent asthma symptoms.

Low self-esteem When a child feels bad about himself or herself and thinks he or she is not as good as other children.

Manage Using medicines and behavior therapy or other ways to treat a health problem, or keep it under control, even if it can't be cured.

Mastoiditis Infection in the bone behind the ear.

MDI/inhaler Puffer; a way to give medicine that gets it into the breathing tubes and lungs.

Medication Pills, drugs, medicine.

Melena Dark blood in the poop (stool).

Metered-dose inhaler/MDI Puffer, inhaler, breathing/asthma medicine.

Miscarriage Losing the baby.

Motivational therapy Using reward charts and letting the child earn points or tokens for good behavior toward getting something they want or doing something special.

Mucus, sputum Snot; phlegm; the slimy liquid that coats the inside of the nose and throat.

Nasal congestion Stuffy, runny nose.

Nasal spray Medicine that you squirt up the nose to help you breathe easier.

Nausea Feeling like throwing up.

Nauseous/nauseated Feeling sick to your stomach.

Nebulizer A machine that turns medicine or water into a mist that the child breathes in.

Night feedings Any liquid other than water given to an infant or toddler at night without brushing or wiping the teeth afterward.

Nocturnal enuresis Wetting the bed at night (peeing in the bed during sleep).

Nostril 1 of 2 holes in the bottom of the nose, where air goes in and out.

Oral Of the mouth.

Oral abscess An infected spot or sore in the mouth, caused by bacteria and filled with liquid/fluid/pus. Similar, in some ways, to a blister on the foot or hand.

Oral hygiene Keeping the mouth and teeth clean.

Oral steroid Pills that stop the breathing tubes from swelling during an asthma attack.

Osteoporosis A disease that makes bones so fragile they can break from just bending over.

Otalgia Ear pain or earache.

Otitis media Ear infection.

Over-the-counter (OTC) Medicine you can get without a prescription.

Oxygen Air.

Peak bone mass The time when bones have the most calcium they will ever have—usually in your early teens and before age 21.

Peak flow Tool to measure breathing. It measures how easy it is for air to go in and out of the lungs.

Peristalsis The way muscles squeeze to move food through your gut, like the way you squeeze toothpaste out of its tube.

Permanent Lasting for a lifetime. Permanent teeth replace baby teeth one by one in your child's mouth. If your child loses a permanent tooth, it *won't* grow back.

Pharmacist A person who has special training to fill prescriptions and teach people about their medicines.

Pharmacy Drugstore.

Pneumonia An infection of the lungs. Many different germs can cause pneumonia.

Pollen The dust from plants.

Precipitants Things that happen before a tantrum and lead to it.

Premature birth (preemie) Born early and not fully developed.

Prescription 'Script,' doctor's order. A note from the doctor that you have to take to the drugstore to get certain kinds of medicine.

Primary teeth Baby teeth.

PRN (as needed) Use only when your child is having the condition/symptom (fever, cough, congestion, etc).

Reaction/side effect A symptom that comes from taking a drug, but isn't part of the treatment. For example, some medicines might make you feel sick to your stomach.

Rectum The last several inches of the large intestine, where stool is stored before passing out of the body.

Referral A note or phone call from a doctor sending you to see someone.

Refill More medicine. The number of refills is the number of times you can get more of the same medicine without getting another prescription from the doctor.

Rehydration formulas Special electrolyte fluids like Pedialyte that a child should drink when he or she is dried out.

Reinforce Things you do that cause something (good or bad) to happen again.

Rescue medication Medicine to help stop an asthma attack right away.

Respiratory distress Serious trouble breathing, like fighting to breathe, breathing fast, muscles around the ribs pull in every time he breathes, a whistling sound, and turning blue around the mouth.

Retractions When the spaces between the ribs suck in from hard breathing.

Reward chart A calendar that the parent uses with the child, marking each success with a star or other sticker, and allowing the child to trade in a certain number of earned stars or stickers for rewards.

Rhinorrhoea Runny nose.

Saliva Spit; the watery liquid in your mouth.

Secondary teeth Permanent teeth; adult teeth.

Secondhand smoke or environmental tobacco smoke (ETS) The smoke that a person breathes out or that comes from burning tobacco in a cigar, pipe, cigarette, etc.

Side effects Symptoms that come from taking a drug and are not part of the treatment. For example, some medicines can make you feel sick to your stomach.

SIDS Short for "sudden infant death syndrome." When a baby younger than 1 year dies during sleep, and doctors can't figure out why. Babies are at higher risk for SIDS if they breathe in secondhand smoke.

Sinus infection An infection of the spaces inside your head, behind your nose (sinuses).

Sippy cup A non-spilling cup (usually with a lid or top) that can be used for liquids with meals, but should not be carried around all day with any liquid other than water in it.

Spacer Extra tube on the inhaler to help the medicine go in right.

Specialist A doctor who is an expert on a subject, like allergies or hearing or feet.

Speech Talking.

Speech therapist A specially trained person who can help children learn to speak and understand words better.

Speech therapy Treatment for people who have trouble talking. There are many different speech problems, and many kinds of speech therapy.

Steroid inhaler A kind of medicine used every day through an inhaler to keep the breathing tubes healthy and keep an asthma attack from happening.

Steroids A medicine that is a pill, liquid, spray you breathe in, or a shot to help asthma and help stop croup. It cuts down inflammation.

Stimulants The safest, best types of medicines for most children with ADHD. They speed up the signals in the child's brain and help them focus. Examples include Adderall, Concerta, and Ritalin.

Stridor A high whistling sound when your child breathes in. It is caused by something blocking the throat or voice box.

Suction bulb Sucks the clogged mucus out of the nose. (This is also called an "ear bulb.")

Supportive Caring, loving, helpful.

Tachycardia When the heart is beating a lot faster than usual.

Tachypnea Breathing a lot faster than usual.

Take every 4 hours as needed Wait 4 hours between doses. For example, if you give it at 8:00 am, then the next dose you can give, if you need to, is at noon.

Take 4 times a day Give in the morning, noon, early evening, and at night before bed.

Take on an empty stomach Give the medicine at least 1 hour before the child eats a meal (breakfast, lunch, dinner), or give the medicine at least 2 hours after the child eats a meal.

Temper tantrum Make a scene, throw a fit, melt down, scream, cry, and kick.

Temperature; fever The temperature is how warm or cold your body is; if the temperature is higher (hotter) than usual, you have a "fever."

Time out The time you take a child out of an activity to allow her to calm down. Try 1 minute of time-out for every year of your child's age.

Trachea Windpipe; airway.

Triggers Things that cause asthma attacks or make asthma worse.

Upper respiratory infection (URI) Cold; the common sickness that gives you a cough, runny nose, and sometimes a fever or other symptoms.

Urine Pee, pee-pee, number 1.

Vaccine A shot or nose spray to keep people from getting sick with illnesses like the flu. In this case, it's commonly called the "flu shot."

Vaporizer A machine that puts cool mist into the air.

Verbalize Use words.

Viral illness Consider using terms such as "cold" or "flu."

Virus A kind of germ that causes infection. Antibiotics do not work against viruses. The body usually needs to get over the virus on its own.

Vomiting Throwing up.

Weight-bearing exercise Activities that you do on your feet—like walking, running, dancing, tennis, or soccer—and other activities like weight-lifting help your bones get strong. (Activities like swimming and biking are healthy and make your heart beat faster, but they aren't weight-bearing exercises.)

Wheeze or wheezing A high-pitched whistling sound when breathing.

Worsening respiratory symptoms Breathing harder, faster, or when the spaces between the ribs start to suck in.

Index

Developmental-behavioral specialist, 193, 194

Developmental delays and communication issues, 187–196

   Ask Me 3 questions for, 187–188

   behavior change, 190–191

   child involvement, 191

   confusing terms and concepts, 189–190

     communication issues, 189–190

   key messages for use, 192

   medical terms and plain language alternatives, 188–189

   patient story, 187

   plain language educational handout on, 193–194

     in Spanish, 195–196

   resources on, 192

   teach-back for, 191–192

Dexamethasone, 178

Diabetes, 27

   low literacy and, 23

Diarrea, vómitos y pérdida de líquidos (deshidratación) (Diarrhea, Vomiting, and Water Loss [Dehydration]), 223–224

Diarrhea

   managing, 222

   vomiting, and water loss (dehydration), 221–222

DIRECT approach, 14–15

Disease, yin-yang of, 84

Disinfect, 155, 156

Distracted driving, 82

Doctors' offices

   creating shame-free care environment in, 17–18

   customization of patient-centered care in, 12

   DIRECT approach in, 14–15

   health literacy assessment tools in, 13–14

   involving all staff, 17

   making changes in practice, 15–17

   need for health literacy in, 11

   red flags of low literacy, 12–13

   safe care in, 11–12

   screening for low literacy in, 13

Don't Rant and Rave on Wednesday (Moser and Melton), 289

Dosing spoons, 244

Double teach-back, 26

Driving, distracted, 82

Drops for measuring liquid medicines, 244

Dry-bed training for bedwetting, 103

E

Ear bulb, clearing baby's nose with, 121

Ear infections, 57–58, 155

   plain language educational handout on, 57–58

     in Spanish, 59–60

   preventing, 58

Ear pain, other causes of, 58

Easy-to-read handouts, tips for creating, 36

Eating, tooth decay and, 266

Educational materials, age-neutral, 26

El cuidado de los dientes de su niño (Caring for Your Child's Teeth), 267–268

Elección de medicinas de venta sin receta para su niño (Choosing Over-the-Counter Medicines for Your Child), 249–250

Electrolyte drink, 205, 221

El uso de medicinas líquidas (Using Liquid Medicines), 245–246

Emergency departments, pediatricians in, 25

Empacho, 163

   treatment of, 163

Encopresis, 162, 167, 170

Enemas, 169

English as a Second Language (ESL), 24

English for Speakers of Other Languages (ESOL), 24

Enuresis

   monosymptomatic nocturnal, 105

   polysymptomatic nocturnal, 105

   primary versus secondary, 105–106

Epiglottitis, acute, 184

Estreñimieno (Constipation), 171–172

Eustachian tube, 58

F

Family issues, health disparities and, 6

Fever, 197–212

   acetaminophen for, 206

   among Latino cultures, 202

   Ask Me 3 questions on, 197–198

   behavioral change, 202–203

   child involvement, 203

   confusing terms and concepts, 199–202

     diagnosis, 199

     management and treatment, 200–201

     prevention and health promotion, 199

     symptoms, 200

   cultural beliefs, 201

     worsening condition, 201–202

Primary care, 32

Provocadores de asma (Asthma Triggers), 77–78

Q

Quality improvement plan, health literacy building into, 15

¿Qué es el déficit de atención con hiperactividad? (What is ADHD?), 91–92

Qué le cuenta su niño de un año? (What Is Your One-Year-Old Telling You?), 195–196

Questions, open-ended, 26

R

Rapid Estimate of Adult Literacy in Medicine (REALM), 13

Reach Out and Read, 25
   model for, 269

Read aloud, 280
   listening to child, 280

Reading, 269–282
   Ask Me 3 questions for, 270–272
   behavior change, 275–276
   child involvement, 276
   confusing terms and concepts, 272–275
      communication issues, 272–275
   facts about, 272
   key messages for use, 277–278
   patient story, 269–270
   plain language educational handout on, 279–280
      in Spanish, 281–282
   referral information, 278
   start reading to your child early, 279–280
   teach-back for, 276–277

Reading aloud, 273

Reading levels, measuring, 40–42

Rectal temperature, taking, 209

Referral, 193, 194

Resfriados (Colds), 149, 153–154

Respiratory syncytial virus (RSV). *See* Bronchiolitis

Respiratory tract infections, secondhand smoke and, 297

Reye syndrome, 156, 201

S

Saline nose drops, 248

Saliva, 183

School, working with, on attention-deficit/hyperactivity disorder (ADHD), 94

School age, health literacy skills for, 7

School-aged children, asthma management and, 68

Secondhand smoke
   exposure to, 297–312
   plain language educational handout on, 305–306
      in Spanish, 307–308

Seizure, managing, 206

Short Test of Functional Health Literacy in Adults (S-TOFHLA), 13–14, 23

Sinus infections, 75, 155

Smoking, sports and, 309

Spanish language plain language handouts
   Asma (Asthma), 73–74
   ¿Cómo se trata el déficit de atención con hiperactividad? (What to Do for ADHD), 95–96
   Cómo tomarle la temperature a su niño (How to take Your Child's Temperature), 211–212
   Diarrea, vómitos y pérdida de líquidos (deshidratación) (Diarrhea, Vomiting, and Water Loss [Dehydration]), 223–224
   El cuidado de los dientes de su niño (Caring for Your Child's Teeth), 267–268
   Elección de medicinas de venta sin receta para su niño (Choosing Over-the-Counter Medicines for Your Child), 249–250
   El uso de medicinas líquidas (Using Liquid Medicines), 245–246
   Estreñimieno (Constipation), 171–172
   Humo de segunda mano (Secondhand Smoke), 307–308
   Infecciones de oído (Ear Infections), 59–60, 207–208
   La fiebre (Fever), 207–208
   La gripe (The Flu), 157–158
   Las rabietas o berrinches (Temper Tantrums), 295–296
   Léale temprano a su niño (Start Reading to Your Child Early), 281–282
   Los adolescentes y el tabaco (Teens and Tobacco), 311–312
   Medicinas recetadas para su niño (Prescription Medicines and Your Child), 241–242
   Orinar o mojar la cama (Bedwetting), 109–110
   Provocadores de asma (Asthma Triggers), 77–78
   ¿Qué es el déficit de atención con hiperactividad? (What Is ADHD?), 91–92
   Resfriados (Colds), 153–154
   Uso de medicinas de venta sin receta con su niño (Using Over-the-Counter (OTC) Medicines With Your Child), 253–254

Special populations, communicating with, 36